Building Bottom-up Health and Disaster Risk Reduction Programmes

Building Bottom-up Health and Disaster Risk Reduction Programmes

Professor Emily Ying Yang Chan
Assistant Dean and Professor,
Faculty of Medicine,
The Chinese University of Hong Kong
Visiting Professor,
Nuffield Department of Medicine,
The University of Oxford

OXFORD
UNIVERSITY PRESS

OXFORD
UNIVERSITY PRESS

Great Clarendon Street, Oxford, OX2 6DP,
United Kingdom

Oxford University Press is a department of the University of Oxford.
It furthers the University's objective of excellence in research, scholarship, and education by publishing worldwide. Oxford is a registered trade mark of Oxford University Press in the UK and in certain other countries

First Edition published in 2018

Published in the United States of America by Oxford University Press
198 Madison Avenue, New York, NY 10016, United States of America

British Library Cataloguing in Publication Data

Data available

Library of Congress Control Number: 2017952352

ISBN978- 0-19-880717-9

POD

Foreword by Professor Tai-fai Fok

Her new book, *Building Bottom-up Health and Disaster Risk Reduction Programme*, reminds me of the humble beginning of the rural health and disaster preparedness programme initiated by Professor Emily Chan at the Faculty of Medicine at The Chinese University of Hong Kong (CUHK) a decade ago when I was then the Faculty Dean.

With the strong support from the Faculty and its Jockey Club School of Public Health and Primary Care, Professor Chan launched the 'CUHK Public Health Humanitarian Initiative' in 2007, based on public health theories and principles. Since then, she and her colleagues have been organizing and bringing colleagues and students in the Faculty and the University to poverty-stricken remote rural China to undertake health and disaster preparedness education activities and research. With the establishment of the Collaborating Centre for Oxford University and CUHK for Disaster and Medical Humanitarian Response (CCOUC) in 2011 as a key joint effort of the two universities, this rural project was re-named the 'Ethnic Minority Health Project' and has evolved into a multi-institution, multidisciplinary, and cross-country endeavour. By the end of 2016, the project has brought close to 500 teachers and students from CUHK and partner universities like University of Oxford, Harvard University, University of Hong Kong, and Peking University to disaster-prone rural communities in China and other Asian countries such as Nepal, Bhutan, and the Democratic People's Republic of Korea.

The work of Professor Chan and her rural health team has epitomized the vision of CUHK and its Faculty of Medicine in nurturing future researchers and professionals imbued with humanistic spirit and advancing knowledge in a translational way by combining research with practice to serve the public good of the local and global communities. Translating theoretical knowledge into applied and practical use is also widely recognized as an essential hallmark of all excellent universities in the twenty-first century. Professor Chan's team has provided an invaluable platform for the university's internationalization effort to promote collaborations in education, research, and community services among renowned academic institutions locally, regionally, and globally.

As an interim chronicle of the persistent work of Professor Chan and her colleagues in the field in the past decade, this book provides insights to combine public health theory and practice in the rural areas in Asia. It will prove to be a key reference for researchers and practitioners in rural health and rural disaster risk reduction work, and will help open up the team's global classroom to a much larger and wider audience across the world who hold dear the humanitarian concern about the well-being of the deprived.

I congratulate Professor Chan on her achievements in the field teaching students and collecting data, as well as back behind the desk consolidating those hard-earned field experience and insights of her team into this book to help disseminate and advance the knowledge in rural health and humanitarian medicine.

Professor Tai-fai Fok
Pro-Vice-Chancellor/Vice-President (Internationalization)
The Chinese University of Hong Kong

Foreword by Professor Sian Griffiths

Two threads interweave within this book—the need to promote better health and address inequalities in poorer rural communities within Asia, while at the same time prepare them for dealing with disasters for which they are at greater risk. While the life expectancy in China has dramatically improved over the last few decades, the gap between more affluent urban areas and many less affluent rural areas has grown. Lifestyle factors, socio-economic influences, and access to services have all played a part, and knowledge of public health skills is an essential part of the necessary armamentarium to promote health. So is an understanding of the threat of natural disaster from the environment. While climate change affects us all, countries in Asia, particularly low- and middle-income countries, face greater risks of disaster. And within these countries, it is the poorer rural areas who are at greatest risk. In addition to national governments committing to action on high-level global agreements such as the Sustainability Development Goals, local communities need to fully engage in local sustained action to be disaster aware and disaster prepared. And to be effective, responses need to be constructed within the framework of promoting better health. Basics such as clean water and better sanitation need to be coupled with hygiene practices such as handwashing. Public heath skills and knowledge need to support frontline workers to be more effective in planning, implementing, and evaluating their interventions.

This book builds on the experience and programmes of the Collaborating Centre for Oxford University and Chinese University of Hong Kong for Disaster and Medical Humanitarian Response (CCOUC). CCOUC was established in 2011 as a non-profit research centre to carry out research, training, and community knowledge transfer in the area of disaster and medical humanitarian response. Its aim has been to be a platform for research, education, and community knowledge transfer in the areas of disaster and medical humanitarian crisis policy development, planning, and response in the Asia–Pacific region. Over the six years since its establishment, CCOUC has worked with many rural communities in China as part of its Ethnic Minority Health Project, as well as in other Asian countries such as Bhutan, Nepal, and the Democratic People's Republic of Korea. This book utilizes the knowledge and experience that has been gained, following the journey from theory of public health and health promotion to practice and implementation, charting both successes and problems encountered as students and researchers from the academic community engage with rural communities and local health workers. The unique experiences of the CCOUC team and their examples of field working are described in order to share the learning and enable others to put theory into more effective practice. The book will be a useful tool for a wide range of people—students, field workers, programme managers, non-governmental organizations (NGOs), and volunteers. I hope it is widely read.

Professor Sian Griffiths
Emeritus Professor and former Director,
JC School of Public Health and Primary Care,
The Chinese University of Hong Kong

Foreword by Professor Jennifer Leaning

'Prevention is better than cure' is one of the key tenets of public health. In the field of medical humanitarian response to disaster, this public health principle is enshrined in the concept of disaster risk reduction. Reducing the risk that a natural hazard may cause harm to ecosystems, populations, and communities requires a broad and detailed range of prevention and mitigation strategies. Disaster risk reduction has emerged as the international community's major approach to the increasingly frequent and intensifying natural disasters confronting societies in the twenty-first century. This approach has been elaborated in the Sendai Framework for Disaster Risk Reduction, which from 2015 to 2030 aims to guide global action in reducing vulnerabilities to disasters and in strengthening capacities for prevention and mitigation of the harms disasters may cause. Health has been recognized as an expected outcome and goal of the Sendai Framework: four out of the seven global targets directly relate to health, including reducing disaster mortality and numbers of people affected.

To design and implement this framework in the context of rural areas in developing countries of Asia and perhaps elsewhere, a bottom-up approach to disaster risk reduction in the context of health is arguably the most practical, efficient, and cost-effective strategy. In these remote and resource-deficient settings, where people are usually cut off from outside assistance in the early days after disasters strike, efforts must be directed at building local capacity to reduce their own vulnerabilities and protect their own health and safety. In this context, as the global agenda is rapidly evolving and new understandings of local resilience are emerging, Professor Emily Chan's new book *Building Bottom-up Health and Disaster Risk Reduction Programmes* is a most timely scholarly contribution.

I have worked with Professor Chan for almost two decades, beginning with her postgraduate days as one of my students at the Harvard School of Public Health. Her promise as a leader and analyst in the field of disaster management and response (as it was known then) was early evident. It has been a distinct pleasure and honour to collaborate with her on many disaster-related research and policy issues over the ensuing years. In recent years, Professor Chan, in her senior roles at the Chinese University of Hong Kong, has established a Centre for Disaster and Medical Humanitarian Response, as a collaborating centre with the University of Oxford (CCOUC). This Centre has responded to a wide range of major disasters in China and elsewhere in Asia, and has developed unique expertise in preparing rural villages in China to assess disaster risks and to respond in feasible and practical ways.

I had the privilege of accompanying Professor Chan and her graduate students on a joint research and education mission to the remote Hongyan Village in Sichuan Province of

China in 2014. This Ethnic Minority Health Project, developed by Professor Chan, places her students in close three–five-day interaction with local residents, going through an intense and enjoyable set of skills-based exercises and conversations. Based on traditional rural village teaching, where minstrels and artists and other people of interest come to a village to promote expressive activities, this teaching format embodies the humanitarian enterprise in action. This immersion in the villages allows students to experience some of the common aspects of humanitarian work in the field. The programme contributes to the global classroom created at CCOUC and establishes the students' understanding that humanitarian responders build a moral lifeline from themselves to the people who are suffering after a disaster. During these field training experiences, the students also help the villagers recognize that disaster is not just a matter of fate. The villagers in their own ways can do something to save themselves and families. This bottom-up approach to capacity-building could serve as a model for such resilience training in many parts of the world.

The work of Professor Chan and her team provides a vigorous response to the current inadequacies in emergency response and disaster risk reduction training witnessed in many parts of Asia, particularly its more remote rural areas. Her programme and her team in Hong Kong are well positioned to provide leadership in promoting strategies and tactics for disaster risk reduction.

This book, a product of years of hard work in the field, provides key concepts and core insights into methods to implement public health theory and practice in the rural areas in Asia. It will help expand the necessary global classroom on these issues and support the humanitarian endeavour to promote the survival and even well-being of those who are poor, but need not be deeply vulnerable to the disasters that lie ahead.

Professor Jennifer Leaning
Professor and Director, François-Xavier Bagnoud (FXB)
Center for Health and Human Rights, Harvard University, USA

Foreword by Mr Darren Nash

In all things we must take care. Most of all, we must take care of each other.

Those people who take part in the research and delivery of disaster and medical humanitarian aid, and in this context enable preparedness for such aid, are among those whom we must take particular care to support and nurture: so as to enable them to continue their good work in the most effective way possible; so that they may learn and pass on skills to individuals and communities; so that they may continue to demonstrate what it truly means to be a global citizen.

This book is a core component to enabling all of these goals, offering unrivalled insights into health and disaster preparedness in rural Asia.

The passion and drive of colleagues and students in this field continues to inspire me. I offer you fellowship.

Fellowship*

I argued with the sea for a while, but it needed no sentry, so I led down.
I sought comfort from the earth for a while, but it
did not take me in, so I stood up.
I berated the sky for a while,
but it heeded no plea, so I turned inward.
I focused my mind for a while, but it held no answers, so I gave up.
I leant into the wind for a while,
but it offered no support, so I was alone.
I fed a witless fire for a while,
but it burnt my hands, so I sought aid.
I joined hands with my fellows, and found the succour I sought.
I should have known.

D. J. Nash, 2015

Mr Darren Nash
Associate Head of Department (Academic Support and Finance)
Nuffield Department of Medicine, University of Oxford, UK

*Nash, D. J. (2016). Fellowship, in *Fellowship*, p.2. Hong Kong: The Chinese University Press.

Preface

As a backdrop of the Sustainable Development Goals (SDGs) (2016–2030), the United Nations pointed out that more than six million children still died before the age of five in 2015. At least 1.8 billion people across the world still consumed drinking water contaminated by faeces, and 2.4 million lacked access to basic sanitation services such as toilets or latrines, while nearly 1,000 children died every day of preventable water- and sanitation-related diarrhoeal diseases. Rural areas fare far worse: children in rural areas are about 1.7 times more likely to die before their fifth birthday than those in urban areas. About 16% of the rural population do not use improved drinking water sources, compared to 4% of the urban population. About 50% of people living in rural areas lack improved sanitation facilities, compared to only 18% of people in urban areas. Just one in three people in rural areas have access to piped drinking water, and one in four still practice open defaecation. These rural health risk issues remain to be resolved under the ambitious, universal, and comprehensive SDGs.

Far too many one-off rural on-site public health knowledge transfer projects fail to deliver results in the long term. Theoretical understanding may be strengthened among NGO practitioners and volunteers to support project planning, monitoring, and evaluations. For NGO frontline workers, especially those who have no or limited public health training, it is of paramount importance that they be equipped with adequate knowledge and skills so that they are able to plan, implement, and evaluate a sustainable field intervention, to approach issues critically, and to execute a well thought-out programme.

Building Bottom-up Health and Disaster Risk Reduction Programmes is an introductory to intermediate level textbook for healthcare professionals and reference book for fieldworkers, volunteers, and students who are interested in promoting health and emergency and disaster risk reduction. Based on public health theories and illustrated by relevant examples, this book introduces how health, emergency, and disaster preparedness education programmes could be organized in remote rural Asia. The book is developed from the experience and insights gained from the long-established Ethnic Minority Health Project of the Collaborating Centre for Oxford University and CUHK for Disaster and Medical Humanitarian Response (CCOUC) in China. In 2009, CCOUC has identified five major health- and disaster-related risks in rural communities for which it has attempted to seek relevant public health interventions. These key issues include waste management, indoor environment, water and hygiene, health promoting habits, and disaster risk literacy. In addition to sharing its experience, the book incorporates new lessons learnt from CCOUC's recent projects in Asian countries like Bhutan, Nepal, and the Democratic People's Republic of Korea. Prevalent and emerging risks identified and relevant cost-effective mitigation procedures are detailed and discussed in the book. Different intervention models and activities are also introduced for application in typical scenarios.

This book carries five major aims: arousing NGO practitioners' awareness of the health and disaster preparedness issues common among rural communities in Asia; providing organizers and volunteers of rural projects with highly practical guidelines for implementation and evaluation of health and emergency and disaster preparedness programmes; providing examples and activity recommendations for on-site public health activities; promoting multidisciplinary collaborations and exchanges; and raising the levels of health and emergency and disaster preparedness in rural Asia.

There are eight chapters in this book. Chapter 1 introduces and explains several basic concepts and elements in public health to provide the conceptual basis for organizing health and emergency and disaster risk reduction programmes at the field level. Examples are given to demonstrate the use of the concepts. Chapter 2 describes the conceptual building blocks introduced in the previous chapter and theoretical models with application examples to guide rural health and disaster preparedness education programmes will be discussed. Chapters 3 and 4 summarize the public health status quo in developing rural Asian regions, highlighting the challenges faced to provide empirical background for organizing health and emergency and disaster risk reduction programmes. Chapter 5 explains some common misconceptions and myths of health promotion, the project cycle of health and disaster preparedness education programmes (i.e. needs assessment, project planning, programme implementation and monitoring, and programme evaluation) and notes for organizers and participants of health and disaster preparedness education programmes will be shared. It integrates the themes in previous chapters with relevant insights gained from actual field experience in Asia, focusing on programme implementation field experience and lessons learnt, as well as the practical challenges and problems encountered in the field in rural Asian settings. It will also discuss the field-policy nexus (i.e. the fulfilment of policy ambitions in such international policy frameworks like the Sustainable Development Goals, Sendai Framework for Disaster Risk Reduction, 2015–2030), and the Paris Agreement for Climate Change by rural field programmes in health and emergency and disaster risk reduction. Chapter 6 highlights five important rural health issues that can be cost-effectively implemented, namely water and health, indoor environment, waste management, health behaviour, and disaster risk-related preparedness. Key messages for education programmes focusing on these areas are presented, together with relevant promotion methods like poster presentation, workshop, drama, performance, game, small group discussion, and souvenirs. Chapters 7, 8, and 9 provide more in-depth background and a forward-looking perspective in rural health for readers and looks into seven emerging areas in rural health, namely technology, migration, older people, border towns, plantations, nomadic groups, and implementation of the health components of major international policy documents in rural settings. Chapter 10 concludes the key discussion of this book.

Acknowledgements

The origin of this work can be traced back to the 'Ethnic Minority Health Project' of the Collaborating Centre for Oxford University and CUHK for Disaster and Medical Humanitarian Response (CCOUC) and its predecessor 'CUHK Public Health Humanitarian Initiative' at the JC School of Public Health and Primary Care (JCSPHPC), Faculty of Medicine, The Chinese University of Hong Kong (CUHK). The decade-long programme organizes and brings colleagues and students in the JCSPHPC to remote rural communities in China to conduct health and disaster preparedness education activities and provides on-site training opportunities for students to put public health theories into practice from my teaching and research. My heartfelt gratitude must be extended to the two universities and their Vice-Chancellors, Professor Andrew Hamilton and Professor Joseph Sung, the former and incumbent Deans of CUHK Faculty of Medicine, Professor Tai-fai Fok and Professor Francis Chan, the former and incumbent Directors of JCSPHPC, Professor Sian Griffiths and Professor Eng-kiong Yeoh, Director of the Wellcome Trust, Professor Jeremy Farrar, Associate Head of Oxford University Nuffield Department of Medicine (NDM), Mr Darren Nash, and Director of the François-Xavier Bagnoud (FXB) Center for Health and Human Rights at Harvard University, Professor Jennifer Leaning, whose vast and incessant support and encouragement have ensured the success and sustainability of this project and the completion of this book amid the ups and downs of its writing process.

I acknowledge with great appreciation the diligent assistance of Mr Chi-shing Wong for preparing the manuscript for submission and the patience of Mrs Nicola Wilson, Mr James Cox, and their colleagues at Oxford University Press. I also wish to thank Professor Samuel Yeung-shan Wong, Professor William B. Goggins III, Professor Colin A. Graham, Professor Vincent Chung-tong Mok, Professor Jean H. Kim, Professor Justin Che-yuen Wu, Professor Peter Horby, Dr Elizabeth Newnham, Ms Sharon Chow, Ms Janet Yiu-wai Chow, Ms Christy Oi-yan-jing Chan, Ms Gloria Kwong-wei Chan, Ms Queenie Wei-ngan Chan, Dr Calvin Ka-yeung Cheng, Dr Eliza Yee-lai Cheung, Mr Cheuk-pong Chiu, Dr Cecilia Yuen-see Choi, Dr Wenwen Du, Mr Eric Man-chi Fu, Professor Gemma Yang Gao, Dr Xue Gao, Ms Hale Hay-lam Ho, Ms Janice Ying-en Ho, Mr Zhe Huang, Professor Kevin Kei-ching Hung, Dr Levina Chandra Khoe, Ms Christine Pui-yan Ko, Ms Dawnie Ho-hei Lau, Ms Clare Ying-wai Lee, Ms Teresa Po-lam Lee, Ms Po-yi Lee, Ms Joyce May-sum Leung, Ms Rachel Ya-yuan Leung, Ms Agatha Kit-ying Lin, Ms Cherry Lee-yung Lin, Mr Kelvin Wai-kit Ling, Mr Kevin Sida Liu, Ms Sharon Tsoon-ting Lo, Mr Jonas Lossau, Ms Carman Ka-man Mark, Ms Nicola Nightingale, Mr Jacky Kwong-yi Ng, Dr Andrew D. Smith, Dr Greta Chun-huen Tam, Mr Zhe Wang, Dr Alvin Ho-cheuk Wong, Ms Carol Ka-po Wong, Mr Terry Wong, Mr Aman Chun-wai Yee, Professor May

Pui-shan Yeung, Ms Tiffany Lok-yan Yeung, Ms Esther Miu-fan Yiu, Mr Marat Tsuen-kweun Yu, Ms Janice So-kuen Yue, Dr Tony Ka-chun Yung, Ms Crystal Yingjia Zhu, Mr Ka-kit Chan, Ms Elizabeth Deacon, Ms Caroline Dubois, Ms Karen Valentine, Ms Tracy Chin-wai Lai, Mr Elgar Chung-po Lam, Dr Johnson Chun-hong Lau, Ms Holly Lai-ho Li, Ms Rebecca Siu-kam Tsui, Professor Chok-wan Chan, Mrs Irene Che-yun Yau Lee, Ms Winnie Chan, Ms Jennifer Ma, Professor Qifu Dai, Professor Jun Mu, family, and all friends who have assisted in the publication of this book for their encouragement, inspiration, support, and assistance at various points in this book project. Further thanks go to colleagues and students at JCSPHPC and CCOUC for their friendship and the joyful memories of fieldwork. As always, special thanks must go to Eric Yau and our children, Ellie and Ernest.

Emily Ying Yang Chan
Professor and Director,
Collaborating Centre for Oxford University and CUHK for
Disaster and Medical Humanitarian Response (CCOUC)
Co-chairperson, WHO Thematic Platform for
Health Emergency & Disaster Risk Management Research Group
Hong Kong

Researchers

Case study and special topic researchers

Gloria Kwong-wai Chan, BSSc (CUHK), MSSc (CUHK), is a professional journalist by training. After spending years in political news reporting in Hong Kong, she joined the international medical humanitarian group Médecins Sans Frontières as the Director of Communications for the organization's communication effort in Hong Kong, China, and Southeast Asia. Her expertise was employed in the frontline of a number of emergencies over the world. Before joining the Collaborating Centre for Oxford University and CUHK for Disaster and Medical Humanitarian Response (CCOUC), she was the Chief Executive of the Hong Kong Medical Association. Ms Chan is currently a Board Member of Médecins Sans Frontières Hong Kong and serves as Assistant Director of CCOUC.

Zhe Huang, BMS (Guangzhou Medical University), MPH (CUHK), is a project officer at CCOUC with a particular focus on climate change and data analysis. He received his Master of Public Health from The Chinese University of Hong Kong, majoring in epidemiology and biostatistics and obtained a Bachelor's degree in public affairs management in Guangzhou Medical University in China. He has participated in field-based assessments and interventions in rural areas in China.

Kevin KC Hung, MBChB, MRCSEd, MPH, EMDM, FHKCEM, FHKAM(EM), FRCEM, is an Assistant Professor in emergency medicine at The Chinese University of Hong Kong. Dr Hung is an emergency medicine specialist with vast experience in conducting rural health needs assessment in the Asia–Pacific region with various NGOs and humanitarian initiatives. He was the founding Director of Hong Kong Jockey Club Disaster Preparedness and Response Institute (HKJCDPRI). Dr Hung is also a Hong Kong Red Cross volunteer and had served as a community health delegate of Japanese Red Cross Society Basic Health Care Emergency Response Unit.

Vivian Sau-wai Lee, BSSc (HKBU), MA (SOAS), has extensive experience in journalism and humanitarian aid. She is a journalist by training and has worked in many of Hong Kong's leading media organizations. After joining the international medical humanitarian organization Médecins Sans Frontières (MSF) in 2003, she has been working in different capacities ranging from field to headquarter positions, in Hong Kong, Asia, and Europe. Among other projects, she was covering communications positions for MSF in Afghanistan (2012–2014), and in Italy for the migrant crisis (2015). Her expertise spans across news reporting, media relations, advocacy, event management, and association management and development. She holds a Master's degree in International and Comparative Legal Studies with School of Oriental and African Studies, University of London.

Kelvin Wai-kit Ling, MPH, has extensive experience in health education and communication, needs assessment, and evaluation and field-based teaching in rural, ethnic minority villages of China and slums in Nairobi, Kenya. He also served as a session co-chair and abstract reviewer to the World Association for Disaster and Emergency Medicine's World Congress on Disaster and Emergency Medicine in Cape Town, South Africa and Toronto, Canada, respectively. He was an Assistant Lecturer at the Collaborating Centre for Oxford University and CUHK for Disaster and Medical Humanitarian Response (CCOUC). His research focuses on conducting household-based trials in rural China that empower villagers to make behaviour change decisions and enhance their health literacy. He holds a Master of Public Health from The Chinese University of Hong Kong and is a registered teacher in Hong Kong.

Kevin Sida Liu, BSc, MSc, MPH, is an assistant lecturer who joined the Collaborating Centre for Oxford University and CUHK for Disaster and Medical Humanitarian Response (CCOUC) and JC School of Public Health and Primary Care, The Chinese University of Hong Kong in 2012 after obtaining his Master of Public Health degree at the same university. He is currently a PhD candidate with research interests in climate change and health. Mr Liu has extensive field experience in conducting health education and needs assessment in underprivileged and disaster-prone communities in the rural areas of China. He also serves as a liaison officer with health authorities in China to coordinate training and research projects at both national and provincial levels.

Sharon Tsoon-ting Lo, MA (University of St Andrews, Scotland), is a Project Officer at the Collaborating Centre for Oxford University and CUHK for Disaster and Medical Humanitarian Response (CCOUC), where she coordinates their engagement with various UN-related international platforms pertaining to health and disaster risk reduction, and at the CUHK Centre for Global Health where she supports the Centre's operation and activities, particularly through the CGH Sustainable Development Goals Series. She is also a Regional Focal Point at the UN Major Group for Children and Youth (UN MGCY), coordinating youth engagement in various UN processes under the 2030 Agenda for Sustainable Development. She founded Youth Empact, an ethnic minority youth empowerment platform, under the Clinton Global University Initiative in January 2016. She won the Collaborating Centre for Oxford University and CUHK Outstanding Disaster Project Award in 2016.

Carman Ka-man Mark, BSc (University of Essex), MPH (CUHK), obtained her Bachelor's degree in Health Studies at the University of Essex in the United Kingdom and received her Master of Public Health from The Chinese University of Hong Kong, majoring in Population and Global Health. She won the Collaborating Centre for Oxford University and CUHK Outstanding Disaster Project Award in 2014. Ms Mark is now a Research Project Officer at the Collaborating Centre for Oxford University and CUHK for Disaster and Medical Humanitarian Response (CCOUC) conducting projects on evaluation of humanitarian intervention and training, and adaptive measures on climate change.

Carol Ka-po Wong, BSSc (CUHK), MIPA (HKU), is a journalist by training and has acquired a Master's degree in International and Public Affairs. She has years of project management experience in NGOs in Hong Kong and overseas, with a focus on public health and disaster managements. Before joining the Collaborating Centre for Oxford University and CUHK for Disaster and Medical Humanitarian Response (CCOUC), Ms Wong had been stationed in the Philippines for almost three years, where her work in the field particularly focused on slum health, disaster preparedness, and response.

Chi-shing Wong, MSc (LSE), is Publication Manager at the Collaborating Centre for Oxford University and CUHK for Disaster and Medical Humanitarian Response (CCOUC) and the copy editor of this book. He has a background in journalism and communication, received his Master's degree in comparative politics at the London School of Economics and Political Science, focusing on democratization, ethnic politics, and nationalism, with regional foci in China and Southeast Asia, and researched on political identity at the University of Oxford. Mr Wong has worked in various teaching, research, and administrative positions in universities.

Tony Ka-chun Yung, BSc (CUHK), MND (U Sydney), APD (Australia), MSDA (Australia), AN (Australia), obtained his Master in Nutrition and Dietetics from the University of Sydney and registered as an Accredited Practicing Dietitian in Australia. He is also a Sports Dietitian and Accredited Nutritionist. He practiced in Grantham Hospital before joining the JC School of Public Health and Primary Care of The Chinese University of Hong Kong in year 2003 responsible for the promotion of nutritional health. He is currently a Senior Lecturer responsible for teachings, tutorials, and researches related to nutrition aspect of public health. His research interests include diet behaviours of vulnerable populations, nutrition issues related to disasters as well as sports nutrition.

Undergraduate and postgraduate research helpers

Ada Ho-yin Fong, BSc (Public Health, 2014–2018)
Eric Man-chi Fu, MBBS-MPH (2012–2019)
Dawnie Ho-hei Lau, MBChB (GPS, 2015–2020)
Hebe Law, MBChB (GPS, 2014–2020)
Mia Mei-yan Lee, BSc (Public Health, 2013–2017)
Karen Ka-ying Li, MBChB (GPS, 2014–2019)

Other co-authors of previous CCOUC training manuals for rural health and disaster preparedness programmes in China

(from which some ideas in the current book originate)
Gloria Kwong-wai Chan
Zhe Huang
Poyi Lee
Kevin Sida Liu
Carol Ka-po Wong
Chi-shing Wong
Tony Ka-chun Yung
Crystal Yingjia Zhu

Table of contents

Abbreviations

AAN	Afghanistan Analysts Network
ADL	activity of daily living
AMV	auxiliary midwife
BPHS	Basic Package of Health Services
CCOUC	Collaborating Centre for Oxford University and CUHK for Disaster and Medical Humanitarian Response
CDC	Center for Disease Control and Prevention
CHARLS	China Health and Retirement Longitudinal Study
CHC	community health centre
CHW	community health worker
COPD	chronic obstructive pulmonary disease
CRED	Centre for Research on the Epidemiology of Disasters
CSMBS	Civil Servant Medical Benefit Scheme
DHO	District Health Office
DMC	disaster management committee
DPRK	Democratic People's Republic of Korea
DRR	disaster risk reduction
DTP3	diphtheria, tetanus toxoid, and pertussis vaccination
EMHP	Ethnic Minority Health Project
EPHS	Essential Package of Hospital Services
FAO	Food and Agriculture Organization
FCHV	female community health volunteer
FGP	family group practice
GDP	gross domestic product
HBM	Health Belief Model
HDI	Human Development Index
HFA	Hyogo Framework for Action
HIV	Human Immunodeficiency Virus
HP	health post
ICT	information and communication technology
IDP	internally displaced person
IDSP	Integrated Diseases Surveillance Programme
IMNCI	Integrated Management of Newborn and Childhood Illness
IOM	International Organization for Migration
MDG	Millennium Development Goals
MoH	Ministry of Health
MoPH	Ministry of Public Health
MSF	Médecins Sans Frontières
NCD	non-communicable disease
NHFPC	National Health and Family Planning Commission
NHM	National Health Mission
NMHP	National Mental Health Programme
NPCB	National Programme for Control of Blindness
NRCMS	New Rural Cooperative Medical Scheme
NRHM	National Rural Health Mission
NVBDCP	National Vector Borne Disease Control Programme
PHC	primary health centre
PHCC	primary healthcare centre
POCUS	point-of-care ultrasound
PRC	People's Republic of China
RHD	rheumatic heart disease
RI	routine immunization
RNTCP	Revised National TB Control Programme
SARS	severe acute respiratory syndrome
SATCM	State Administration of Traditional Chinese Medicine
SDG	Sustainable Development Goal
STI	sexually transmitted infection
TB	tuberculosis
TPB	Theory of Planned Behaviour
TT	tetanus toxoid

UCS	Universal Coverage Scheme
UN	United Nations
UNDP	United Nations Development Programme
UNICEF	United Nations Children's Fund
URBMI	Urban Residence Basic Medical Insurance
USAID	United States Agency for International Development
WASH	water, sanitation, and hygiene
WHO	World Health Organization

About the author

Emily Ying Yang Chan, MBBS (HKU), BS (Johns Hopkins), SM PIH (Harvard), MD (CUHK), DFM (HKCFP), FFPH, FHKAM (Community Medicine), FHKCCM, serves as Professor and Assistant Dean (Development), Faculty of Medicine, and Associate Director (External Affairs and Collaboration), JC School of Public Health and Primary Care, The Chinese University of Hong Kong (CUHK); Director, Collaborating Centre for Oxford University and CUHK for Disaster and Medical Humanitarian Response (CCOUC), Centre for Global Health (CGH) and Centre of Excellence (ICoE-CCOUC), Integrated Research on Disaster Risk (IRDR); Visiting Professor, Oxford University Nuffield Department of Medicine; Senior Fellow, Harvard Humanitarian Initiative, and Visiting Scholar, FXB Center, Harvard University; Honorary Professor, Li Ka Shing Faculty of Medicine, University of Hong Kong; Fellow, Hong Kong Academy of Medicine; Co-chairperson, WHO Thematic Platform for Health Emergency & Disaster Risk Management Research Group; and member, Asia Science Technology and Academia Advisory Group (ASTAAG). She received her academic training at Johns Hopkins Universtiy, Harvard T.H. Chan School of Public Health, London School of Hygiene and Tropical Medicine, University of Hong Kong and CUHK. Her research interests include disaster and humanitarian medicine, health needs and programme impact evaluation of evidence-based medical and public health interventions in resource-deficit settings, climate change and health, global health, and violence and injury epidemiology. She also has extensive experience as a frontline emergency relief practitioner in the mid-1990s, spanning across 20 countries and received the National Geographic Chinese Explorer Award from the *National Geographic* magazine in 2016.

Chapter 1

Introduction: An example of programme development

CCOUC Ethnic Minority Health Project

Globally, China's rural population faces the highest natural disaster risk (see Fig. 1.1). People living in these disaster-prone rural communities are often characterized by being ethnic-minority-based, living in extreme poverty (less than US$1.25/person/day), and lacking technical 'know-how' or resources for disaster preparedness. After disasters, these rural communities are often left to manage their own post-disaster health risks and have to face the post-disaster development challenges alone.

1.1 Context of the project

According to the national census in 2010, 670 million (constituting 50.05% of China's total population) lived in rural areas in China. The Collaborating Centre for Oxford University and CUHK for Disaster and Medical Humanitarian Response (CCOUC), a joint academic unit between the University of Oxford and The Chinese University of Hong Kong (CUHK), has developed he Ethnic Minority Health Project (EMHP) in 2009 to examine health outcomes, disaster impact, and medical humanitarian issues in remote, extreme poverty, disaster-prone non-Han ethnic minority villages in China (CCOUC, n.d.). Over the years, the project indicated that the majority of residents are left behind older people, children of limited education level (primary school), and in many of the ethnic minority-based areas, residents still face language barriers to understand Mandarin, the lingua franca of China. Even in communities with younger populations who had received formal education, health risk and disaster awareness are often very limited. CCOUC's survey results showed 40% to 50% of the communities perceived their health as being poor and rural health infrastructure generally remains rudimentary.

The primary goal for EMHP is to identify evidence-based solutions to support bottom-up resilience building efforts in health and disaster preparedness in remote and rural communities. Five major project objectives include: (1) empowering vulnerable communities in rural and remote settings to prepare and mitigate the adverse impact of natural disasters; (2) bringing science and technical 'know-how' developed in academic settings to field practices; (3) developing rural and remote community capacity through collaborative field training; (4) raising global awareness of issues related to disaster impact and preparedness among remote communities in developing countries; and (5) documenting empirical findings to

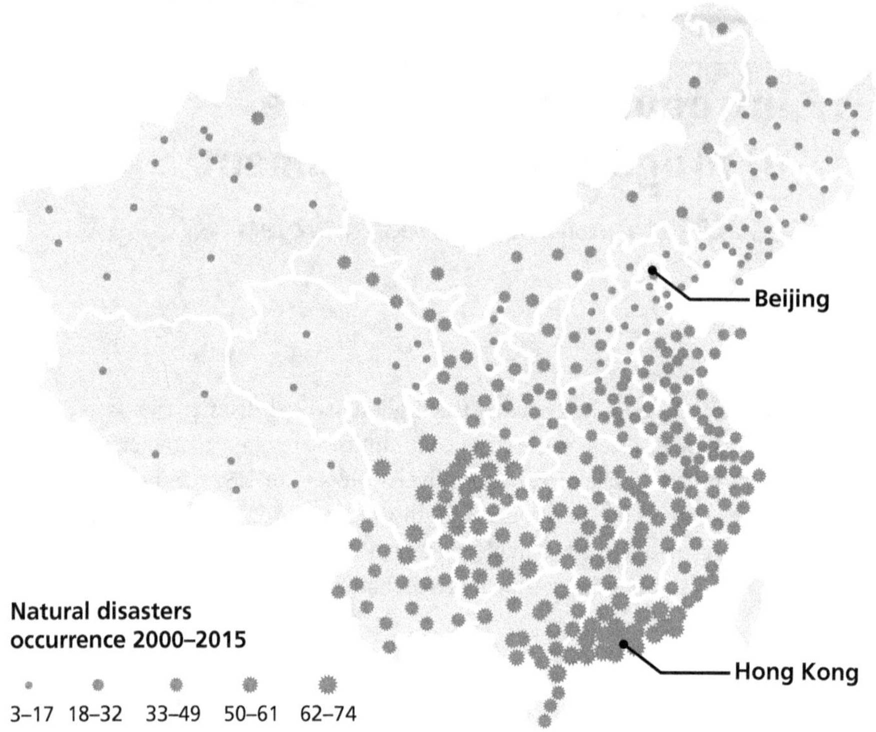

Fig. 1.1 Natural disasters in China 2000–2015.

Reproduced with permission from Centre for Research on the Epidemiology of Disasters, EM-DAT: The Emergency Events Database - Université catholique de Louvain (UCL) - CRED, D. Guha-Sapir, Brussels, Belgium, 'Country Maps', http://emdat.be/country-maps#overlay-context=map-archive, accessed 07 Mar. 2017, Copyright © 2017 Université catholique de Louvain - Centre for Research on the Epidemiology of Disasters.

support the future development of related intervention for other rural, community-based health projects.

1.1.1 Site selection and needs assessment

Site selection for the EMHP project is based on four key principles: geographical remoteness, ethnic minority representation, economic vulnerability, and disaster proneness. Hence, the EMHP targets remote, rural, ethnic minority-based communities in China that live in extreme poverty (less than US$1.25/person/day). By December 2016, the project team has established more than 16 project village sites across eight provinces in China. Throughout these years, the project has enabled the training of more than 700 public health, medical, and related professionals, as well as outreached to more than 18,000 villagers in remote communities of the northwest Ancient Silk Road, the southwest Ancient Tea Horse Trail, the southwest border adjacent to the infamous Thailand-Laos-Myanmar Golden Triangle, the Tibetan Plateau, the Loess Plateau of the Yellow River, the origin of the Yangtze River, and the northeast 'Rust Belt'. Figure 1.2 shows the distribution of project villages and Figure 1.3 the summarized figures of the project.

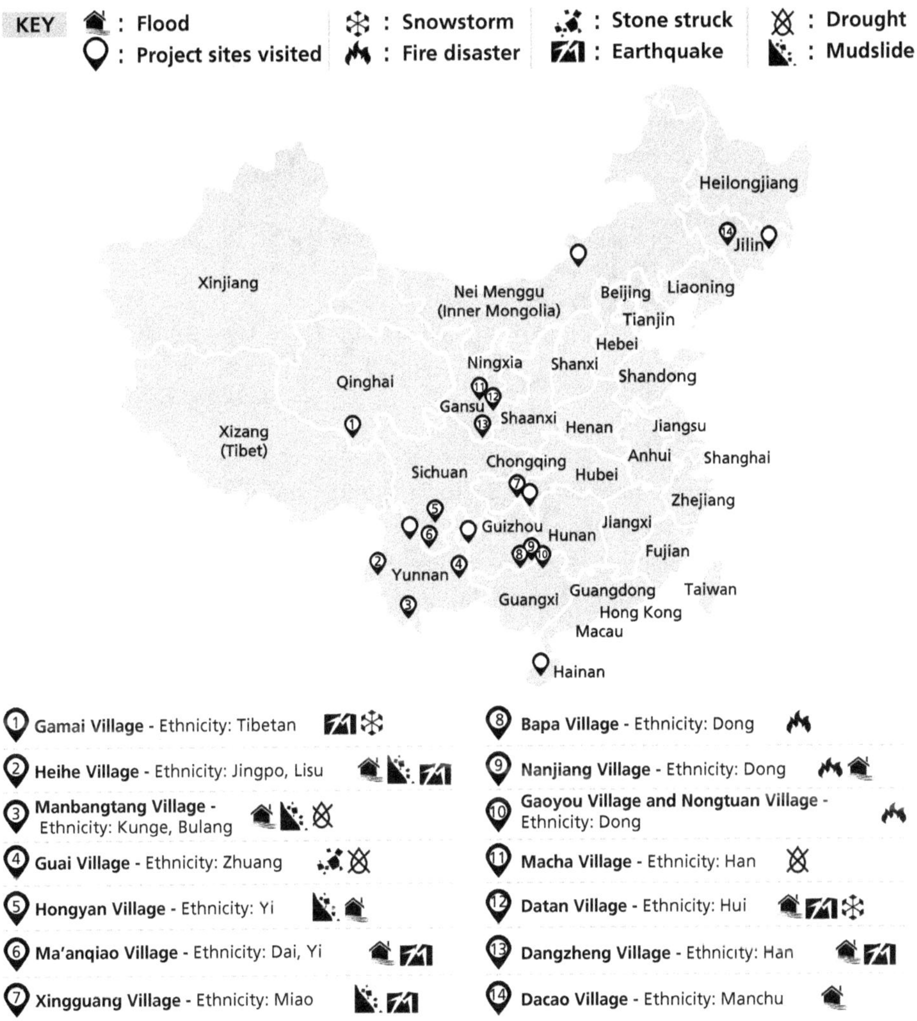
KEY
: Flood
: Project sites visited
: Snowstorm
: Fire disaster
: Stone struck
: Earthquake
: Drought
: Mudslide
Heilongjiang
Jilin
Xinjiang
Nei Menggu
(Inner Mongolia)
Beijing
Liaoning
Tianjin
Hebei
Ningxia
Shanxi
Shandong
Qinghai
Gansu
Shaanxi
Henan
Jiangsu
Xizang
(Tibet)
Anhui
Shanghai
Sichuan
Chongqing
Hubei
Zhejiang
Guizhou
Hunan
Jiangxi
Fujian
Yunnan
Guangxi
Guangdong
Taiwan
Hong Kong
Macau
Hainan
1 Gamai Village - Ethnicity: Tibetan
2 Heihe Village - Ethnicity: Jingpo, Lisu
3 Manbangtang Village - Ethnicity: Kunge, Bulang
4 Guai Village - Ethnicity: Zhuang
5 Hongyan Village - Ethnicity: Yi
6 Ma'anqiao Village - Ethnicity: Dai, Yi
7 Xingguang Village - Ethnicity: Miao
8 Bapa Village - Ethnicity: Dong
9 Nanjiang Village - Ethnicity: Dong
10 Gaoyou Village and Nongtuan Village - Ethnicity: Dong
11 Macha Village - Ethnicity: Han
12 Datan Village - Ethnicity: Hui
13 Dangzheng Village - Ethnicity: Han
14 Dacao Village - Ethnicity: Manchu

Fig. 1.2 Project sites of the CCOUC Ethnic Minority Health Project in China.

1.1.2 Project structure

The project team collaborates with multidisciplinary partners and the community leaders to identify specific health risks and disaster-preparedness solutions that might be relevant and useful for their local situations. In-depth health needs assessments are conducted in selected sites through household interviews, focus groups, and environmental analysis. Information will be collected related to general socioeconomic, demographic health status, as well as community- and household-based disaster preparedness (in terms of availability of household disaster kits, knowledge of oral rehydration solution (ORS) preparation, food and water security, proneness to infectious

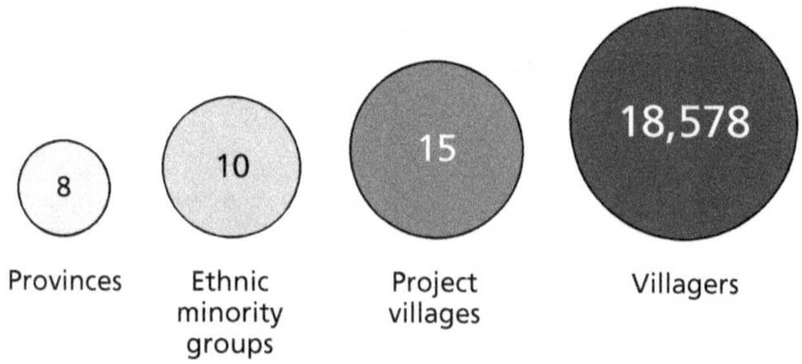

Fig. 1.3 The CCOUC Ethnic Minority Health Project in numbers.
Reproduced by kind permission of Emily Ying Yang CHAN, Copyright © 2017 Emily Ying Yang CHAN.

diseases, as well as their access to healthcare services). Each of the project sites would ensure a project time commitment of 18 to 24 months and the project cycle can be categorized into four main phases, namely site selection, needs assessment, health intervention, and impact evaluation (see Fig. 1.4). Each phase, including site selection, requires paying at least one visit to the village; time in-between visits ranges from three months to one year.

1.2 Main areas for interventions

Five main interventions in health and disaster preparedness (water and health, indoor environment, waste management, health behaviour, and disaster preparedness and risk reduction) were chosen and implemented for EMHP since 2009. The project team has gained many valuable insights for building this bottom-up health and disaster risk reduction programme in remote areas in China. The following are some

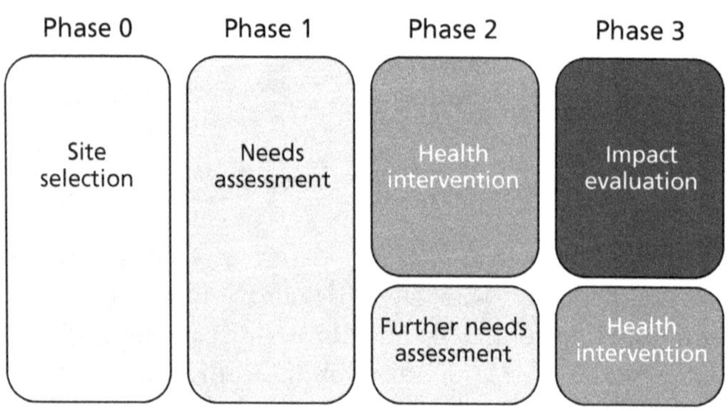

Fig. 1.4 Project structure of the CCOUC Ethnic Minority Health Project in China.
Reproduced by kind permission of Emily Ying Yang CHAN, Copyright © 2017 Emily Ying Yang CHAN.

key findings that might be relevant as reference for programme developers or policy-makers who may be interested in the context.

1.2.1 Water and health

Globally, the World Health Organization (WHO, 2000) estimates that more than 2.2 million people died from diarrhoea in 1999. WHO (2008) suggested clean and safe drinking water can prevent 1.4 million of children dying from diarrhoea annually. A more recent global assessment of risk factors for ill health highlighted that unsafe water and poor sanitation still accounted for 0.9% of all years of disability-adjusted life years (DALYs) in 2010 (Lim *et al.*, 2012). In China, water-related health problems include inadequate protection of water sources, lack of basic hygiene infrastructure (e.g. toilets), lack of knowledge in drinking water management, as well as suboptimal personal hygiene practices.

Inadequate protection of the water source

In many rural villages in China, although water shortage has been addressed by better infrastructure support in recent years, water quality and safety still pose significant risks of waterborne diseases. Drinking water in rural villages may be polluted by various human factors (e.g. cross-contamination when the same water sources are used by both livestock and humans, poor selection of sanitation locations, or lack of awareness of personal hygiene practices).

Lack of basic hygiene infrastructure (e.g. toilets)

CCOUC study found that toilet availability in remote areas is generally low. Forty-three per cent of rural residents did not have a fixed place for urination and defaecation. Unprocessed and directly exposed human excretion provides a breeding ground for vectors (e.g. flies, mosquitoes, and rodents), thereby increasing the likelihood of the outbreak of vector-borne communicable diseases. In addition, research indicated the incidence of gastrointestinal diseases among areas with readily available toilet facilities is lower than those without proper facilities (Zhong, 2007). However, field observations indicted that availability of toilet facilities and good personal hygiene practice among villagers might not be correlated.

Lack of knowledge on drinking water management

Suboptimal water quality maintenance may result from erroneous risk perception and the lack of proper knowledge. For example, many rural residents may perceive mountain water as clean and, thus, CCOUC field assessments found that half of the villagers preferred to drink unboiled water. In communities which experience water scarcity, people were also found to drink untreated long-stored rainwater for the concern that boiling water may evaporate precious water resources.

Lack of proper personal hygiene habits

Even with infrastructure advancement, basic hygiene promotion remains a core component to protect public health in rural context. However, even with media and policy campaigns, reports from CCOUC project sites showed 30% of villagers did not have a habit of regular handwashing before a meal. The prevalence of regular tooth brushing and bathing were also found to be low in rural China.

1.2.2 Indoor environment

With modernization and urbanized living in rural communities, the indoor environment presents significant risks to health and disaster preparedness. Fire hazards resulted from suboptimal electricity installation, air pollution generated by cooking fuel, lack of separation of livestock and human living quarters, and burning waste indoors (plastics, electronic waste such as batteries, and so on) cause major health risks.

Indoor air pollution caused by incomplete combustion of cooking fuel

Long-term exposure to the thick smoke generated by the incomplete combustion of solid fuel may trigger different respiratory diseases and cancers. WHO (n.d. and 2014) indicates that household indoor air pollution from cooking with solid fuels led to 7.7% of the global mortality and the premature deaths of about 4.3 million, particularly in low- and middle-income countries, in 2012. In China, studies found women with prolonged exposure to cooking fumes were 4.1 times more likely to suffer from lung cancer than their non-exposed counterparts (Shi *et al.*, 2005). In rural areas, the risk is particularly high as villagers cook primarily with solid fuel (e.g. firewood or cow dung).

No fixed place for keeping livestock and human living quarters

In rural areas, it is common to see livestock roaming freely in and out of the living rooms, kitchens, and even bedrooms of some rural houses. Although most sheds for keeping livestock have locks, CCOUC found more than 90% of farm households would leave their sheds unlocked during the daytime to facilitate feeding. Not only do the livestock carry a strong odour, but also cause problems for household hygiene (e.g. animal faeces and pests are readily found around the house), and may increase communicable disease risk to rural residents (WHO, 2006).

1.2.3 Waste management

With economic development and an increase of disposable household income, consumption patterns of rural people have changed considerably. Research showed that 140 million tonnes of waste were produced by rural villages in China in 2000, with an average rate of 0.8 kg per person per day (Sun *et al.*, 2008). If the current rate of rural–urban economic development and consumption pattern is to be continued, waste is estimated to increase at an annual rate of 10% in China.

Lack of knowledge on waste management

For villages with good transport support and better economic conditions, waste management are done centrally and collected waste transported to the landfills nearby. Yet, for villages without the economic or logistic capacity to manage the ever-increasing amount of waste, less than 10% of the village communities are aware of the concept ‘Reduce,

Reuse, and Recycle' and 82.3% of the villagers had the habit of burning waste indiscriminately (including plastics/batteries) indoors at home with no awareness of the potential health impacts associated with such practices.

Improper handling of pesticide-related waste

Use of pesticides is a common farming practice in rural China. The labelling, storage, and recycling of pesticides must be handled cautiously (Wang *et al.*, 2011). Improper management of pesticides can cause acute and chronic toxication, which is hazardous to the environment and threatening to human health. However, from field observations, there are limited awareness and concerns in rural communities with pesticide-related waste and pollution.

1.2.4 **Health behaviour**

Smoking

According to the Chinese Adult Tobacco Survey in 2015, the smoking rate among the Chinese population was 27.7%. Among males, 52.1% were current smokers, with a higher rate in rural areas (55.4%) when compared with that in urban areas (49.0%) (China CDC, 2015). Although no significant difference in prevalence of smoking was found compared to 2010 (51.6% among males), a declining trend was observed for smoking in public places (e.g. offices, schools, and healthcare facilities) during 2010–15, implying a reduced exposure to second-hand smoke in the community (China CDC, 2015).

Health impact of alcoholism

In China, drinking rates for males and females were 84.1% and 29.3%, respectively, in which up to 65.3% of the drinkers fell into the category of health drinking status. In addition, the survey co-published by the China Health Care Association, the Chinese Medical Association, and other units entitled 'Survey on healthy drinking status among Chinese citizens' indicates that Chinese citizens have serious gaps in their knowledge regarding alcohol consumption, particularly with regard to consumption quantity, legal drinking ages, and the control of one's tendency to drink ('Healthy Drinking in China' Organizing Committee, 2008). Only 0.51% of drinkers possessed accurate knowledge about drinking. More than 30% of drinkers did not agree with the statement 'excessive drinking brings harm to health and the quantity and content of alcohol should be controlled'. Another national survey found that the average annual alcohol intake was 3 litres among persons aged 18 years or above in 2012, while 9.3% of drinkers had excessive drinking behaviour (NHFPC, 2015).

Lack of knowledge and management of chronic diseases

Chronic illnesses are commonly regarded as 'urban diseases' or 'diseases for the rich' in the country. In 2015, the prevalence of chronic illnesses in urban and rural areas was 26.3% and 22.7%, up from 19.3% and 18.6% in 2002, respectively (Li *et al.*, 2005; NHFPC, 2016). The mortality rate of cerebrovascular disease and heart disease in rural areas have increased drastically, from 115.20 and 73.43 in 1995 to 153.63 and 144.79 per 100,000 in 2015, respectively (NHFPC, 2016). CCOUC's survey indicates that only half of the 43.4% of villagers who needed long-term medication for their chronic illnesses could afford regular medication. Reasons identified by focus groups showed villagers' limited resources, as well as the common attitude that 'if I can stand it, I do not need a doctor' are the two main underlying reasons for such phenomena. When affected individuals finally decided to seek medical help, their health conditions often became untreatable, and the treatment effectiveness were often severely compromised.

1.2.5 Disaster preparedness and risk reduction

China has a large population, complex geographical and metrological conditions, as well as a mosaic of communities in various stages of socioeconomic development within its vast territory. It is also one of the countries which endure almost all types of natural disasters globally. About 50% of the 1.4 billion population in China are living in natural disaster-prone areas and more than 200 million people are affected by disasters annually. Before the Millennium, natural disasters had led to a high death toll and injuries in China, along with substantial economic loss: more than 200 million individuals were affected by disasters annually on average and the direct economic loss was more than RMB 100 billion (Blaikie *et al.*, 1994). Since 2000, despite the further development of disaster response systems following the outbreak of severe acute respiratory syndrome (SARS) in 2003 and several major earthquakes (e.g. the Wenchuan earthquake in 2008), bottom-up disaster preparedness and health risk reduction efforts in rural China are still limited.

Geographical, economic, and living conditions

About half of China's population resides in disaster-prone areas. The socioeconomic and education levels of these areas are relatively low, hence rural residents often suffer from higher risk in life and property losses in disasters when compared with their urban counterparts. In addition, ethnic minorities (non-Han Chinese in China) typically reside in remote areas, have limited access to timely external assistance, and can only rely on their capability and preparedness at the early stages of disaster relief. A CCOUC study in Datan Village of Gansu Province found that previous disaster exposure was significantly associated with villagers' perception of living in a high disaster risk area, but not their level of disaster preparedness (Chan *et al.*, 2014)."

Lack of awareness on disaster preparedness and risk reduction at household and individual levels

Only 20–30% of villagers in CCOUC project sites believe that they have the ability to keep their family members and themselves safe and less than 80% of households living in disaster-prone communities (with disaster occurrence within five years before the interview) have ever thought about preparing for disasters. Global climate change has rendered China more vulnerable to extreme weather and climate-related natural hazards.

Approaches for disaster preparedness and risk reduction are thus becoming increasingly urgent matters to ensure the well-being and community resilience of rural citizens.

Effectiveness of bottom-up disaster resilience intervention

A CCOUC study in Hongyan Village of Sichuan Province found that health intervention participants managed to gain knowledge from interventions and were nine times more likely to know the correct composition and retain relevant knowledge of oral rehydration solution (ORS) and disaster preparedness kit ownership 12 months after the intervention (Chan *et al.*, 2017). More results will be discussed in later chapters.[1]

Note

1 For updated information about the EMHP, see CCOUC website at http://ccouc.org/home-5

References

Blaikie, P., Cannon, T., Davis, I., & Wisner, B. (1994). *At Risk: Natural Hazards, People's Vulnerability, and Disasters.* London, UK: Routledge.

Chan, E. Y. Y., Guo, C., Lee, P., Liu, S., & Mark, C. K. M. (2017). Health Emergency and Disaster Risk Management (Health-EDRM) in remote ethnic minority areas of rural China: the case of a flood-prone village in Sichuan. *Int J Disaster Risk Sci.* doi:10.1007/s13753-017-0121-1 [Online].

Chan, E. Y. Y., Kim, J. H., Lin, C., Cheung, E. Y. L., & Lee, P. P. Y. (2014). Is previous disaster experience a good predictor for disaster preparedness in extreme poverty households in remote Muslim minority based community in China? *J Immigr Minor Health*, **16**, 466–72.

Chinese Center for Disease Control and Prevention (China CDC) (2015). [*The 2015 Chinese Adult Tobacco Survey*]. Available at: http://www.tcrc.org.cn/UploadFiles/2016-03/318/201603231215175500.pdf (accessed 20 July 2017) (Chinese). [Online].

Collaborating Centre for Oxford University and CUHK for Disaster and Medical Humanitarian Response (CCOUC) (n.d.). Ethnic minority health project. Available at: http://ccouc.org/home-5 (accessed 20 February 2017) [Online].

'Healthy Drinking in China' Organizing Committee (2008). [*Healthy Drinking in 25 Provinces of China Survey Report 2007*]. China: Author (Chinese).

Li, L. M., Rao, K. Q., Kong, L. Z., *et al.* (2005). [A description on the Chinese national nutrition and health survey in 2002]. *Chinese Journal of Epidemiology*, **26**, 478–84 (Chinese).

Lim, S. S., Vos, T., Flaxman, A. D., *et al.* (2012). A comparative risk assessment of burden of disease and injury attributable to 67 risk factors and risk factor clusters in 21 regions, 1990–2010: a systematic analysis for the Global Burden of Disease Study 2010. *Lancet*, **380**, 2224–60.

Ministry of Health of the People's Republic of China. Centre for Health Statistics and Information (2009). [*An Analysis Report of the Fourth National Health Services Survey in China in 2008*]. Beijing, China: Peking Union Medical College Press (Chinese).

National Health and Family Plaining Commission of China (NHFPC) (2015). [*The National Nutrition and Chronic Disease Survey 2015*]. Available at: http://www.nhfpc.gov.cn/jkj/s5879/201506/4505528e65f3460fb88685081ff158a2.shtml (accessed 20 July 2017) (Chinese). [Online].

National Health and Family Plaining Commission of China (NHFPC) (2016). *2016 China Health and Family Planning Statistical Yearbook.* Beijing, China: Peking Union Medical College Press.

Shi, H. L., He, Q. C., Dai, X. C., & Zhou, B. S. (2005). [Study on risk factors of lung cancer in non-smoking women]. *Chinese Journal of Lung Cancer*, **8**, 280–3 (Chinese).

Sun, H. M., Zhang, J. F., & Liu, G. Z. (2008). [Exploring solid waste recycling in rural China]. *Journal of Agricultural Resources and Environment*, **6**, 29–31 (Chinese).

Wang, C., Zhang, W., & Guo, Y. H. (2011). [Hazard classification and labelling for pesticide packing and transport]. *Agrochemicals*, 7, 534–8 (Chinese).

World Health Organization (WHO) (n.d.). Mortality from household air pollution. Available at: http://www.who.int/gho/phe/indoor_air_pollution/burden/en/ (accessed 20 February 2017) [Online].

World Health Organization (WHO) (2000). *The World Health Report 2000: Health Systems: Improving Performance*. Geneva, Switzerland: WHO.

World Health Organization (WHO) (2006). *The Control of Neglected Zoonotic Diseases: A Route to Poverty Alleviation*. Geneva, Switzerland: WHO.

World Health Organization (WHO) (2008). How does safe water impact global health? Available at: http://www.who.int/features/qa/70/en/ (accessed 24 January 2017) [Online].

World Health Organization (WHO) (2014). Burden of disease from household air pollution for 2012. Available at: http://www.who.int/phe/health_topics/outdoorair/databases/HAP_BoD_results_March2014.pdf?ua=1 (accessed 20 February 2017) [Online].

Zhong, G. M. (2007). [Progress in water and sanitation improvement in China and its effectiveness for gastrointestinal infection control]. *Journal of Environment and Health*, **11**, 927–9 (Chinese).

Further reading on the ethnic minority health project

Centre for Research on the Epidemiology of Disasters (2016). Country Maps. Available at: http://emdat.be/country-maps#overlay-c=map-archive (accessed 7 March 2017) [Online].

Chan, E. Y. Y. (2005). [*Sans Frontières under the Sun*]. Hong Kong, China: Hong Kong Economic Times Press (Chinese).

Chan, E. Y. Y. (2012). [Stories in Wenchuan earthquake response]. In: Zhou, Y., & Li, W. Y. (eds) [*Notes from Médecins Sans Frontières*], pp. 120–3. Changsha, China: Hunan Science and Technology Press (Chinese).

Chan, E. Y. Y. (2013). Health needs of older people after earthquake. In: Guest, C., Ricciardi, W., Kawachi, I., & Lang, I. (eds) *Oxford Handbook of Public Health Practice*, 3rd Edition, p. 42. Oxford, UK: Oxford University Press.

Chan, E. Y. Y. (2015a). [*Public Health and Liberal Studies: Analysis of Cross-Module Issues*]. Hong Kong, China: Hong Kong Educational Publishing Company (Chinese).

Chan, E. Y. Y. (2015b). [Urban disaster preparedness in Hong Kong]. In: Ma, Z. J. (ed.) [*A Hundred Thousand Why (New Vision Edition): Disasters and Preparedness I*], p. 10. Hong Kong, China: Commercial Press (Chinese).

Chan, E. Y. Y., Chan, G. K. W., Wong, C. K. P., Huang, Z., & Wong, C. S. (2016). *Relationship between Disasters and Public Health from a Hong Kong Perspective*. Hong Kong, China: Collaborating Centre for Oxford University and CUHK for Disaster and Medical Humanitarian Response.

Chan, E. Y. Y., Chan, G. K. W., Wong, C. K. P., Huang, Z., Yung, T. K. C., & Liu, S. D. (2016). [*Health and Disaster Preparedness in Rural China: Advanced Training Manual*]. Hong Kong, China: CCOUC and WZQCF (Chinese).

Chan, E. Y. Y., Chan, G. K. W., Wong, C. K. P., *et al.* (2016). [*Globalization: Climate Change and Human Health*]. Hong Kong, China: Collaborating Centre for Oxford University and CUHK for Disaster and Medical Humanitarian Response. (Chinese).

Chan, E. Y. Y., & Gao, Y. (2013). [The current situation of healthcare and disaster preparedness needs in remote rural ethnic minority areas in China: insights from public health research and services]. *Injury Medicine*, **1**, 1–3 (Chinese).

Chan, E. Y. Y., Kim, J. H., Lin, C., Cheung, E. Y. L., & Lee, P. P. Y. (2014). Is previous disaster experience a good predictor for disaster preparedness in extreme poverty households in remote Muslim minority based community in China? *Journal of Immigrant and Minority Health*, **16**, 466–72.

Chan, E. Y. Y., & Li, W. (2016). Role of government and NGOs. In: Wolfson, N., Lerner, A., & Roshal, L. (eds) *Orthopedics in Disasters: Orthopedic Injuries in Natural Disasters and Mass Casualty Events*, pp. 47–59. Berlin, Germany: Springer-Verlag Berlin Heidelberg.

Chan, E. Y. Y., Liu, K. S., Lee, P. Y., Ling, K. W. K., & Wong, C. S. (2016). *Training Manual on Health and Disaster Preparedness in Rural China*. Hong Kong, China: CCOUC and WZQCF.

Chan, E. Y. Y., & Southgate, R. J. (2014). Responding to chronic disease needs following disasters: A rethink using the Human Security approach. In: Hobson, C., Bacon, P., Cameron, R. (eds) *Human Security and Natural Disasters* (Routledge Humanitarian Studies series), pp. 74–93. Tokyo, Japan: Routledge.

Chan, E. Y. Y., Zhu, C. Y. J., Lee, P. Y., & Liu, K. S. (2015). [*Training Manual on Health and Disaster Preparedness in Rural China*]. Hong Kong, China: CCOUC and WZQCF (Chinese).

Chapter 2

Public health principles for health and disaster risk reduction programmes

Public health is a multidisciplinary subject which not only concerns health on an individual level, but also the protection and improvement of the community's health as a whole. This chapter discusses a number of basic concepts in public health to support conceptualization and building of health and emergency and disaster risk reduction programmes at the field level.

2.1 Definition of health and public health

According to the World Health Organization (WHO), 'health' covers the physical, mental, and social well-being of individuals (Constitution of the World Health Organization, 1946; see Fig. 2.1). In addition to disease pattern monitoring and risk factor identification that are associated with negative health, the definition also encompasses the positive dimension of individual well-being (such as health improvements, disease prevention, and well-being enhancement efforts).

Public health concerns health at the individual, community, and global levels. It is a subject that includes clinical medicine, physical, and social sciences, ethics, and law to examine the well-being of human in a society. It may be defined as 'the science and art of preventing disease, prolonging life and promoting health through organized efforts of society' (Acheson, 1988, p. 1).

Although public health and clinical medicine are different, they are interconnected subjects. Clinical medicine focuses on an individual level while public health targets issues at the population level. The nexus lies in their applications of research methods and principles of evidence-based medicine to conduct research and decision-making to embrace patient-centred values in the practice of healthcare.

2.2 Three domains of public health

Subjects within public health might be categorized into three major domains, namely health protection, health improvement, and health services (see Fig. 2.2) (Lewis *et al.*, 2015).

Health protection targets the prevention and control of infectious diseases from environmental risks (such as the quality of the air, drinking water and food, and natural, chemical and technological emergencies). Examples of health protection in public health activity ranges from environment management (air quality monitoring, rodent and pest

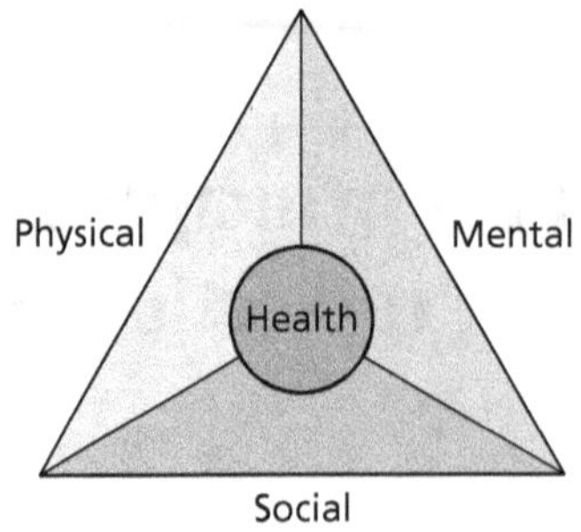

Fig. 2.1 A representation of the definition of health by the World Health Organization (WHO).
Source: data from World Health Organization. *Constitution of the World Health Organization*, http://apps.who.int/gb/bd/PDF/bd47/EN/constitution-en.pdf?ua=1, accessed 01 Feb. 2017, Copyright © 1946 World Health Organization.

control, food safety and restaurant hygiene management), occupational health protection, and infectious disease protection efforts (such as vaccination, quarantine, vector control measures). *Health improvement* refers to activities that improve well-being and reduce health inequalities. Effective actions and approaches always involve multisectoral collaborations (in the fields of housing and education, for instance, and the working environment

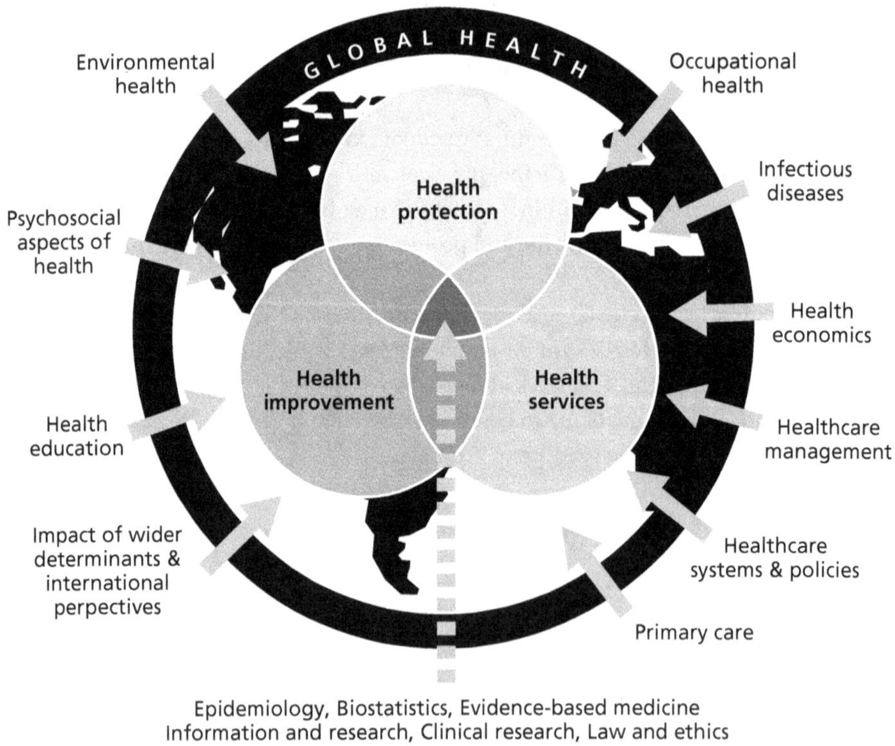

Fig. 2.2 The three domains of public health.

and family/community networks), such as the promotion of balanced diet, sex education, smoking cessation, hiking campaigns, and so on. *Health services* focus on health service-related organization, management, and policy development. Legal and management principles can be used to support service development and resource allocation.

2.3 Determinants of health

Theories and frameworks have been developed to describe factors that may influence health outcomes. Among the health determinants frameworks, the Dahlgren–Whitehead rainbow diagram of health determinants categorizes different health determinants into conceptual layers (Dahlgren and Whitehead, 1991; see Fig. 2.3).

Individual/personal determinants, such as age, sex, gene/hereditary factors, are regarded as *non-modifiable factors* and constitute as the innermost part of the rainbow diagram. The factors in the remaining layers are *modifiable factors* that can be modified and thus final health outcomes are very often affected by these determinants. The second layer comprises individual *lifestyle and behavioural determinants* such as daily diet, physical exercise, smoking, and drinking. Personal habits can be modified and their related health risks may be reduced through education and information provision. The third layer encompasses *society, network, and community* determinants that may influence health outcomes, including peers, social context, and network. *Socioeconomic* factors, the fourth layer, influence health outcomes through working and living environments. Transportation, location, and the local

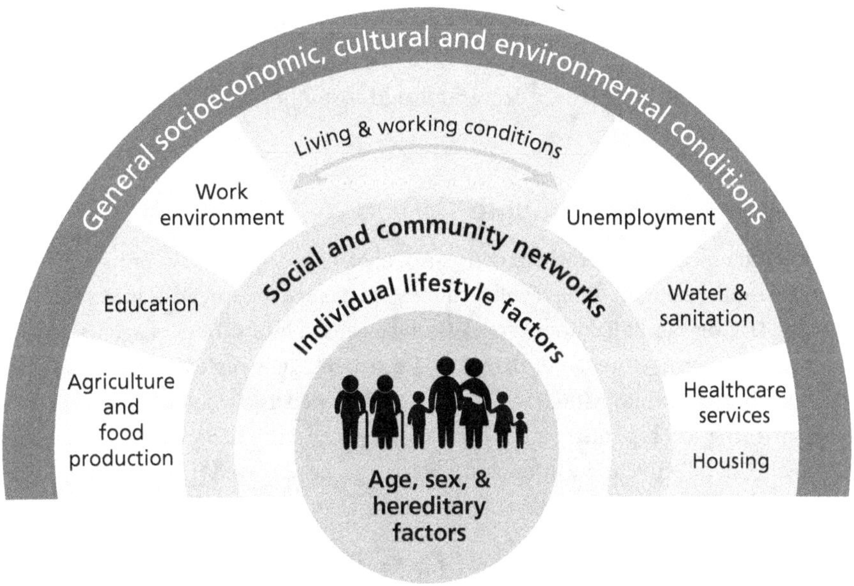

Fig. 2.3 A rainbow diagram of health determinants.

Reproduced with permission from Dahlgren G and Whitehead M. *Policies and strategies to promote social equity in health.* Copyright © 1991 Institute for Future Studies, Stockholm, http://www.iffs.se/media/1326/20080109110739filmZ8UVQv2wQFShMRF6cuT.pdf, accessed 01 Feb 2017.

culture surrounding the use of facilities surrounding these environments may have profound impacts on individuals' health. The outermost layer of determinants are named as *macro-determinants*, such as global, socioeconomic, cultural, and environmental factors that affect a country and the world. In summary, the Dahlgren–Whitehead health determinant model demonstrates a significant proportion of health determinants are modifiable. Public health practice and policy advocacy should aim to examine and target determinants according to relevant conceptual theories and models.

2.4 Disease prevention

A classical disease prevention framework (i.e. a hierarchy of prevention) consists of three levels of disease prevention (Leavell and Clark, 1958): *primary prevention* aims to prevent disease or injury from occurring and it includes efforts to ensure health protection and health improvement. Health protection can be achieved by programme organization (e.g. vaccination programmes), legislation, and health policy and law enforcement (e.g. banning of indoor smoking and drunk driving). Health improvement focuses on health education and promotion to reduce and prevent health risk. *Secondary prevention* refers to measures that may reduce disease impact. For example, screening of a high-risk population (such those at risk of cancer) is an example of secondary prevention. Chances of cure may increase with early screening as it may prevent disease progression and symptom development. *Tertiary prevention* helps individuals/patients to reduce disease complications and disabilities. It highlights that even if a disease cannot be cured, proper rehabilitation will reduce disease-related ability loss and improve quality of life for the affected individuals. In principle, primary prevention efforts usually target the general population or cover the largest proportion of preventable health impacts. Secondary prevention targets high-risk groups, and tertiary prevention addresses the health needs of those who are already affected by disease.

2.5 Epidemiological triangle

The epidemiological triangle, which consists of agents, hosts, and environment, describes the three essential elements which will facilitate and change the spread of infectious disease (see Fig. 2.4). Common infectious diseases can be caused by a variety of agents/pathogens such as bacteria, virus, fungi, and parasites. These pathogens replicate inside the body of a host and clinical symptoms/diseases might be developed as a result of toxins released by these agents. The accompanied pathophysiological process might damage normal cells and their functions. Effective prevention and control can be achieved if connections between any two elements may be disrupted with this triangle.

2.5.1 Communicable diseases and infection control

Communicable diseases are clinical conditions that may be transmitted within a host community. There are three basic principles in communicable disease control. First, boosting host's immune system (e.g. vaccination and use of prophylactic medicine) may help reduce

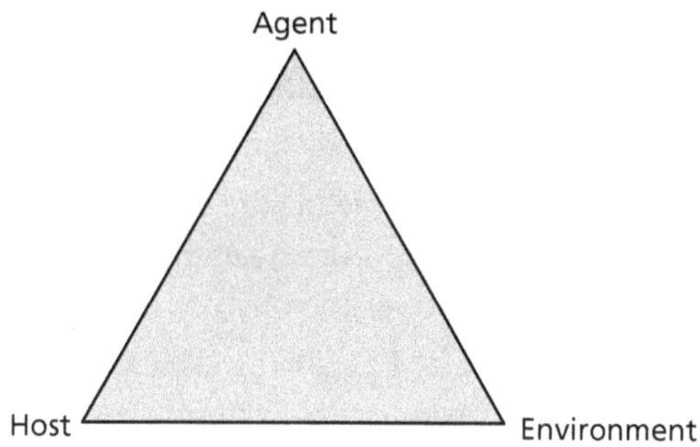

Fig. 2.4 The epidemiological triangle.

adverse clinical manifestations and disease proliferation. Second, measures that may eliminate the source of infection (e.g. sterilization, isolation, patient treatment, and the removal of pathogen breeding grounds) should be developed. Last, but not least, prevention strategies (good personal, environmental, and food hygiene) that will block specific transmission route of the targeted infectious diseases should be established (Box 2.1).

2.5.2 **Non-communicable diseases and control**

Non-communicable diseases (NCDs) are medical conditions that do not spread among host community. In the twenty-first century, personal habits, and living conditions evolve rapidly with the advanced global economy and social development. Coupled with the changing of disease pattern and population ageing around the world, NCD prevalence has significantly increased in both developed and developing countries. Globally, approximately 36 million people lose their lives annually to NCDs or their related complications. With 80% of these deaths taking place in countries of low and middle income and are the main cause of death in all regions except Africa, NCDs currently account for 43% of the global health burden. It is predicted that in 2020, NCDs will be responsible for 60% of the global health burden and 73% of deaths.

There are two main types of NCD, and they can be grouped according to their temporality—acute and chronic. *Acute* NCDs are short-term clinical incidents such as stroke, myocardial infarction, injuries/accidents, and overdose of drugs and alcohol. *Chronic* NCDs are continuous diseases which exert a long-term effect on health. The four main common NCDs in the twenty-first century include cardiovascular disease, cancer, chronic respiratory disease, and diabetes mellitus. Mental health issues are also significant global chronic NCDs, with a prevalence rate ranging between 4% and 26%. Not only are mental health conditions (such as depressions) one of the underlying causes for self-harm and suicide, they are also known to be associated with an increased risk for cardiovascular diseases and diabetes mellitus. *Injury*, unintentional and intentional, represents another significant non-communicable healthcare burden in the twenty-first century (Haagsma *et al.*, 2015). Although overall injury-caused mortality and morbidity have decreased with time, two-thirds of deaths globally were resulted from unintentional causes and one-third

Box 2.1 Transmission routes of infectious diseases

The transmission routes can be broadly divided into seven categories:

1. **Contact transmission**: direct contact with patients or their body fluids or contact with contaminated objects. Examples are scabies, head lice, hand-foot-and-mouth disease (HFMD), and acute infectious conjunctivitis.
2. **Droplet transmission**: the infected person produces droplets when they cough, sneeze, or speak that contain pathogens. Examples include influenza, the common cold, and severe acute respiratory syndrome (SARS). These diseases can be controlled by vaccination, good personal (e.g. frequent handwashing) and environmental hygiene, as well as maintenance of indoor air ventilation.
3. **Airborne transmission**: patients spread the pathogens when they cough and sneeze. The pathogens can stay in the air for a period of time and enter human bodies via the respiratory tract. An example is tuberculosis. When patients cough, sneeze, and speak, germs will be spread into the air. People, particularly the immunocompromised, may get infected. To control the spread of tuberculosis, BCG vaccination, rapid treatment, good personal and environmental hygiene, and good indoor air ventilation are helpful strategies.
4. **Vector transmission**: the term *vector* refers to tiny organisms such as mosquitoes, house dust mites, and ticks. They can transfer the pathogens from an infected person to another person. Examples are dengue fever, malaria, and Japanese encephalitis. Transmission of these diseases requires mosquitoes. Disease control can be achieved by elimination of mosquito breeding grounds and spraying of pesticides. Personal preventive measures include wearing pale, long-sleeved tops and long trousers, using insect repellent and mosquito nets, and taking prophylactic medicine before going to areas where malaria is prevalent.
5. **Blood-borne** and **body fluid transmission**: pathogens can be spread from the infected person to others by blood and body fluids. Examples include hepatitis B, hepatitis C and Human Immunodeficiency Virus (HIV)/Acquired Immunodeficiency Syndrome (AIDS). Transmission routes include sexual contact, needle sharing and mother-to-child vertical transmission. Quitting drugs and safe sex practices (such as using condoms) can control disease spread by blocking the transmission route
6. **Foodborne transmission**: ingestion of contaminated food. Examples are food poisoning, cholera, and shigellosis. Control measures include good personal and environmental hygiene, and safe food handling practices.
7. **Congenital transmission**: also known as vertical transmission. The disease is spread from an infected mother to her foetus. An example is congenital Acquired Immunodeficiency Syndrome (AIDS). Control measures include antenatal and neonatal screening, safe delivery practices, and postnatal management.

was from intentional injury. Road injury, self-harm, falls, and interpersonal violence are the main causes of death for the past decades. Except for burn-related injuries, males are more likely to sustain injury than females globally. Due to the difference in context, pattern differences are reported between developed and developing regions, as well as urban and rural injury environments (Jacobsen, 2014).

According to the concept of 'determinants of health', an individual's likelihood of developing illnesses can vary with many factors. Among them, personal lifestyle choices (smoking, lack of exercise, alcohol abuse, unhealthy diet, and so on) are found to be closely associated to NCD development. These unhealthy lifestyles will lead to physiological changes that could increase the risk of developing NCDs. For example, having a diet that is high in salt, sugar, and fat may lead to the three 'H = hyper diseases' (hypertension, hyperglycaemia, and hyperlipidaemia). These conditions increase the chance of obesity, cardiovascular diseases, diabetes, and hypertension. Nevertheless, as the development of these NCDs tends to take a long duration and people seldom experience the direct relationship between lifestyle and these diseases (e.g. smoking and lung cancer, and between alcoholism and liver cancer), the awareness and active management of health risks remain low.

2.6 Health promotion

Health promotion is a core component of public health and plays a leading role in health improvement. The First International Conference on Health Promotion, held in Ottawa, Canada in 1986, produced the *Ottawa Charter for Health Promotion* which defined health promotion as 'the process of enabling people to increase control over, and to improve, their health'. It also advocated regarding health as a resource for everyday life rather than the objective of living (WHO, 1986). The purpose of health promotion is to reduce health inequalities and ensure people have equal opportunities and resources in order to maximize health. Health promotion includes the provision of a stable and supportive environment to give the general public access to health messages. It also includes education on life skills to empower individuals to make choices that are conducive to their health (Box 2.2). Apart from promoting health behaviour, successful health promotion also requires collaborative implementations measures by the government, health service institutions, non-governmental organizations, voluntary organizations, and the media.

There are many ways to promote health, but programmes should always take into account the social background of targets and the local culture. For example, in urban areas of China, three levels of the health education network—city, district, and street—are designed to create a Healthy City. In rural areas, the 'National Health Promotion Project for Hundreds of Millions of Chinese Farmers' mainly targets villagers, farmers, and migrant workers. The project may have multiple objectives that include the increase of the childhood vaccination rate, reduction of the number with iodine deficiency, improvement of tobacco control, and prevention and control of infections like schistosomiasis, Acute Immunodeficiency Syndrome (AIDS), avian flu, and hepatitis. Successful health promotion requires collaborative and concerted efforts in a society (Box 2.3).

Box 2.2 WHO on health promotion

WHO has proposed five major steps in health promotion.

1. **Build healthy public policy**: place health on the agenda of policymakers in all sectors and directs them to be conscious of the impact on public health of their decisions and accept their responsibilities for health.
2. **Create supportive environments**: create a society which adopts the principle of taking care of each other, communities, and the environment.
3. **Strengthen community actions**: implement concrete and effective community action in priority setting, strategy planning, and programme implementation. Community development draws on existing human and material resources in the community to enhance self-help and social support and to develop flexible systems for reinforcement of public participation in health issues.
4. **Develop personal skills**: support personal and social development through providing information, health education, and life skills enhancement, health promotion. People can exercise more control over their health and the environment and be able to make decisions beneficial to health. Action is needed through schools and families, as well as professional, commercial, and voluntary bodies.
5. **Reorient health services**: move the health sector in a health promotion direction, beyond its responsibilities for providing clinical and curative services to support the needs of individuals and communities for a healthier life.

Box 2.3 Health promotion = health education?

Many practitioners regard health promotion and health education as similar approaches but they are in fact different. WHO defines health promotion as 'the process of enabling people to increase control over, and to improve, their health. It moves beyond a focus on individual behaviour towards a wide range of social and environmental interventions', while health education is 'any combination of learning experiences designed to help individuals and communities improve their health, by increasing their knowledge or influencing their attitudes'. Education is a major component of health promotion, and formal health education programmes may influence attitudes, knowledge, and behaviour as to enable the stakeholders to make informed decision about their lifestyles or health-related choices. People's actions and knowledge are also affected by norms, context, and ranges of information routes other than health education campaigns. Of note, as health education does not include policy recommendations and actions that change infrastructure, environment, or social policy. Health promotion efforts rarely rely on health education alone for potential success.

2.7 Healthy Settings

Settings offer structure (infrastructure), resources (staff), and access to people. When engaging in activities related to health promotion, important consideration should be made to ensure appropriate settings are selected for such efforts. Some examples of typical health promotion settings include workplaces, schools, primary care, prisons, and universities. The Healthy Settings movement came out of the WHO strategy of 'Health for All' in 1980. Building on the *Ottawa Charter for Health Promotion* in 1986, the Sundsvall Statement of 1992 called for the creation of supportive environments with a focus on settings for health, while the Jakarta Declaration in 1997 emphasized the value of settings for implementing comprehensive strategies and providing an infrastructure for health promotion. Today, various settings are used to facilitate the improvement of public health throughout the world.

'Healthy Villages' is a holistic approach to address critical environmental health problems in rural areas and is a concept first proposed by the WHO Eastern Mediterranean Regional Office (EMRO) in 1989, in a Technical Consultation on Urban Environmental Health, which was held in the WHO Eastern Mediterranean Regional Office in Alexandria, Egypt (WHO, 1990, 1994). The basis of the Healthy Villages programme is similar to the Healthy Cities programme, but applied in rural areas as opposed to urban ones (Khosh-Chashm, 1995). Although health may be defined differently by rural residents, the generally accepted definition of a 'Healthy Village' includes a community with low rates of infectious diseases, access to basic healthcare services, and a stable and peaceful social environment. According to Howard *et al.* (2002), there are five main health-affecting components that might need to be addressed to develop a 'Healthy Village'. This includes environment, awareness of individuals and community about health, personal hygiene, healthcare, and diseases. As of 2009, Healthy Village initiatives were implemented actively only in the WHO African Regional Office and EMRO, two of the six regions of WHO. The concept is not being actively pursued in the WHO Western Pacific Region (WHO, n.d., 2009). WHO has developed the concept in *Healthy Villages: A guide for communities and community health workers* (Howard *et al.*, 2002) and describes five main factors affecting the health of a village:

- Environment: this includes work, living environment, and community structure. A clean environment can prevent the spread of diseases. It can also promote mental well-being. An open-minded society which encourages the resolution of conflicts via dialogue can make people healthier.
- Awareness of health issues: if people do not understand the causes of diseases and how to improve health, they cannot decide how to allocate resources and fight for external assistance. Therefore, awareness of health issues among individuals and the community is the basis of improving community health.
- Personal hygiene: personal hygiene is an important element of health improvement and the maintenance of the benefits brought by health interventions. If people do not know how to manage wounds, there may be infection or more severe complications

even for a minor injury. If people do not wash their hands after using the toilet, store drinking water appropriately, clean their clothes and utensils, and bathe properly, attempts to prevent the spread of disease will not be effective even with drinking water and sanitation facilities.

- Healthcare: everyone suffers from diseases in their lifetime. They need medical services when they fall ill. Hence, the accessibility to healthcare services has an important influence on people's health.
- Diseases: faecal–oral diseases and vector-borne diseases affect a large population annually and may cause death occasionally. Clean drinking water, good personal hygiene, and effective pest control are effective ways to improve community health.

The Ethnic Minority Health Project of CCOUC aims to increase both an understanding of the need for personal hygiene and an awareness of health issues in villages.

2.8 Health system

According to the WHO's definition, *health system* includes all units, individuals, and behaviours that aim to improve, resume, and maintain a population's health status. A health system can be conceptualised into six main components (de Savigny and Adam, 2009). The first is *leadership and governance*, which concerns the oversight, coalition, regulation, and policy of the health system of a country or a region. The second element is the *healthcare financing structure*, which concerns the appropriate acquisition, allocation, and utilization of resources, as well as risk management, all of which are prerequisites to a well-functioning health system. The third component is the *health workforce*. Healthcare practitioners with different specialization, including doctors, nurses, pharmacists, physiotherapists, and nutritionists, are needed to address the healthcare needs of the community. The fourth component is *medical product and technology*, which includes various medical products, vaccines, medical technologies, and safety protocols and guidelines that can ensure quality, effective, and safe medical care. The fifth domain is about *information and research*. Health information exchange and management, as well as the application of new research findings in medical science, can greatly improve people's health. A smoothly run health system can effectively disseminate reliable and timely information to the community and practitioners. The sixth component is *service delivery*. A healthcare system includes three levels of care to cover the wide scope of health services (see Fig. 2.5). A quality health system can deliver appropriate and comprehensive healthcare services, from primary care, specialist treatment to recovery.

2.9 Pathway of care

Pathway of care is a conceptual framework that illustrates how health needs may be addressed over an individual's progression in his/her journey for a health condition or a

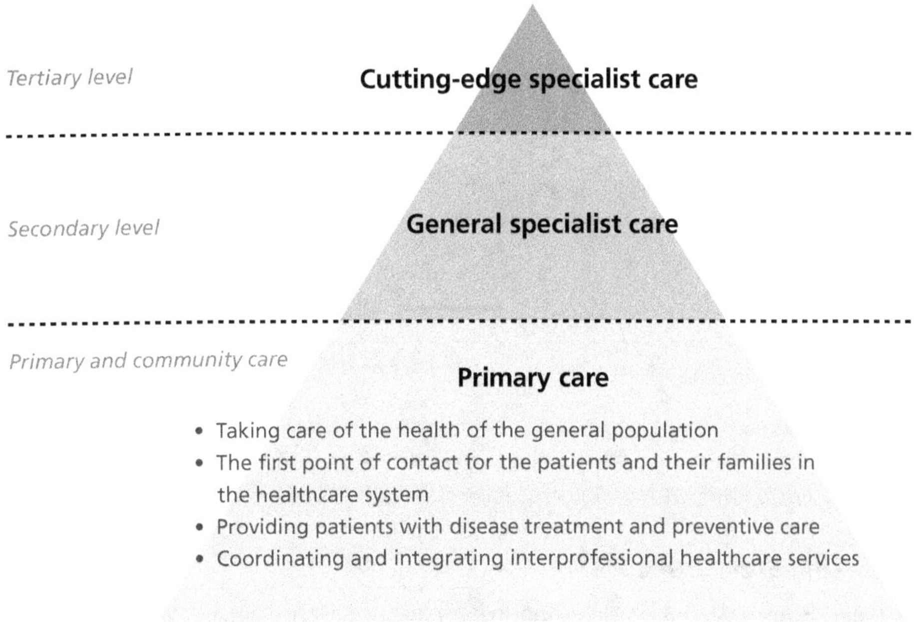

Fig. 2.5 Three levels of care in a healthcare system.

disease. In modern societies, an individual would usually encounters activities/interventions that aim to protect health, prevent disease, and promote general well-being. If a health condition or disease develops, the individual will then undergo diagnosis, treatment, and palliative care (see Fig. 2.6). As public health emphasizes prevention along the pathway of care model, related comprehensive healthcare services can still be provided under limited resources.

While the management of medical conditions involves a spectrum of services targeting various elements along the pathway of care. In rural communities, medical groups and health workers with limited technical capacity and resources might consider providing technical knowledge transfer and community capacity training to local staff so as to ensure the possibility of public health activities and clinical case follow-up along the pathway after treatment. Community partnerships and collaborations can promote local ownership and technical transfer for the sustainability of health service along the pathway of care beyond the immediate disaster relief period.

For example, for chronic disease, even if medical and health programmes do not include the provision of treatment, health practitioners may consider various entry points along the pathway of care, such as: (1) carrying out health education and health promotion on chronic diseases to empower patients with knowledge to enhance their well-being and to reduce potential disease complications on their own; (2) identifying potential referral facilities where services and clinical management support of chronic

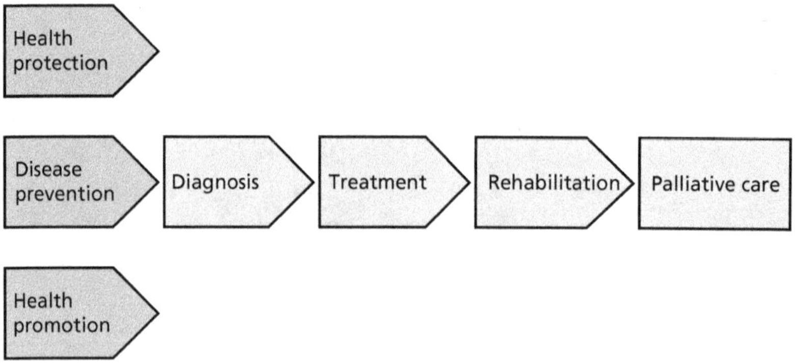

Fig. 2.6 Pathway of care.

diseases may be provided; (3) facilitating referral with good clinical record keeping; and (4) coordinating with various relief services to minimize avoidable complications.

2.10 Disaster concepts

Disasters can usually be divided into three phases conceptually, namely (1) pre-impact phase, (2) impact phase, and (3) post-impact phase. The *pre-impact phase* is the period of time before the onset of a disaster. This is the phase with the greatest potential for negative health impact prevent and the goals may be achieved by implementing two categories of measure: disaster preparedness and mitigation. *Disaster preparedness* refers to activities that can ensure the readiness of timely and efficient response when a hazard strikes. Actions are pre-planned and can be taken at the community and individual levels to minimize the physical and mental damages to individuals arising from disasters. *Mitigations* are measures that can reduce health risks posed by hazards. Both natural and built environments may degenerate a natural hazard into disaster if appropriate mitigation measures to insulate the population from hazard exposure. The *impact phase* refers to the period during and immediately after a disaster. *Disaster response* describes actions taken in reaction to a disaster during the impact phase. In addition to search and rescue operations, disaster response also includes initial rapid needs assessments to ensure the effectiveness of these operations. The *post-impact phase* follows the impact phase, when the relief effort has been stabilized and long-term rehabilitation and recovery programmes kick in. *Disaster recovery* encompasses measures taken by national leaders and community stakeholders to help the disaster victims resume their 'normal' state of living before the disaster struck. Mitigation measures may also be taken in this phase to reduce the health risk posed by the disaster to the affected population.

2.11 General public health impact of natural disasters

Five general public health consequences might result after a natural disaster. These include: (1) overwhelmed local response capacity with a sudden surge in mortality and morbidity;

(2) damaged health and community infrastructure that disrupted regular clinical service and health-maintaining service provision; (3) harmful effects on the environment and population; (4) distressed psychological well-being and social context of affected community; and (5) long-term adverse consequences (Chan, 2017).

2.12 **Disaster management principles**

In general, disaster management includes the following five principles: (1) *Prevention* refers to reducing disaster risks and preventing disasters from happening. This may include hazard elimination, infrastructure strengthening, education, and so on; (2) *Preparedness*, which aims to develop community resilience through activities such as community training, contingency plan development, and drills and exercises for potential hazards in response, rescue, and recovery phases; (3) *Detection and alert* is the ability to monitor, identify, and forecast disasters, as well as disseminate relevant information in a timely manner on related hazards to the public; (4) *Response* involves mobilizing different emergency services to rescue and provide relief to disaster victims; and (5) *Recovery* means facilitating relief, rehabilitation, and reconstruction to allow the victims to return to their normal living contexts (Lewis *et al.*, 2015; see Fig. 2.7).

2.13 **General public health response to disasters**

There are three basic principles that underline general public health response to any disaster or crisis. These are to: (1) secure the basic resources required for human beings to maintain health; (2) determine the current and likely health threats to the affected community, taking into account of the local environmental, cultural, and religious context, and available community resources and knowledge, which may enable health-maintaining behaviours; and (3) identify and provide the resources required to address the first two principles.

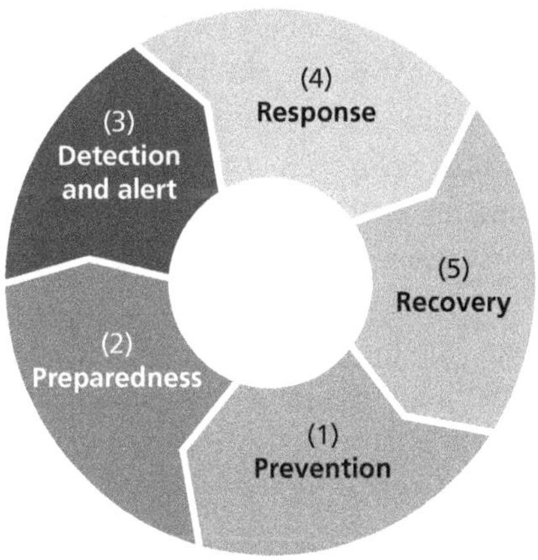

Fig. 2.7 Disaster management cycle proposed by WHO.

Of note, the five basic requirements for health maintenance include: (1) clean water and sanitation; (2) food and nutrition; (3) shelter and clothing; (4) health services; and (5) information (Bolton, 2006; Chan, 2017). Each of these domains has its own standards, technical challenges, key respondents, and stakeholders who intend to address health needs in suboptimal contexts such as disasters and extreme environments (Box 2.4). Various stakeholders should take note of additional information and technical reference in their specialist fields.

2.14 Disaster health literacy

Disaster health literacy is the capacity of an individual to comprehend, understand, and respond appropriately to health and disasters risks. With a high level of disaster health literacy, people have better capacity to build bottom-up resilience through taking proper actions to protect their well-being when crisis/disaster strikes. The promotion of community disaster health literacy will enhance bottom-up resilience and self-care during time of crisis. For example, during heatwaves and cold spells, if elders, children, and people with chronic health conditions are aware of their own health risks and take appropriate

Box 2.4 The Sphere Project

The Sphere Project is a voluntary initiative involving a variety of humanitarian agencies, including national and international non-governmental organizations (NGOs), International Federation of Red Cross and Red Crescent Societies (IFRC), United Nations (UN) agencies, host governments, and local disaster-affected communities. It was initiated in 1997 by a group of humanitarian NGOs and the International Red Cross and Red Crescent Movement, following the 1994 Rwanda crisis which demonstrated the need to establish certain humanitarian standards. This led to the publication of the first edition of the Sphere handbook in 2000. The fourth edition is expected to be finalized in 2018 (The Sphere Project, 2016). The project aims 'to help improve the quality of assistance to people affected by disaster or conflict, as well as the accountability of humanitarian agencies and states towards their constituents, donors and affected populations' (The Sphere Project, 2012). Its guiding values are based on two sets of documents: international humanitarian initiatives, human rights and refugee law, and the Code of Conduct for The International Red Cross and Red Crescent Movement and NGOs in Disaster Relief (IFRC & International Committee of Red Cross [ICRC], n.d.). Regarding the standards for disaster and humanitarian action, the Sphere Project provides a set of minimum standards for humanitarian actors to plan, manage, and implement interventions within the four key sectors for survival in emergencies: water supply and sanitation; nutrition and food aid; shelter and clothing; and health services.

actions to protect their own health, needs of hospitalization and death associated with these climatological hazards may be reduced.

2.15 Health Emergency and Disaster Risk Management (H-EDRM)

Since 2015, the four landmark global United Nations agreements adopted in 2015-16, namely Sendai Framework for Disaster Risk Reduction 2015-30, 2030 Sustainable Development Goals (SDGs), Paris climate agreement and New Urban Agenda (Habitat III) have all recognized health as an outcome and a goal of disaster risk reduction. The broad intersection of health and disaster risk reduction is captured in the concept of Health Emergency and Disaster Risk Management (H-EDRM), which encompasses various fields (Chan and Murray, 2017; Lo *et al.*, 2017). The focuses of H-EDRM research include:

- an all-hazards approach that incorporates the full spectrum of hazards;
- a holistic all-needs approach, including physical, mental, and psycho-social health and well-being;
- research and interventions facilitated during all phases of a disaster;
- disaster risk identification for populations with specific health needs such as children, people with disabilities, and older people; and
- research on and the building of health resilience in all communities.

2.16 Conclusion

This chapter presents the key building blocks to examine, understand, and establish public health and disaster risk reduction programmes in the rural context. The next chapter will discuss some key principles and theories that help to conceptualize health promotion and related activities.

References

Acheson, D. (1988). *Public Health in England: The Report of the Committee of Inquiry into the Future Development to the Public Health Function*. London, UK: Her Majesty's Stationery Office.

Bolton, P. (2006). Managing disasters and other public health crises. In: Pencheon, D., Guest, C., Melzer, D., & Gray, J. A. M. (eds.), *Oxford Handbook of Public Health Practice*, 2nd Edition, pp. 249–56. New York, NY: Oxford University Press.

Chan, E. Y. Y. (2017). *Public Health Humanitarian Responses to Natural Disasters* (Routledge Humanitarian Series). London, UK: Routledge.

Chan, E. Y. Y., & **Murray, V.** (2017). What are the health research needs for the Sendai Framework? *Lancet*. Published Online 2017 June 19. doi: 10.1016/S0140-6736(17)31670-7.

Constitution of the World Health Organization, 22 July 1946, T.I.A.S. No. 1,808.

Dahlgren, G. & Whitehead, M. (1991). *Policies and Strategies to Promote Social Equity in Health* (working paper). Stockholm, Sweden: Institute for Further Studies. Available at: http://www.iffs.se/media/1326/20080109110739filmZ8UVQv2wQFShMRF6cuT.pdf (accessed 7 January 2017) [Online].

de Savigny, D. & Adam, T. (eds) (2009). *Systems Thinking for Health Systems Strengthening*. Geneva, Switzerland: Alliance for Health Policy and Systems Research, WHO. Available at: http://apps.who.int/iris/bitstream/10665/44204/1/9789241563895_eng.pdf?ua=1 (accessed 7 January 2017) [Online].

Haagsma, J. A., Graetz, N., Bolliger, I., *et al.* (2015). The global burden of injury: incidence, mortality, disability-adjusted life years and time trends from the Global Burden of Disease study 2013. Available at: http://injuryprevention.bmj.com/content/early/2015/10/20/injuryprev-2015-041616.full.pdf+html (accessed 27 January 2017) [Online].

Howard, G., Bogh, C., Goldstein, G., *et al.* (2002). *Healthy Villages: A guide for communities and community health workers*. Geneva, Switzerland: WHO. Available at: http://www.who.int/water_sanitation_health/hygiene/settings/hvintro.pdf (accessed 7 January 2017) [Online].

International Federation of Red Cross and Red Crescent Societies, International Committee of Red Cross (n.d.). *The Code of Conduct for the International Red Cross and Red Crescent Movement and Non-Governmental Organisations (NGOs) in Disaster Relief*. Available at: http://www.ifrc.org/Global/Publications/disasters/code-of-conduct/code-english.pdf (accessed 26 January 2017) [Online].

Jacobsen, K. H. (2014). *Introduction to Global Health*, 2nd Edition. Boston, MA: Jones & Bartlett Learning.

Khosh-Chashm, K. (1995). Healthy cities and healthy villages: how to tackle health and environmental problems in urban and rural areas. *Eastern Mediterranean Health Journal*, **1**, 103–1.

Leavell, H. R. & Clark, E. G. (1958). *Preventive Medicine for the Doctor in his Community: An Epidemiologic Approach*, 2nd Edition. New York, NY: McGraw-Hill.

Lewis, G., Sheringham, J., Bernal, J. L., & Crayford, T. (2015). *Mastering Public Health: A Postgraduate Guide to Examinations and Revalidation*, 2nd Edition. Boca Raton, FL: CRC Press.

Lo, S. T. T., Chan, E. Y. Y., Chan, G. K. W., Murray, V., Ardalan, A., & Abrahams, J. (2017). Health Emergency and Disaster Management (H-EDRM): developing the research field within the Sendai Framework paradigm. *Int J Disaster Risk Sci*. doi: 10.1007/s13753-017-0122-0

The Sphere Project (2012). *The Sphere Project: humanitarian charter and minimum standards in disaster response*. Available at: https://www.sphereproject.org/download/5049f50b33a50/ (accessed 26 January 2017) [Online].

The Sphere Project (2016). The next Sphere Handbook: much more than just an update. Available at: www.sphereproject.org/news/the-next-sphere-handbook-more-than-just-a-revision/ (accessed 26 January 2017) [Online].

World Health Organization (WHO) (1986). *The Ottawa Charter for Health Promotion*. Available at: http://www.who.int/healthpromotion/conferences/previous/ottawa/en/ (accessed 7 January 2017) [Online].

World Health Organization (WHO) (n.d.). Regional activities: approaches as implemented in the WHO regions. Available at: http://www.who.int/healthy_settings/regional/en/index.html (accessed 26 January 2017) [Online].

World Health Organization (WHO) (1990). *Environment Health in Rural and Urban Development and Housing: A Collaborative Framework and Strategy for WHO Technical Cooperation in the Eastern Mediterranean Region*. Alexandria, Egypt: WHO Regional Office for the Eastern Mediterranean.

World Health Organization (WHO) (1994). *Report of the second WHO/EMRO Healthy Cities Conference, Hammamet, Tunisia* (Document No.: WHO-EM/PEH/466/E/L/07.94/115). Alexandria, Egypt: WHO/EMRO.

World Health Organization (WHO) (2009). WHO community based initiative: healthy village programme. Available at: http://www.emro.who.int/cbi/cbi_hvp.htm (accessed 18 September 2009) [Online].

Chapter 3

Health promotion planning approaches, human behavioural change models, and health promotion theories

Public health practitioners used different theories and models to conceptualize thoughts and behaviours (Rimer and Glanz, 2005). This chapter discusses how health messages or education can be communicated and potentially applied in a specific context/environment (legislation, cultural/religious context) for field-based promotion planning. A number of commonly applied theoretical human behavioural models, namely the Health Belief Model, Transtheoretical (Stages of Change) Model, Theory of Planned Behaviour, Social Cognitive Theory, and Complex Intervention Design, will also be discussed.

3.1 Overview

Health might be considered as an individual or collective responsibility in a society. Approaches based on individual responsibilities will focus on activities or initiatives which enable informed choice (through information sharing), empowerment (e.g. deregulation to allow individual to make choices), or decision-making (e.g. choice of healthcare). However, health approaches which emphasize collective responsibilities will encourage legislation, regulation, and population-wide measures to protect health against health risks and harmful behaviours.

3.1.1 Prevention paradox

When engaging in population-based initiatives in health, the common paradox for health practitioners will be to decide whether to target people at the greatest risk of a disease/condition, or to focus on lowering the general health risk across the whole population. Rose (1981) argued that although universal-based programmes which aim to address the risk of the overall population will have the greatest overall impact in a community, 'a preventive measure that brings large benefit to the community offers few benefits to each participating individual'. A targeted approach may thus be more attractive, because health promotion activities under this approach may be more visible in benefiting the high-risk groups (Hunt and Emslie, 2001).

Overall, when planning for health promotion activities, it is important to first identify the target group and differentiate the health risks, such as pure harm (e.g. smoking), mixed risks (with harm and benefits, e.g. as alcohol or certain food use), or harm (which affects second parties or others, e.g. drunk driving and unprotected sexual intercourse), and to consider the intervention taking into account of prevention paradox.

3.2 Health communication

Effective health communication is essential to health promotion. McGuire (1989) highlights five core components (source, message, channel, receiver, and destination) which underline the planning of behaviour-changing health messages for a community. The message might be verbal or non-verbal, and can be addressed horizontally (good behaviour that might simultaneously improve a few aspects of health, e.g. handwashing might reduce diarrhoea, food hygiene, and so on), or vertically (for a specific health problem). Factors associated with successful community health communication include: be seen/heard, attract attention, be understood, be accepted, and change of behaviour. More related discussion can be found in Chapters 6 and 7.

3.3 Approaches in health promotion

Interventions targeting health risk might be implemented at different levels. It might address the individual level (e.g. target high-risk sociodemographic subgroups, patients) through professionally oriented services. At the policy level, a typical programme might involve policy implementation to shift culture or behaviour; distribution/redistribution of resources (incentives, or remove barriers which obstruct good health-promoting behaviour); as well as community development which includes health.

Top-down approaches may also include legal banning and restrictions of availability, usage, sales, advertisement, and information, and fiscal measures like taxation and subsidies. Enabling environment and context (e.g. smoking ban) might need to be created for the top-down approaches. The success of top-down approaches might require efforts to overcome implementation challenges, which include shared values, motivation, skills of the relevant staff, guidance available, and time commitment of the project. Chapter 6 will discuss some examples of how a health promotion programme might be developed at the *bottom-up* level.

3.4 Approaches in health promotion planning

There are number of health promotion planning models, and the three main models, namely MAP-IT, preceed–proceed, and P-Process, are discussed in this section.

3.4.1 MAP-IT

The *MAP-IT* approach is developed by United States Department of Health and Human Services (2001) and is the acronym for Mobile, Assess, Plan, Implement, and Track. Chapter 6 shares how this planning approach was used for planning of the CCOUC

Table 3.1 Five planning steps of the MAP-IT approach and its application to the planning of the 'Healthy Village' model

Planning steps	Description
1	**Mobilize** individuals and organizations that care about the health of the community into a coalition
2	**Assess** the areas of greatest need in the community, as well as the resources and other strengths that you can help in address those areas
3	**Plan** the approach: start with a vision of where the programme want to be as a community; then add strategies and action steps to help the programme achieve that vision
4	**Implement** the plan with concrete action steps that can be monitored and will make a difference
5	**Track** progress over time

Reproduced from United States Department of Health and Human Services (2001). *Healthy people in healthy communities: A community planning guide using Healthy People 2010*, http://atfiles.org/files/pdf/healthycom.pdf, accessed 06 Mar. 2017, Office of Disease Prevention and Health Promotion, Office of Public Health and Science, US Department of Health and Human Services, Rockville, MD, USA.

EMHP project described in Chapter 1. Table 3.1 describes the five planning steps within the framework.

3.4.2 Precede–proceed model

The *precede–proceed* eight-phased planning model serves as a comprehensive guide for the planning and evaluation of health promotion programmes (Gielen *et al.*, 2008; McKenzie *et al.*, 2016; Porter, 2016)[1]. Theoretically underpinned by their socioecological model to cover contextual determinants of health, Green and Kreuter emphasized a participatory approach that involved target audiences in the identification and assessment of community needs.

Precede (*p*redisposing, *r*einforcing, and *e*nabling *c*onstructs in *e*ducational/*e*cological *d*iagnosis and *e*valuation) has four phases of systematic assessments, namely:

Phase 1: social assessment;

Phase 2: epidemiological, behavioural, and environmental assessment;

Phase 3: educational and ecological assessment; and

Phase 4: administrative and policy assessment.

Social assessement includes situational analysis with a focus on quality of life indicators such as subjective happiness or perceived self-esteem. In addition to identifying the community health issues from vital statistics or credible reports, phase 2 traces behavioural, environmental, as well as genetic determinants that may affect target audience's health. More important and changeable issues can be ranked by a prioritization matrix. In phase 3, pre-existing knowledge, attitudes, values, and beliefs (predisposing factors) of the target audience, the types of feedback loop or reward mechanism for encouraging or discouraging the continuation of a behaviour (reinforcing factor), and the skills and resources required to facilitate or hinder the desired changes (enabling factor) are the key factors to be considered.

Health promotion models mentioned in the subsequent sections (e.g. the social cognitive theory and the theory of planned behaviour) may also be incorporated in phase 3 to address the three key determinants of health and to design health messages with reference to the profile of the target audience. Aligning different strategies and priorities identified in phase 1 to 3 with the intended interventions is the key component of phase 4. Moreover, the assessment of organizational factors (including resource constraints or power relationships) is also important to ensure the intervention programme is effectively implemented and sustained.

Proceed (policy, regulatory, and organizational constructs in educational and environmental development) also involves four phases, namely:

Phase 5: implementation;

Phase 6: process evaluation;

Phase 7: impact evaluation; and

Phase 8: outcome evaluation.

In the proceed phases, the assessment insights of precede are analysed and strategically implemented. Through systematic implementation (phase 5) of the programme, phases 6 to 8 review how the programme has been conducted and if the desired objectives have been achieved (see also Box 3.1).

3.4.3 **P-Process**

Similar to the precede–proceed model, the *P-Process model* is a long-established planning tool to serve as a roadmap for field professionals and practitioners to design and plan health communication programmes (Health Communication Capacity Collaborative, 2013)[2]. P-Process may be useful to target programmes that aim at social and behaviour change communication (such as HIV/AIDS campaigns, family planning promotion, and environmental protection). Throughout the planning journey, P-Process focuses on the use of behaviour change theories, stakeholder participation, and capacity strengthening (see also Box 3.2).

As a strategic, iterative five-step process, P-Process has the following components:

Box 3.1 Theory in practice: Non-communicable disease prevention in the Himalayas

When designing a field health promotion programme on non-communicable disease (NCD) prevention in the Himalayan context (e.g. Kingdom of Bhutan), the social assessment in phase 1 of the precede–proceed model should be carefully conducted. Quality of life indicators that have social and policy relevance are essential. For instance, in line with the Gross National Happiness framework, the specific aspects (in terms of different indicators) of the people's happiness level in the Kingdom of Bhutan (phase 2) can first be considered.

An ecological assessment (phase 3) that considers the cultural and religious contexts is equally important. Given the belief in Tibetan Buddhism (predisposing factor), the dietary advice on less calorie intake, for example, has to be contextually crafted—a sole focus on less red meat consumption, for instance, will not be effective—as does advice on taking exercise. An emphasis on being more physically active, for instance, can be encouraged through organizing community-based campaigns featuring the Bhutanese's favourite national sport: archery (enabling factor). Schools can also be an optimal setting when schoolchildren are the target audience. In phase 4, the endorsement of the programme by, and support from, the royal family of the Kingdom of Bhutan will be crucial to ensuring programme sustainability and smooth implementation (phase 5).

Step 1—Inquire

Step 1 involves baseline assessment to understand the scope of health issues and identify the most suitable target audience. Situational analysis will identify health problems, and the facilitators and barriers for behaviour change. The problem statement will summarize the overall goal and programme objectives.

Step 2—Design strategy

A project strategic plan will be developed in step 2, where the communication objectives, specific selection of target audience, intended communication channels, programme positioning, and the monitoring and evaluation plan are planned in details. Key stakeholders, if possible, should be involved as early as possible to allow involvement and ownership of the target audience. The use of health promotion theories may guide the intervention design.

Step 3—Create and test

Printed (e.g. leaflets or posters) or mass media materials (e.g. songs or videos) may be used as communication tools. A participatory approach is assumed and sufficient training sessions should be organized to allow community members to contribute their local insights on the product design. Comments on feasibility and applicability of the intended health

Box 3.2 Theory in practice: Separate collection of plastic waste in rural China

Through a detailed situational analysis (step 1) in a rural, ethnic minority-based village in in Guizhou province, the southwestern region of China, it was discovered that wasteburning was the usual waste management practice and plastic the most common type of waste. Most of the households did not possess waste collection bins. Despite strong concerns over the burning odours, villagers did not realize what could be done to alleviate their worries about the potential harm from waste burning. Face-to-face interviews showed that floor sweeping was a common practice in the village and the responsible person was also the one who managed the household waste. The interviewees also suggested that alternatives be provided should they need to use less plastic carrier bags. Survey results showed that all participants were receptive to the idea of providing household-based plastic waste collection bins in the village.

Collating all the relevant information, a health promotion campaign on encouraging villagers to separate their plastics from general waste and put them into the plastic waste collection bins provided was organized after close discussions with these key household waste managers (step 2). A household-to-household interpersonal communication strategy was adopted given the context of this ethnic-based 'society of acquaintances'.

In step 3, co-designing and co-producing communication products with the villagers, including local designs of canvas tote bags as substitutes, was a long, yet important and rewarding process. Despite the considerable time required for the process, the pre-testing and finalization of the products showed it could be done in a smooth manner if the target audience was involved right from the design stage.

Recruitment and training of local translators and helpers will be a crucial step in the implementation stage (step 4). Similarly, a careful and detailed documentation of the implementation processes provides valuable data for assessment of process evaluation (step 5).

promotion messages should be collected from the users. Pre-testing and subsequent revisions are important before finalizing and producing the communication products.

Step 4—Mobilize and monitor

Step 4 describes the implementation process and the progress of the programme can be monitored throughout against this plan. Training of field-based practitioners or local helpers is important to ensure the programme is delivered appropriately. Any adjustment to the programme should also be documented with justifications and arguments.

Step 5 Evaluate and evolve

As a summative assessment, the intervention and programme effects can be checked against the outcome measures outlined in the strategic plan in step 2. In order to evaluate the effectiveness of the programme, a qualitative approach using focus groups or in-depth interviews with the target audience is encouraged. The programme outcomes and success stories should then be effectively disseminated to the local community, donors, and other key stakeholders and partners. In terms of future planning, a programme-level evaluation should be conducted for a possible scale-up.

3.5 **Models of behavioural changes and theories of health promotion**

3.5.1 **Health Belief Model**

The Health Belief Model (HBM) is one of the most widely used health behaviour theories. It was developed to improve outcomes in response to the failure of free TB health screening programmes (Hochbam, 1958; Hochbam *et al.*, 1952). The key concepts in the theory include perceived susceptibility, perceived severity, perceived benefits, perceived barriers, cues to action, and self-efficacy. The HBM shows these factors affect people's intention to take action to prevent, monitor, and control health problems (Lewis *et al.*, 2014; Rimer and Glanz, 2005). The concepts and their relationship to health behaviours are illustrated in Figure 3.1.

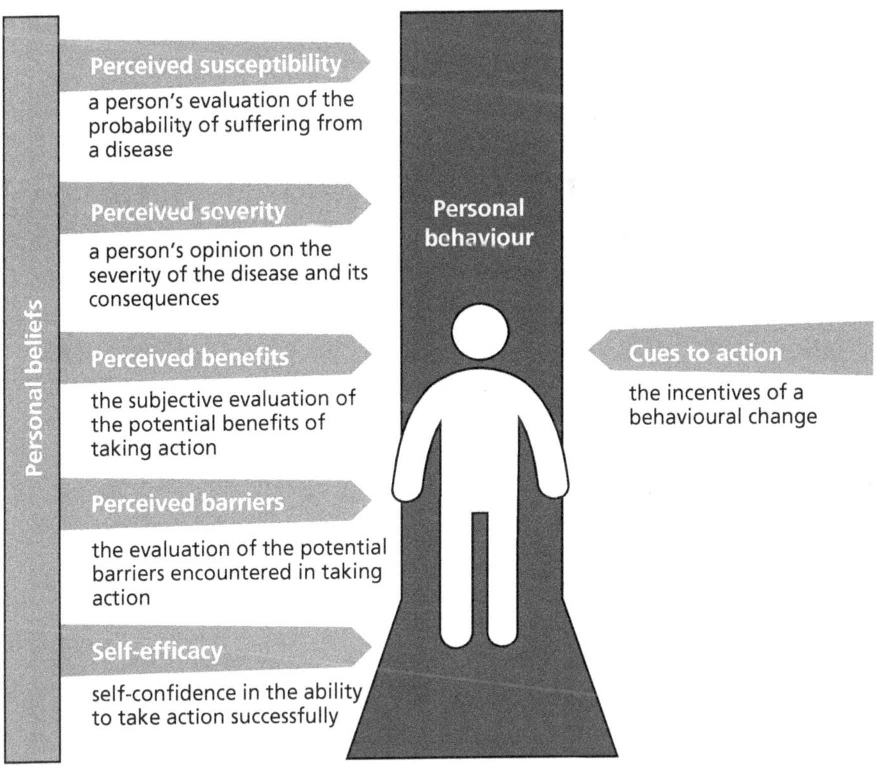

Fig. 3.1 Health Belief Model.

The effects of alcohol consumption provide a useful example that helps explain the concepts of the health belief model:

1. Perceived susceptibility: the drinker thinks about how likely s/he will develop diseases due to drinking (e.g. whether drinking will cause cirrhosis);
2. Perceived severity: how the drinker perceives the severity of the disease s/he may develop due to drinking (e.g. whether they acknowledge cirrhosis is a severe disease);
3. Perceived benefit: the potential benefits the drinker expects to have because of quitting alcohol (e.g. whether the drinker agrees that quitting alcohol can reduce expenses and improve health);
4. Perceived barrier: the potential barriers in quitting drinking that the drinker foresees (e.g. whether quitting causes inconvenience in his/her social interaction with friends);
5. Cues to action: the cues to action, in this case quitting drinking, can be external such as advice from family, check-up results, and the persuasion of healthcare professionals. The internal cues can be the self-perceived worsening of the health condition; and
6. Self-efficacy: the drinker's perception of his/her ability to quit.

Apart from the cues to action, the concepts are all the personal beliefs of the drinker. Intervention, therefore, can be designed to focus on their misconceptions (see Box 3.3; see also Fig. 3.2).

Box 3.3 An example of applying the Health Belief Model to health interventions

The promotion of alcohol abstinence is a useful example of HBM. Health workers may focus on increasing the 'perceived benefits' of the action to villagers in order to increase their intention to quit. For instance, health workers can increase the willingness of villagers to give up drinking through dramas which show how money saved from abstaining from drinking may be used to pay for the education of their children. In addition, health workers may invite experts to give talks and illustrate the diseases caused by alcohol abuse by showing related medical illustrations and photos to increase the level of 'perceived severity'.

This model is most useful to apply for simpler preventive behavioural changes (e.g. screening participation), predicting behaviour patterns, and to monitor effectiveness of related health interventions. However, there are limitations to apply the HBM model to conceptualize the change of complex long-term behaviour, such as alcohol dependence and circumstances associated with boarder contextual factors that affect behaviour, such as social norms.

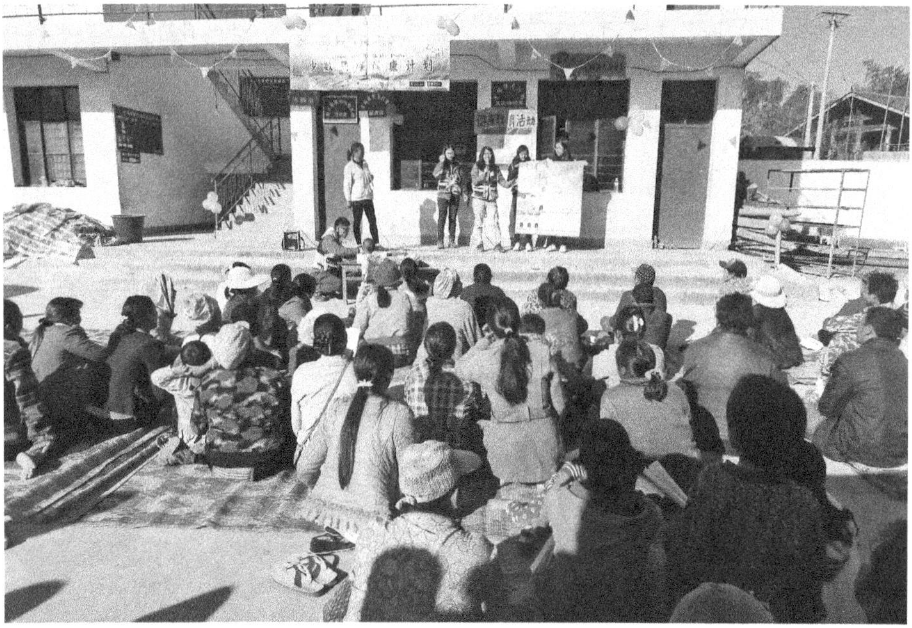

Fig. 3.2 A health education project team in action in a rural village.
Reproduced by kind permission of Emily Ying Yang CHAN, Copyright © 2017 Emily Ying Yang CHAN.

3.5.2 **Transtheoretical (Stages of Change) Model**

The Transtheoretical (Stages of Change) Model integrates key constructs in different theories, including theories in psychotherapy and behavioural change, and this is why it is so-named (Prochaska and Velicer, 1997; Rimer and Glanz, 2005). The key idea of the model is that a behavioural change involves a series of stages. A person will experience the following five stages in changing behaviour:

1. Precontemplation: the individual does not intend and does not have any motivation to change his/her behaviour in the foreseeable future (usually within six months).
2. Contemplation: the individual intends to change his/her current behaviour in the coming six months. They realize the advantages and disadvantages brought by behavioural change but do not have any idea of how to achieve it.
3. Preparation: the individual is prepared to take action within 30 days. They usually have plans and have done some preparation work, like participating in health education talks and consulting doctors for their opinion.
4. Action: the individual has implemented a significant change in lifestyle over the past six months and is willing to maintain the change.
5. Maintenance: the individual's change in behaviour has lasted for at least six months and they are willing to maintain the change and prevent a relapse.

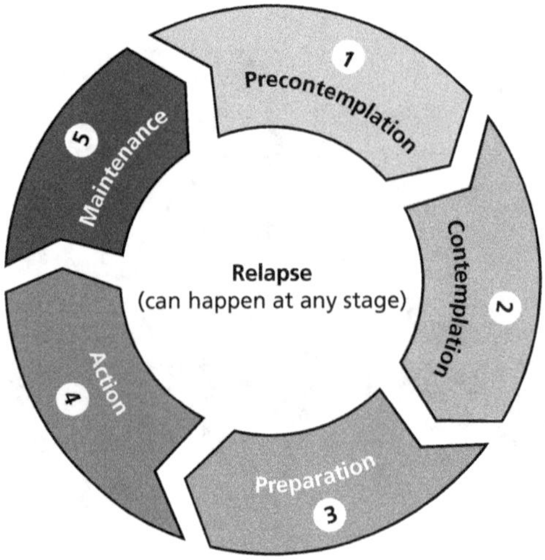

Fig. 3.3 Transtheoretical (Stages of Change) Model.

In the process, however, episodes of the previous behaviour may recur. Relapse can happen at any stage and, if they do, the individual needs to go through the stages from the start to effect a change. For instance, if a person gives up the plan after all the preparation work, s/he will return to the precontemplation stage from the preparation stage. Hence, the path of a change in the model is circular but not linear. This is illustrated in Figure 3.3.

Before health interventions, health promotion practitioners should examine the following behavioural patterns to understand which stage of change they are in. The following questions use drinking as an illustration:

- Have you ever thought of quitting alcohol? (Precontemplation)
- Have you thought quitting alcohol in the near future? (Contemplation)
- Do you have plans for refraining from alcohol? (Preparation)
- Are you quitting drinking? (Action)
- Have you abstained from alcohol and you are now maintaining abstinence? (Maintenance)

Knowing the stages of change target groups are undergoing allows the project team to design appropriate messages, strategies, and the content of its intervention (see also Box 3.4).

3.5.3 Theory of Planned Behaviour

The Theory of Planned Behaviour (TPB) explains the concept of behavioural intention. It investigates the relationship between behaviour and three factors, namely belief, attitude, and intention (Ajzen, 1991).

Box 3.4 An example of applying the Transtheoretical (Stages of Change) Model to health interventions

Again, using the promotion of alcohol abstinence as an example, if health workers assume most of the target group are at the precontemplation stage and might not understand the adverse health impact of alcohol, the educators can aim at transiting the villagers to the contemplation stage by educating them about the harms of excessive drinking to personal health. For villagers at the contemplation stage, they can be encouraged to make concrete action plans, such as deciding when to start the reduction of alcohol consumption.

This model is useful to apply for the changing of complex long-term behaviour such as tobacco addiction and alcohol dependence. It is useful to help practitioners to tailor specific interventions to patients/target group according to their expectations, as well as to organize interventions according to stages of change of the population subgroup of interest. This model, however, might face challenges for community-based interventions (which might have a mosaic pattern of stages of change behaviour among its members).

Behavioural intention is determined by three main elements: the person's attitude towards the behaviour; how one perceives the social norm; and his/her perceived behavioural control (see Fig. 3.4).

- Attitude towards behaviour: a person's view on a certain behaviour and his/her evaluation of its outcome.
- Subjective norm: whether the person thinks the behaviour is accepted by others (particularly significant others/family members) and whether s/he is willing to comply with the perceived social norm.

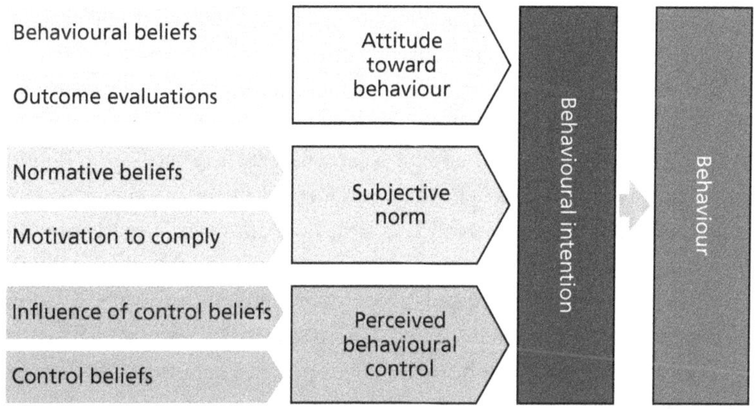

Fig. 3.4 Theory of Planned Behaviour.

- Perceived behavioural control: the person's perceived ability to control certain behaviour and whether s/he thinks there are other factors that facilitate/impede the behaviour. If the perceived behavioural control is high, the person will have a higher tendency to carry out that action. Similarly, if s/he can identify more facilitators, s/he may be more likely to initiate the behavioural change.

The following questions use alcohol consumption as an example to illustrate how to understand the view of the target audience by applying the TPB (see also Box 3.5).

- Are you at risk of alcohol abuse?[3] (Behavioural intention)
- Do you agree that alcohol abuse is acceptable? (Attitude towards behaviour)
- Do you agree that the majority of society approves of this behaviour? (Subjective norm)
- Do you agree that you can control your use of alcohol? (Perceived behavioural control)

3.5.4 Social Cognitive Theory

Social Cognitive Theory proposes that individuals are under the influence of their social environment. The thoughts and behaviour of a person are affected by the opinions, thoughts, behaviour, advice, and support of the people surrounding them. Reciprocally, the person also exerts influence on his/her surroundings. This theory tries to explain how people adjust their behaviour by control and reinforcement to achieve maintainable goal-directed behaviour. The key concepts in the theory include reciprocal determinism, behavioural capacity, expectation, self-efficacy, observational learning, and reinforcement (Bandura, 1986; see Fig. 3.6; see also Box 3.6).

Reciprocal determinism is the core of social cognitive theory. It refers to the dynamic interaction between personal factors, environmental factors, and behaviour. Behavioural capacity refers to the ability to behave in a certain way with the necessary knowledge and skills. In order to adopt a particular behaviour, it is essential to know what to do and how to do it. Expectation refers to the expected outcomes of the behaviour. People evaluate the outcomes of behaviour before taking action and these expected outcomes will affect whether the person adopts the behaviour. Self-efficacy is the ability to overcome barriers to adopt a new behaviour. Observational learning is learning through observing others' performances and their outcomes. Reinforcement concerns the response after a behavioural change and if it will affect whether a person repeats that behaviour. Reinforcement can either be positive or negative. Positive reinforcement means giving rewards which increases the possibility for the person to repeat the behaviour. Negative reinforcement warns the person and prevents repetition of the behaviour. For example, a warning will be given when drivers go beyond the speed limit. Reinforcement can also be categorized into internal and external reinforcement. Internal reinforcement refers to self-reward, while external reinforcement applies to how the environment encourages or discourages the repetition of a behaviour.

Box 3.5 An example of applying the Theory of Planned Behaviour to health interventions

The promotion of alcohol abstinence provides a useful example of the theory of planned behaviour. Team members can modify the 'subjective norm' in villages to increase the chance of quitting. For example, they can invite the significant others of villagers who should quit drinking to write about how they would like their partners to quit drinking. The team then give the written statement to the drinkers to let them know what their partners think. This can increase their motivation to quit. In addition, team members can also increase the villagers' 'perceived behavioural control' to enhance their incentives. For instance, they can lay stress on the fact that drinking is solely a personal choice and not necessarily related to maintaining friendships. This may increase the confidence of drinkers in their behavioural control (Fig. 3.5).

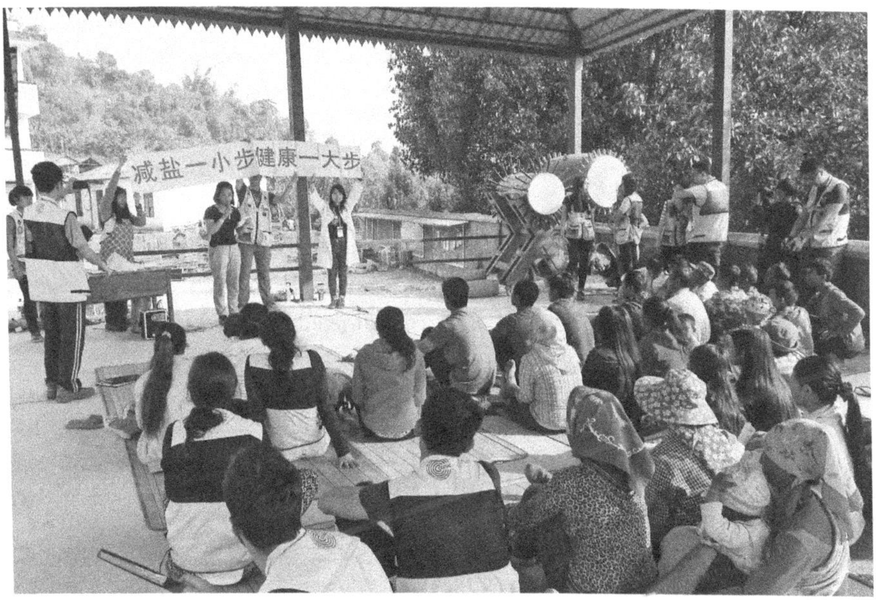

Fig. 3.5 A project team's rehearsal in the village before the actual intervention activity.
Reproduced by kind permission of Emily Ying Yang CHAN, Copyright © 2017 Emily Ying Yang CHAN.

The model helps to understand the contextual challenges (i.e. a person's belief of what others expect) that a health behavioural change might require of an individual. It stresses self-efficacy. But similar to the stages of change model, it might not be the most effective in examining changes for the whole community, which has a diverse pattern of subjective social norms and self-efficacy.

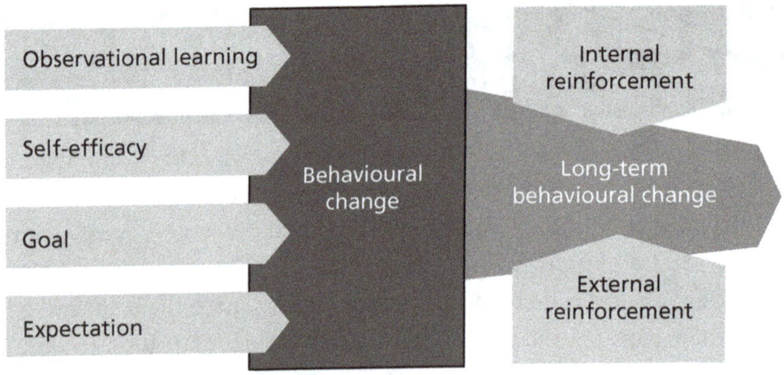

Fig. 3.6 Social Cognitive Theory.

3.5.5 **Complex interventions**

Complex interventions refer to interventions which comprise of several interacting elements and health promotion increasingly adopts complex interventions design as its evaluation strategy in recent years (Campbell *et al.*, 2000; Craig *et al.*, 2008; MRC; 2000). According to the MRC (2000), the complexity of the set of interventions is affected by the following factors:

- The number of and interactions between components within the experimental and control interventions;
- The number and difficulty of behaviours required by those delivering or receiving the intervention;
- The number of groups or organizational levels targeted by the intervention;
- The number and variability of outcomes; and
- The degree of flexibility or tailoring of the intervention permitted.

Box 3.6 An example of applying the Social Cognitive Theory to health interventions

This example uses the promotion of alcohol abstinence. By showing the 'expectation', or expected outcome, of abstinence, health workers can boost the motivation of villagers to quit alcohol. Money saved as a result of abstinence may be considered as is one 'expectation'. Health workers may explain that, in addition to saving money, quitting alcohol may also help to avoid the medical expenses resulted from the treatment of alcohol-related diseases. Similarly, the team can apply the principle of 'observational learning' to motivate the villagers to take the first step. For instance, examples of successful cases can be used to illustrate that it is possible to give up alcohol.

Complex solutions recognize behavioural, social, and environmental factors may affect personal belief and behavioural uptake. At the field implementation level, multidisciplinary efforts are usually preferred but might be difficult to track the results due to all the interactive effects.

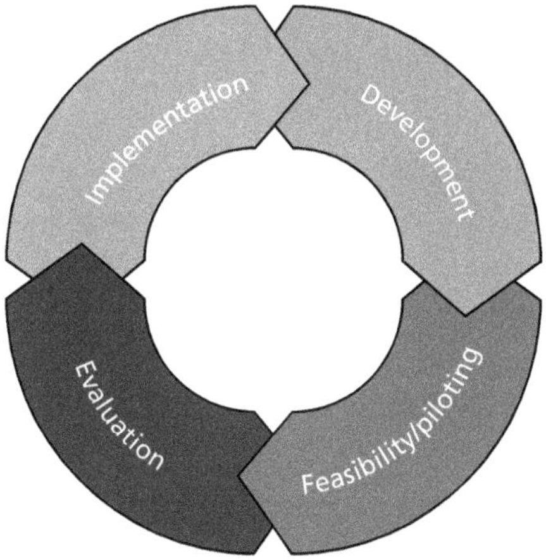

Fig. 3.7 Medical Research Council complex interventions framework (2008).
Adapted with permission from Medical Research Council. *Developing and evaluating complex interventions: new guidance*, https://www.mrc.ac.uk/documents/pdf/complex-interventions-guidance/, accessed 01 Feb. 2017, Copyright © 2008 Medical Research Council.

Examples of complex interventions designed to assess cognitive behavioural therapy include projects that aim to improve symptoms of depression (individual); school-based obesity intervention (group); the electronic medical record project in public hospitals (institutional); and community-based cardiovascular health intervention (community). Application of the framework of complex interventions requires a good understanding of the concept (see Fig. 3.7).

3.6 **Intervention strategies**

A number of intervention strategies may support health promotion. In general, these strategies might be categorized into seven groups (McKenzie *et al.*, 2016), namely:

1. Health communication strategies
2. Health education strategies
3. Health policy/enforcement strategies
4. Environmental change strategies
5. Health-related community service strategies
6. Community mobilization strategies
7. Others

While it is beyond the scope of this book for detailed discussions of these strategies, it is important to highlight that these strategies are not independent of each other. More often than not, multiple strategies and efforts are required to maximize impact. For rural and remote Asian communities, the most common approach for bottom-up health and disaster resilience-building efforts might be related to health communication and education.

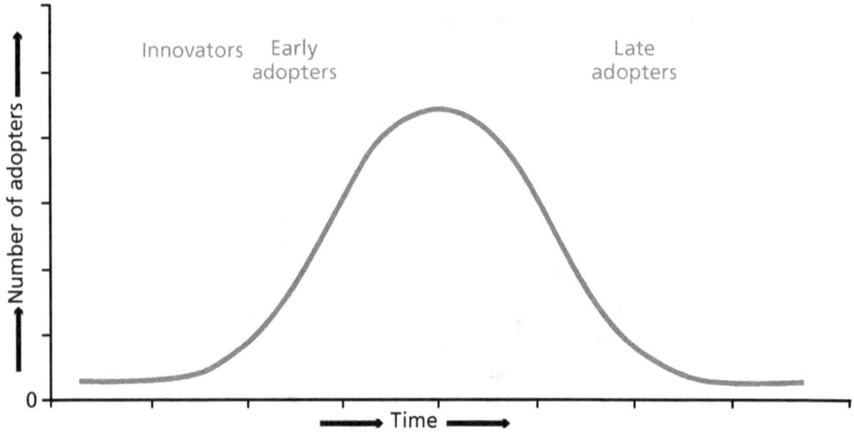

Fig. 3.8 Innovation diffusion curve.

For health communication and education strategies, it is important to highlight the concept of diffusion theory and the idea of cumulative adoption which explains the general pattern of diffusion of new ideas/innovation/knowledge to the population for a realistic appreciation of the potential tracking, monitoring, and evaluation of the efforts (Rogers, 2003; Goldman, 1998; McKenzie *et al.*, 2016; see Figs 3.8 and 3.9).

"Chapters 6 and 7 will discuss these two approaches in more detail."

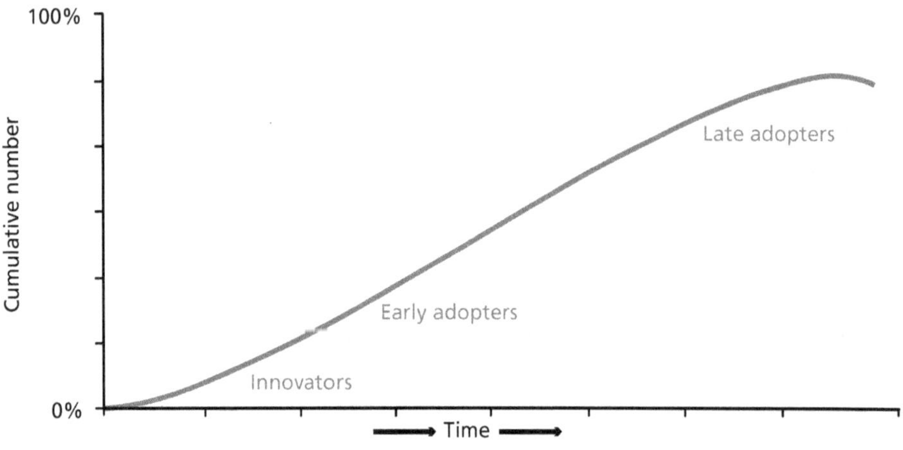

Fig. 3.9 Cumulative adoption curve of innovation.

3.7 Conclusion

Theories and models in health promotion may help disseminate evidence-based solutions to promote health. Although these theories and models can help to conceptualize human thought and behaviour the decision about which theory or model should be used depends on the intervention objectives and the local situation. The next two chapters will describe the public health context in a number of Asia-Pacific countries.

Notes

1. This model has been widely used around the globe in the past four decades. Lawrence Green and colleagues developed the precede model in 1974 and Marshall Kreuter joined him in 1991 to add the proceed part.
2. The model was developed by the Johns Hopkins Bloomberg School of Public Health Center for Communication Programs in 1982 and revised in 2013.
3. The definition of alcohol abuse should be clarified with the intended audience.

References

Ajzen, I. (1991). The theory of planned behavior. *Organizational Behavior and Human Decision Processes*, **50**, 179–211.

Bandura, A. (1986). *Social Foundations of Thought and Action: A Social Cognitive Theory*. Englewood Cliffs, NJ: Prentice-Hall.

Campbell, M., Fitzpatrick, R., Haines, A., *et al.* (2000). Framework for design and evaluation of complex interventions to improve health. *BMJ*, **321**, 694–6.

Craig, P., Dieppe, P., Macintyre, S., *et al.* (2008). Developing and evaluating complex interventions: the new Medical Research Council guidance. *BMJ*, **337**, 979–83.

Gielen, A. C., McDonald, E. M., Gary, T. L., & Bone, L. R. (2008). Using the precede-proceed model to apply health behavior theories. In: Glanz, K., Rimer, B. K., & Viswanath, K. (eds), *Health Behavior and Health Education: Theory, Research, and Practice*, 4th Edition, pp. 407–33. San Francisco, CA: Jossey-Bass.

Goldman, K. D. (1998). Promoting new ideas on the job: Practical theory-based strategies. *The Health Educator*, **30**, 49–52.

Health Communication Capacity Collaborative (2013). *The P-Process: Five steps to strategic communication*. Baltimore, MD: Johns Hopkins Bloomberg School of Public Health Center for Communication Programs. Available at: http://ccp.jhu.edu/documents/P_Process_5_Steps.pdf (accessed 11 January 2017) [Online].

Hochbaum, G. (1958). *Public Participation in Medical Screening Programms: A Socio-Psychological Study*. Washington DC: United States Public Health Service.

Hochbaum, G., Rosenstock, I., & Kegels, S. (1952). *Health Belief Model*. Washington, DC: United States Public Health Service.

Hunt, K. & Emslie, C. (2001). Commentary: the prevention paradox in lay epidemiology-Rose revisited. *Int J Epidemiol*, **30**, 442–6.

Lewis, G., Sheringham, J., Bernal, J. L., & Crayford, T. (2014). *Mastering Public Health: A Postgraduate Guide to Examinations and Revalidation*, 2nd Edition. Boca Raton, FL: CRC Press.

McGuire, W. J. (1989). Theoretical foundations of campaigns. In: Rice, E. R. & Atkin, C. K. (eds), *Public Communications Campaigns*, 2nd Edition, pp. 43–65. Newbury Park, CA: SAGE.

McKenzie, J. F., Neiger, B. L., & Thackeray, R. (2016). *Planning, Implementing & Evaluating Health Promotion Programs: A Primer*, 7th Edition. Boston, MA: Pearson Education.

Medical Research Council (MRC) (2000). *A Framework for Development and Evaluation of RCTs for Complex Interventions to Improve Health* [discussion document]. Medical Research Council, London, United Kingdom. Available at: https://www.mrc.ac.uk/documents/pdf/rcts-for-complex-interventions-to-improve-health/ (accessed 11 January 2017) [Online].

Porter, C. M. (2016). Revisiting precede-proceed: a leading model for ecological and ethical health promotion. *Health Educ J*, 75, 753–64.

Prochaska, J. O. & Velicer, W. F. (1997). The transtheoretical model of health behavior change. *Am J Health Promot*, **12**, 38–48.

Rimer, B. K. & Glanz, K. (2005). *Theory at a Glance: A Guide for Health Promotion Practice*, 2nd Edition. Bethesda, MD: National Cancer Institute, National Institutes of Health, U.S. Department of Health and Human Services. Available at: https://www.k4health.org/sites/default/files/NCI%20Theory%20at%20a%20Glance.pdf (accessed 11 January 2017) [Online].

Rogers, E. M.. (2003). *Diffusion of Innovations*, 5th Edition. New York, NY: Free Press.

Rose, G. (1981). Strategy of prevention: lessons from cardiovascular disease. *BMJ*, **282**, 1847–51.

United States Department of Health and Human Services (2001). *Healthy People in Healthy Communities: A Community Planning Guide Using Healthy People 2010*. Available at: http://www.healthypeople.gov/Publications/HealthyCommunities2001/healthycom01hk.pdf (accessed on 12 September 2009) [Online].

Chapter 4

Public health in rural Asia I

This chapter discusses the current status of health outcomes and context for the populations living in Islamic Republic of Afghanistan (Afghanistan), Kingdom of Bhutan (Bhutan), Kingdom of Cambodia (Cambodia), People's Republic of China (PRC), Republic of India (India), Republic of Indonesia (Indonesia), Democratic People's Republic of Korea (DPRK), and Lao People's Democratic Republic (Lao PDR). Together with Chapter 5, these two chapters attempt to provide an empirical background for the understanding of how healthcare services are being organized in rural context of these countries. A brief description of natural disaster pattern is also included.

4.1 Introduction

In the twentieth century, more people lived in rural than urban settings in the world. However, by 2014, more than half (53.6%) of the world's population lives in urban areas and the percentage will continue to rise and reach two-thirds (66.4%) in 2050 (United Nations (UN), 2014, 2015; World Heart Foundation, 2012). Asia is vast, populous, and immensely diverse. Rural health in Asia varies from country to country. About half (47.5%) of Asian population were urban dwellers in 2014 and the rate of urbanization is expected to be the fastest compared to all other continents, in which approximately 65% live in urban settings. Projected between 2014 and 2050, seven of the ten countries with the largest declines in the rural population are from Asia, with the top five coming from China, India, Indonesia, Thailand, and Bangladesh. The top five most populous urban agglomerations in 2030 will all be located in Asia, namely Tokyo (37.2 million), Delhi (36.1 million), Shanghai (30.8 million), Mumbai (27.8 million), and Beijing (27.7 million).

Given the fast pace of urbanization, the total rural population is naturally assumed to decline. For instance, China is expected to have 300 million fewer rural residents. Nonetheless, this assumption is not completely correct as some countries in Asia are observed to have an increasing rural population. The largest rise in the rural population in Asia comes from the Philippines with more than 13 million increase between 2014 and 2050, whereas Tajikistan, Cambodia, Pakistan, and Nepal are also on the global top 50 list for the largest rural population increase.

4.1.1 To urbanize or not to urbanize

Urbanization offers opportunities for better mobility, economic prospects, as well as access to improved education and healthcare services. However, more health risk factors are associated with urbanized lifestyles. As in the case of megacities in China, the fast pace of work and stressful urban lifestyles may change diet and physical activity patterns, which may increase the risks for developing non-communicable diseases (NCDs) (Gong *et al.*, 2012). Environmental risk factors including air pollution, occupational hazards, or traffic injuries may also heighten risks of different disease burdens. However, in spite of less modern development and well-equipped facilities, rural dwellers share a stronger sense of community and belonging than urban residents. The close-knit neighbourhoods serve as an important source of physical and psychological support and this social capital is a crucial community asset in maintaining the mental well-being of rural dwellers, which may be less frequently noticed in urban settlements (Boyd *et al.*, 2008).

4.1.2 Different facets of health issues

In general, people living in rural areas are reported to experience poorer health status with significant health differentials than their urban counterparts (Smith *et al.*, 2008). Yet, published studies have found mixed results in terms of NCDs, cancer incidence, and mental health disorders. For example, the multifactorial Type II diabetes mellitus is one of the few exceptions with a more consistent heavier burden in urban areas compared to rural contexts. However, if factors associated with mortality patterns are compared, management of diabetes tends to be poorer and the mortality risks of dying from diabetes in rural areas are higher, despite having lower number of diabetic cases (Bragg *et al.*, 2017). Obesity, however, makes no distinction for any rural–urban differentials in some Asian countries. For example, the prevalence of obese adults was high in both urban and rural India. However, with the existing malnutrition in some parts of rural India, it makes both overnutrition and undernutrition a plausible 'double burden' to tackle (Singh *et al.*, 2014).

4.2 Countries' profiles and discussion

The following sections highlight the general and rural health status in eight countries of in the Asia–Pacific region (see Fig. 4.1).

In both Chapters 4 and 5, key health indicators are used to describe the health of the country's population. *Life expectancy* is one of the most representative indicators showing the overall health status of the population. Immunization coverage of *diphtheria, tetanus toxoid, and pertussis (DTP3)*, and *measles-containing vaccine (MCV1)*, the most basic vaccines for infants and children, shows the strength of a country's health system. A strong health system should guarantee follow-ups with children at appropriate times to ensure a high coverage of three doses of DTP vaccine, while a weaker health system may not be able to do so. Another set of indicators is regarding the mortality rates of

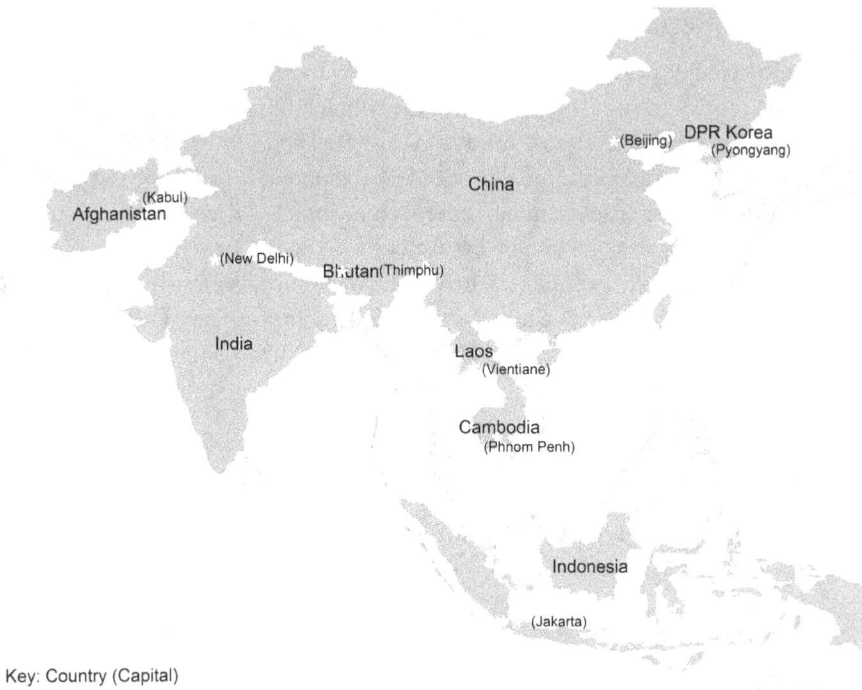

Fig. 4.1 Locations of countries discussed in Chapter 4, including Afghanistan, Bhutan, Cambodia, China, India, Indonesia, Democratic People's Republic of Korea, and Laos in Asia.

mothers and children—including *maternal mortality, neonatal mortality*, and *under-five child mortality*. The provision of mother and child care is a basic component in any primary healthcare system, thus these indicators reflect the performance of a country's primary healthcare service and infrastructure. The health financing indicators, such as *total expenditure on health*, show how important the health expenditure is to a country's economy and how the healthcare expenses are financed—the *government's expenditure* indicates the respective government's commitment on healthcare, and the *private expenditure* shows the burden that the population has to bear in terms of healthcare costs. *Physician density* indicates the resources of the health system in terms of the supply of medical personnel. Information sources used in these two chapters include websites of the respective Ministry of Health (MoH), World Health Organization (WHO), and the World Factbook published by the Central Intelligence Agency. With regard to the rural context delineation of the selected country, a brief discussion will accompany the country profile with regard to how the health system was developed, general health status, rural–urban gaps in healthcare, public health and primary care system, disease control, and health promotion, as well as disaster trends and situations. Case examples from countries in these chapters are also featured in the thematic topic discussions in Chapters 8 to 10.

4.3 Islamic Republic of Afghanistan

The Islamic Republic of Afghanistan (Afghanistan), which ranked 169th out of 188 countries and territories with a Human Development Index (HDI) value of 0.479 in the low human development category in 2015, is a rural-based country with low socioeconomic status and political instability (United Nations Development Programme [UNDP], 2016). In the past decade, it has substantially improved its infant and maternal mortality rates. While its health indicators remain below average for low-income countries, Afghanistan suffers from ongoing civil conflict and frequent natural disasters which often result in high mortality, disruption of livelihoods, and infrastructure damage (WHO, 2016, May). In 2016, humanitarian assistance represented to be about US$9.3 million (UN, 2016) (see Table 4.1).

4.3.1 Development of a health system

Before 2001, non-governmental organizations (NGOs) were the main health service providers in Afghanistan. Ministry of Public Health (MoPH) had very limited engagement and management of service delivery. Rural areas and insecure regions were often unserved

Table 4.1 Afghanistan: Basic facts and key health indicators

Total population (2015)	32.5 million
Proportion of rural population (2015) (World Bank, n.d.-e)	73%
Life expectancy (years) (2015)	61.9 (female); 59.3 (male); 60.5 (both sexes)
Diphtheria tetanus toxoid and pertussis (DTP3) immunization coverage among one-year-olds (2015)	78%
Measles-containing vaccines (MCV1) immunization coverage for infants (2015) (WHO, 2016, December 1, WHO-UNICEF estimates; WHO & United Nations Children's Fund [UNICEF], 2016, July 6a)	68%
Neonatal mortality rate (per 1,000 live births) (2015)	35.5 [19.2–6.4]
Under-five mortality rate (probability of dying by age five per 1,000 live births) (2015)	91.1 [69.6–118.8]
Maternal mortality rate (per 100,000 live births) (2015)	396 [253–620]
Total expenditure on health as % of GDP (2014)	8.18%
General government expenditure on health as % of total expenditure on health (2014)	35.84%
Private expenditure on health as % of total expenditure on health (2014)	64.16%
Physicians density (per 1,000 population) (2013)	0.266

Source: data from World Health Organization. *Key country indicators – Afghanistan: key indicators*, http://apps.who.int/gho/data/node.cco.ki-AFG?lang=en, accessed 16 Feb 2017, Copyright © 2016 World Health Organization.

or underserved as most health services were concentrated in urban areas (Afghanistan Ministry of Public Health, 2015).

In 2003, the MoPH gained the support from donors and decided to take a stewardship role. The government developed the Basic Package of Health Services (BPHS) in 2003 and the Essential Package of Hospital Services (EPHS) (UN, 2016). The EPHS aimed to improve health services, facilities, staff, equipment, and drugs in hospitals. Both BPHS and EPHS are contracted out to the NGOs commissioned by the government. The contracting out strategy intended to allow the MoPH to focus on its institutional development and governance of health system (Afghanistan Ministry of Public Health, 2016).

BPHS and EPHS provide around 2,300 health facilities, and the 34 hospitals in provincial capitals are BPHS facilities. Besides the public sector, there is also a large growing private sector in which the providers are mostly informal and not regulated (Afghanistan Ministry of Public Health, 2016).

The national health policy for 2015–2020 focuses on governance, institutional development, public health, health services, and health workforce. Afghanistan spends approximately US$55 per capita per year in its total health expenditure, with 20–25% covered by development partners and 4–6% by the government budget. The out-of-pocket spending is high at 70% and the population is at high risk of catastrophic expenditure and impoverishment. Of note, the heavy dependence on donors in health financing is unsustainable in the long term (Afghanistan Ministry of Public Health, 2015).

4.3.2 General health status

Afghanistan reported an under-5 mortality rate of 91.1 per 1,000 live births in 2015 (see Table 4.1) and total fertility rate of 5.1 per woman in 2012 (WHO, n.d.). As of 2015, life expectancy for female and male was projected to be 62 and 59 respectively (see Table 4.1). Life expectancy at birth for both sexes increased by 5 years over the period of 2000–2012 when the WHO region average was reported to have an average increase of 3 years in the same period (WHO, n.d.). Lower respiratory infection was the leading cause of death in 2012, accounting for 11.6% of the total number (WHO, n.d.). In 2012, death due to malaria was reported to be 0.1 per 100,000 population (WHO, n.d.) and NCDs accounted for 37% of all deaths (WHO, 2014b). The insecurity issue also takes a toll on Afghans' health (WHO, 2016, May).

4.3.3 The rural–urban gap in healthcare

When compared with urban pattern, the maternal mortality rate in rural areas remains very high in Afghanistan. One major reason is the inequitable access to health services and health workforce. Due to conflicts and instability, most health workers opt to work in urban areas to reduce the risks of being victims of crimes and terrorism in rural communities (Afghanistan Ministry of Public Health, 2016). Unequal distribution of qualified health workers and the lack of female health providers are obstacles for the effective use of healthcare, especially by women (Afghanistan Central Statistics Organization, 2014).

A large gap in the healthcare provision between the urban and rural populations exists (Afghanistan Central Statistics Organization, 2014). For maternity care, the proportion of urban women (72%) who have received antenatal care from a skilled provider is higher than rural women (55%). Urban women (32%) generally have four or more antenatal care visits than rural women (14%). Urban mothers who give birth with assistance from a skilled provider (79%) or in a health facility (76%) double that of their rural counterparts (42% and 40%, respectively). Moreover, the percentage of urban women receiving a postnatal check-up within two days of delivery (48%) is also higher than rural women (28%) and it increases with education and wealth (Afghanistan Central Statistics Organization, Afghanistan Ministry of Public Health, & ICF International, 2016).

4.3.4 **Public health and primary healthcare system**

While MoPH has a stewardship role regarding the health of the whole population, other government ministries and agencies are also involved in people's health. Key stakeholders in rural areas include bilateral and multilateral development partners, NGOs, professional associations, regulatory bodies, and the private sector (Afghanistan Central Statistics Organization *et al.*, 2016).

The Afghanistan government commits to primary healthcare in the national health policy. The implementation of the BPHS and EPHS is an achievement in rebuilding the health system and the BPHS offers a platform for stakeholders for developing strategic health policies and goals, and to minimize the inefficiencies and duplications in the health system (Afghanistan Ministry of Public Health, 2016). With the financial and technical assistance from developmental partners, the BPHS/EPHS covers around 65% of the population with a compromised quality of service delivery. However, the service provision remains is very limited to the 35% who live in insecure areas or areas with difficult terrain in the country. A survey indicated ongoing armed conflicts remained one of the main barriers to accessing healthcare, which had resulted in subsequent deaths (Médecins Sans Frontières, 2014). Moreover, population living in high disaster risk areas faces constant displacement risks (WHO, 2016, May).

4.3.5 **Disease control and health promotion**

Afghanistan is vulnerable to infectious disease outbreaks. Infectious diseases accounted for more than 60% of the use of outpatient services and lead to more than half of all deaths. Tuberculosis remains a key public health problem, with about 58,000 cases reported and 13,000 deaths annually. More than 75% of the population lives in areas at risk of malaria transmission. Immunization coverage remains low, with approximately 50% of one-year-olds were fully immunized. Around 20% of women and children have never been immunized against diseases and poor immunization coverage continues to challenge the well-being of the population in Afghanistan (WHO, 2016, May). Obstacles for the implementation and maintenance of disease control include weak and fragmented disease control programmes, national insecurity, geographic inaccessibility, and ongoing population due to natural disasters and the impact of climate change (WHO, 2016a).

Even transforming from a disease warning surveillance system to an integrated disease surveillance and response system, Afghanistan faces the challenge of maintaining the improvement and achievements in detection, prevention, and response to epidemics of emerging infections. Strengthening of the epidemiological and laboratory surveillance capacities at the peripheral level, as well as enhancing the capacity for informed decision-making on the prevention and control of emerging health threats at the local level are urgently needed. (WHO, 2016a). In addition, public awareness towards NCDs is generally low, and health promotion programmes are constantly underfunded (Afghanistan Ministry of Public Health, 2016). As the major healthcare provider remains the public sector, there is an absence of formal assessment in the healthcare quality and lack of guidelines and training for the prevention and control of the most common NCDs. Tests and procedures available for early detection, diagnosis, and monitoring at the primary care level are very limited (WHO, 2016a).

Overall, enhancement in access, coverage, and quality of health services has been attempted for rural population over the past 15 years. The decrease in infant mortality is related to the improved access and expansion of basic preventive and treatment services. The number of health facilities increased fivefold from 496 in 2002 to more than 2,000 in 2012. Reduction in maternal mortality is attributable to combination of health policies and strategies, including setting a higher age of first marriage; promoting the use of contraceptives; increasing immunization coverage; expanding antenatal, postnatal, and delivery care; and recruiting more community health workers and midwives, as well as increasing access to the BPHS (Afghanistan Ministry of Public Health, 2016).

Afghanistan is reported to have one of the highest child malnutrition levels globally. Some 39% of all the children under five years old are malnourished and a high prevalence of vitamin and mineral deficiencies exist among women and children.

4.3.6 Disaster trends and situations

From 2000 to 2016, floods and earthquakes are reported to be the most common types of natural disaster in Afghanistan. The deadliest disaster in Afghanistan during that period was an epidemic in April 2002, causing 2,500 deaths. The disaster which was reported to have the greatest number of affected people was a drought in May 2000, where 2.58 million people were affected. The greatest economic damage was resulted from a 2011 drought, leading to a loss of US$142 million (CRED, 2017).

4.4 The Kingdom of Bhutan

The Kingdom of Bhutan (Bhutan) is a land-locked country with a small population in the Himalayas. According to UNDP (2016), Bhutan's HDI value for 2015 was 0.607, positioning it at 169 out of 188 countries/territories and in the medium human development category. However, Gross National Happiness, the core theme of Bhutan's social development, puts people's physical, mental, cultural, and spiritual needs at the top priority and influences the health system (WHO, 2014). The Bhutan government's adoption of

Table 4.2 Bhutan: Basic facts and key health indicators

Total population (2015)	774,800
Proportion of rural population (2015) (World Bank, n.d.-e)	61%
Life expectancy (years) (2015)	70.1 (female); 69.5 (male); 69.8 (both sexes)
Diphtheria tetanus toxoid and pertussis (DTP3) immunization coverage among one-year-olds (2015)	99%
Measles-containing vaccines (MCV1) immunization coverage for infants (2015) (WHO, 2016, December 1, WHO-UNICEF estimates)	97%
Neonatal mortality rate (per 1,000 live births) (2015)	18.3 [11.9–26.6]
Under-five mortality rate (probability of dying by age five per 1,000 live births) (2015)	32.9 [24.0–44.5]
Maternal mortality rate (per 100,000 live births) (2015)	148 [101–241]
Total expenditure on health as % of GDP (2014)	3.57%
General government expenditure on health as % of total expenditure on health (2014)	73.19%
Private expenditure on health as % of total expenditure on health (2014)	26.81%
Physicians density (per 1,000 population) (2012)	0.259

Source: data from World Health Organization. *Key country indicators—Bhutan: key indicators*, http://apps.who.int/gho/data/node.cco.ki-BTN?lang=en, accessed 16 Feb 2017, Copyright © 2016 World Health Organization.

free universal health coverage has proved successful in reducing poverty, morbidity, and mortality. The country has made remarkable progress in the prevention and control of infectious diseases, as well as improvement in maternal and child health (WHO, 2014a) (see Table 4.2).

4.4.1 **Development of the health system**

From a country with nearly non-existent modern Western healthcare in the 1960s, Bhutan has transformed remarkably to its current system within 15 years. Since 1961, when Bhutan embarked on its modernization journey, the country has reduced its reliance on a traditional medicine system and started to develop a modern allopathic healthcare system (Bhutan Ministry of Health [MoH], 2014a).

The healthcare system is mainly financed by the government's general revenues (Bhutan MoH, 2014b) and health services are provided free-of-charge to over 90% of the citizens. The constitution protects every Bhutanese citizen from catastrophic health expenditures (Bhutan MoH, 2014a) and Bhutan's annual allocation of more than 6% of the total government budget to the health sector has demonstrated the government's strong political commitment to health (WHO, 2014a). The government also created the Bhutan Health

Trust Fund in 1997 to build self-reliance and develop financial sustainability in the health system. It aims at increasing the availability of essential drugs and vaccines, as well as improving the quality of primary healthcare (Bhutan MoH, 2014b).

Overall, the health system is decentralized for which central government manages the overall planning, while local government identifies the needs and implements policies and programmes accordingly. It has a three-tiered healthcare delivery system, with primary healthcare provided at the basic health units; secondary healthcare at the district hospitals; and tertiary healthcare at the regional and national referral hospitals. The government introduced a referral system which operates via seven categories of health facilities. For specialized services not available in Bhutan, the state supports referral expenditure outside the country. To reduce the increasing pressure on the public health facilities, the government has allowed the privatization of selective diagnostic services since 2012. However, the government still possesses the exclusive rights for clinical services (Bhutan MoH, 2014a).

4.4.2 General health status

Bhutan reported an under-5 mortality rate of 32.9 per 1,000 live births in 2015 (see Table 4.2) and total fertility rate of 2.2 per woman in 2013 (WHO, n.d.). As of 2015, life expectancy projected for female and male was both around 70 (see Table 4.2). Life expectancy at birth for both sexes increased by 8 years over the period of 2000-2012 when the WHO region average was reported to have an average increase of 5 years in the same period (WHO, n.d.). Ischaemic heart disease was the leading cause of death in 2012, accounting for 8.2% of the total number (WHO, n.d.). In 2012, no death was resulted from malaria (WHO, n.d.) and NCDs accounted for 56% of all deaths (WHO, 2014b).

4.4.3 The rural–urban gap in healthcare

The majority of the poor (92%) live in rural areas (WHO, 2014a). As all the hospitals of Bhutan are situated in urban areas, most health workers (75%) are concentrated in urban areas. The proportion of rural residents with a three-hour walking distance from home to the nearest health facility is almost six times greater than that of urban residents. Even with free healthcare services, the rural population still has to spend a large amount of time and/or money on transportation to health facilities, which is almost triple of that in urban households (Bhutan MoH, 2014a).

Infant and under-five mortality rates are higher in rural Bhutan when compared with urban contexts. Higher infant and child mortality rates are correlated to poverty and a lower level of mothers' education. The under-five mortality rate in rural areas is double that of urban areas (Bhutan National Statistics Bureau, 2011). Rural women, in general, have less access to health services. Compared to mothers in urban areas (95%), a much lower proportion of rural mothers (66.3%) gave birth at a health facility. Rural women have a lower chance of receiving antenatal and postnatal care (Bhutan MoH, 2014a), poorer reproductive health, and less knowledge about family planning. They are also more vulnerable to HIV and human papillomavirus (HPV) infections. Less than half of rural women and more than two-thirds of urban women received counselling about HIV in 2010 (Bhutan MoH, 2014b). In 2012, a lower proportion of girls living in rural areas (17.3%) were immunized against HPV compared to their urban counterparts (10.7%).

4.4.4 Public health and primary healthcare system

Average life expectancy increased significantly from 37 years in 1960 to 70 in 2015. Meanwhile, Bhutan still has a number of communicable diseases to combat, such as dengue, human immunodeficiency virus (HIV), and TB, as well as tropical diseases. NCDs show a rising trend due to people's changes in lifestyle. In addition, Bhutan is vulnerable to climate change and natural disasters (WHO, 2014a). As the demand for healthcare services increases and the country's income level improves, there is a risk of a gradual decrease in financial support on free universal health coverage from traditional partners and international funding initiatives. This requires a review on health financing and strengthening of health systems to maintain the basic health services (WHO, 2014a).

Free universal health coverage, the government's political commitment on health, and overall socioeconomic development are key determinants of the improved health status of the Bhutanese population. High coverage of the expanded immunization programme has led to a remarkable decrease in vaccine-preventable diseases and no case of poliomyelitis has been reported since 1986. Other public health achievements include a significant improvement in maternal and child health, reduction in prevalence and mortality of major infectious diseases (namely tuberculosis (TB) and malaria), and elimination of endemic goitre and leprosy, as well as an increase in the coverage and access to safe drinking water and improved sanitation (WHO, 2014a).

Bhutan's health system provides comprehensive care, through 31 hospitals, 235 basic health units and subposts, 52 indigenous units, and 562 outreach clinics in 2016 (Bhutan MoH, 2016).

4.4.5 Disease control and health promotion

Basic health units, outreach clinics, and mobile health units connect communities with health services, especially for remote populations (WHO, 2014a). Community healthcare services, including health promotion, disease prevention, child immunization, and assisted delivery, are delivered at the family level, especially in rural areas. Village health workers, health assistants, and nurses provide such services at homes, communities, outreach centres, and subposts. Primary healthcare services are provided at the health centres located near communities. Curative, health promotion, and disease prevention services are provided at health centres and at communities by nurses and health assistants. Secondary healthcare services are provided at district hospitals. Doctors and health teams are responsible for providing preventive, curative, and rehabilitative care. District hospitals can also serve as referral centres for primary healthcare facilities, while tertiary healthcare services are provided at regional referral hospitals and national referral hospitals (Bhutan MoH, 2014b).

Bhutan has made laudable progress in improving maternal and child health. To attain safe maternal and child health, the Bhutan government has actively educated family planning, provided free and equitable access to vaccination free-of-charge, and encouraged breastfeeding nutrition. Bhutan has provided the HPV vaccine since 2009 and the pentavalent DTP–Hib–HepB vaccine since 2011. Since 2005, the MoH has worked to increase the coverage of institutional delivery to 66% and anticipated to achieve 100% in the near future. District medical officers are responsible to train all health workers up to the midwifery standards revised in 2004. Facilities at basic health units are improved with heating, indoor toilets, and number of delivery beds. Standards for reproductive and child health services are developed and adopted, including Integrated Management of Newborn and Childhood Illness (IMNCI), neonatal care, breastfeeding, contraceptive services, management of abortion, and management of sexually transmitted infections (STIs) (WHO, 2014a).

Basic health units provide youth-friendly health services while district hospitals provide counselling on teenage pregnancies, contraception, abortion, and management of post-abortion complications, sexual abuse, treatment of STIs, and menstrual disorders. Adolescents can also receive counselling, testing, and advice on prevention on maternal transmission of HIV as well as information and treatment for nutrition, mental health, and substance abuse. Governmental and non-governmental organizations provide flexible outreach services, such as health checks and community health camps. Regular education on maternal and reproductive is widely implemented in the rural communities. The MoH and the Ministry of Education cooperate to promote reproductive health to teenagers at secondary schools (WHO, 2014a).

In regard to the ageing population, the government also has started to develop healthy ageing programmes. A group of retired senior government officials formed the Royal Society of Senior Citizens' Association to plan policies and strategies. The National Pension and Provident Fund was introduced to provide old age retirement benefits (WHO, 2014a).

4.4.6 **Disaster trends and situations**

From 2000 to 2016, Bhutan experienced five major disasters, including two earthquakes, two floods, and a storm. The deadliest was a flood in August 2000, which caused 200 deaths. The disaster reported to have the greatest number of affected people was an earthquake in September 2011, where 20,016 people were affected. The greatest economic damage was resulted from a 1999 wildfire, leading to a loss of US$3.5 million (CRED, 2017).

4.5 **Kingdom of Cambodia**

According to the 2008 General Population Census of Cambodia, while 80.5% of the 13.4 million people (in an annual growth rate of 1.54) in the Kingdom of Cambodia (Cambodia) live in rural settings, less than 20% reside in an urban area (Cambodia National Institute of Statistics, Cambodia Directorate General for Health & ICF International, 2015, September). According to the population pyramid of 2015, less

Table 4.3 Cambodia: Basic facts and key health indicators

Total population (2015)	15.6 million
Proportion of rural population (2015) (World Bank, n.d.-e)	79
Life expectancy (years) (2015)	70.7 (female); 66.6 (male); 68.7 (both sexes)
Diphtheria tetanus toxoid and pertussis (DTP3) immunization coverage among one-year-olds (2015)	89%
Measles-containing vaccines (MCV1) immunization coverage for infants (2015) (WHO, 2016, December 1, WHO-UNICEF estimates)	81%
Neonatal mortality rate (per 1,000 live births) (2015) (World Bank, n.d.-b)	14.8 [10.1–21.6]
Under-five mortality rate (probability of dying by age five per 1,000 live births) (2015) (World Bank, n.d.-c)	28.7 [19.6–41.4]
Maternal mortality rate (per 100,000 live births) (2015) (World Bank, n.d.-a)	161 [117–213]
Total expenditure on health as % of GDP (2014)	5.68%
General government expenditure on health as % of total expenditure on health (2014)	22.04%
Private expenditure on health as % of total expenditure on health (2014)	77.96%
Physicians density (per 1,000 population) (2012)	0.169

Source: data from World Health Organization. *Key country indicators—Cambodia: key indicators*, http://apps.who.int/gho/data/node.cco.ki-KHM?lang=en, accessed 16 Feb 2017, Copyright © 2016 World Health Organization.

than 10% of the population age over 60 and more than 30% are under 15 years of age (Population pyramids of the world from 1950 to 2100: Cambodia 2015, n.d.). In the medium human development category, Cambodia's HDI value in 2015 was 0.563, ranked 143rd out of 188 countries and territories (UNDP, 2016). (see Table 4.3).

4.5.1 Development of the health system

Since the independence of Cambodia in 1953, its healthcare system has developed in several layers. During the 1980s, when Cambodia was still regarded as 'the Kingdom of Cambodia', development of healthcare mainly focused on basic elements such as reconstruction, rehabilitation, and training for health professionals. By 1993, the country progressed to establish its first Royal Government, where the government took authority and developed its first Ministry of Health (MoH).

As the main governance body in the healthcare sector, the MoH aims to provide well-being through tackling issues such as the quality and accessibility of healthcare. In recent years, the MoH has taken several initiations such as the *Health Sector Strategic Plan 2008–2015*. Focusing on three specific areas of maternal and children's health, communicable diseases, and NCDs, this plan intends to develop health services, improve resource and financial allocation, and ensure equity across the country (WHO Regional Office for Western Pacific [WHO WPRO] & Cambodia MoH, 2012). While the *Health Coverage Plan* in 1996 successfully established a healthcare network which developed the health centres and hospitals, the delivery of services was guided by two policies: Law on the Management of Private Medical, Paramedical and Medical Aid Services in 2000, and the Policy on Public Service Delivery in 2006 (WHO WPRO & Cambodia MoH, 2012).

Cambodia delivers healthcare through two sectors: public and private. Within the public sector, it is further divided into two categories based on two levels: the health centres which provide basic packaged services, and the referral hospitals which provide complementary packaged services. Nevertheless, the private sector is very limited in terms of service capacity (WHO WPRO & Cambodia MoH, 2012).

In Cambodia, out-of-pocket payment accounts for 95% of the country's health expenditure (World Bank, n.d.-d). As health expenditure in Cambodia is highly dependent on out-of-pocket payment, rural populations who cannot afford the cost may have to cope by borrowing money and selling assets. Those who can afford it would often pay through their savings and earnings. These limited payment methods for healthcare services are built on the issue of poverty. Several measures have been taken by the government to ease the burden on the rural community, especially for those poor and vulnerable. It includes the Health Equity Fund, which provides services that meets the patients' food, transportation, and other costs related to accessibility for the eligible poor. In addition, this Fund has also standardized user fees for services within the schemes. The government has also developed the voucher scheme allowing payment of services to be done through vouchers rather than cash.

4.5.2 General health status

Cambodia reported an under-5 mortality rate of 28.7 per 1,000 live births in 2015 (see Table 4.3) and fertility rate of 2.9 per woman in 2013 (WHO, n.d.). As of 2015, life expectancy for female and male was projected to be 71 and 67 respectively (see Table 4.3). Life expectancy at birth for both sexes increased by 12 years over the period of 2000-2012 when the WHO region average was reported to have an average increase of 4 years in the same period. Ischaemic heart disease was the leading cause of death in 2012, accounting for 10.1% of mortality (WHO, n.d.). In 2012, death due to malaria was reported to be 1.7 per 100,000 population (WHO, n.d.) and NCDs accounted for 52% of all deaths (WHO, 2014b). Issues on malnutrition and access to healthcare remain prevalent problems (WHO WPRO & Cambodia MoH, 2012).

4.5.3 The rural–urban gap in healthcare

As of 2014, 80% of the population resides in rural households, 20% live in urban settings. Although statistics also reflect and increase of urbanization, living in an urban area does not reflect one's economic status. In 2011, poverty incidence is the highest among urban residents in comparison to those living in rural settings. Regarding access to healthcare facilities, while 27% of those residing in an urban setting would visit private clinics, only 16% of those living in rural areas would do so (Schelzig, 2014).

Cambodia has recently implemented its country's urban–rural partnership strategy for 2014–2018 to reduce poverty and vulnerability among the different populations. This strategic programme also aims to develop rural areas and improve the rural–urban linkages. Through building infrastructure, it will improve accessibility and expand opportunities to obtain healthcare services. In addition, tourism growth has aided Cambodia in urbanizing its countryside (WHO WPRO & Cambodia MoH, 2012).

4.5.4 Public health and primary healthcare system

Within the rural population, health centres often act as the gatekeepers of healthcare services. Therefore, health centres aim to provide primary healthcare services to the different groups of population in Cambodia. As Cambodia is on an epidemiological transition from communicable diseases to NCDs, the country has experienced a double disease burden. Since 2005, the health centres have offered three important types of preventive services: contraception, antenatal care, and tetanus vaccination. At the same time, many of these health centres also provide consultation, primary diagnosis, and chronic disease management for the rural community (WHO WPRO & Cambodia MoH, 2012).

4.5.5 Disease control and health promotion

In Cambodia, the 10 leading causes of morbidity include: acute respiratory infection, diarrhoea, malaria, cough, gynaeco-obstetric issues, tuberculosis, road accidents, measles, dengue haemorrhagic fever, and dysentery. Communicable diseases make up 83% of the reported disease burden. Dominating all age groups, 67% happens among older people and 96% among the age group between 0–5 years. More significantly, it has been noted that the trend on NCD is rising, as 53% of deaths each year are caused by NCDs (WHO WPRO & Cambodia MoH, 2012).

The government aims to control these factors through implementing the Health Strategic Plan and the Millennium Development Goals (MDGs). Since the end of the MDG era, the incidence of communicable diseases has improved as there has been a significant decrease in HIV/AIDS incidence from 1.9% in 1997 to 0.7% in 2008. In addition, the malaria mortality rate has dropped from 4.0 in 2005 to 2.4 in 2010 and the tuberculosis rate has also attained a significant decrease. More significantly, Cambodia is undergoing a fast epidemiological transition to NCDs. However, due to the inadequate manpower and healthcare resources there is a lack of expertise in this field and no service delivery model has been developed yet (WHO WPRO & Cambodia MoH, 2012).

4.5.6 Disaster trends and situations

From 2000 to 2016, Cambodia experienced 22 natural disasters, with floods as the most common type of disaster. The deadliest was a flood in July 2000, causing 347 deaths. The disaster with the greatest number of affected people is the same flood in July 2000, where 3.45 million people were affected. The greatest loss was caused by a flood in August 2011 (US$521 million) (CRED, 2017).

4.6 People's Republic of China

People's Republic of China (PRC or China) has the largest population in the world, approximating 1.4 billion. Its HDI value for 2015 was 0.738, positioning it at 90 out of 188 countries and territories in the high human development category (UNDP, 2016). According to statistics in 2014, the proportion of rural population to the whole population was 45.2% (National Bureau of Statistics of China, 2015) and socioeconomic disparity existed between urban and rural areas. Since China's economic reform in 1978, the health system of China also underwent several stages of reform. Although the issues of agriculture, rural areas, and farmers become some of the priorities in the development strategy in China there are still challenges ahead (see Table 4.4).

Table 4.4 China: Basic facts and key health indicators

Total population (2015)	1.40 billion
Proportion of rural population (2015) (World Bank, n.d.-e)	44%
Life expectancy (years) (2015)	77.6 (female); 74.6 (male); 76.1 (both sexes)
Diphtheria tetanus toxoid and pertussis (DTP3) immunization coverage among one-year-olds (2013)	99%
Measles-containing vaccines (MCV1) immunization coverage for infants (2015) (WHO, 2016, December 1, WHO-UNICEF estimates; WHO & United Nations Children's Fund [UNICEF], 2016, July 6b)	99%
Neonatal mortality rate (per 1,000 live births) (2015)	5.5 [4.3–6.9]
Under-five mortality rate (probability of dying by age five per 1,000 live births) (2015)	10.7 [9.0–12.7]
Maternal mortality rate (per 100,000 live births) (2015)	27 [22–32]
Total expenditure on health as % of GDP (2014)	5.55%
General government expenditure on health as % of total expenditure on health (2014)	30.0%* [55.79% (WHO, 2016e)]
Private expenditure on health as % of total expenditure on health (2014)	32.0% [44.21% (WHO, 2016e)]
Physicians density (per 1,000 population) (2014) (National Health and Family Planning Commission of China, 2015)	1.74

*Total health expenditure in China includes government health expenditure, social health expenditure, and out-of-pocket health expenditure, wherein social health expenditure refers to the expenditure from all sectors of society apart from all levels of government, including social health insurance, commercial health insurance, social donation, and so on. In 2014, government health expenditure accounts for 30.0% of total health expenditure, social health expenditure 38.1%, and out-of-pocket health expenditure 32.0%.

Source: data from World Health Organization. *Key country indicators China: key indicators*, http://apps.who.int/gho/data/node.cco.ki-CHN?lang=en, accessed 16 Feb 2017, Copyright © 2016 World Health Organization.

4.6.1 Development of the health system

Before economic reform in 1978, China had a planned and collective economy; the health system was mainly financed by government and all healthcare services were provided by the public sector. However, due to the nearly free medical services, individual out-of-pocket health expenses were low. The transformation to a market economy in the late 1970s had led to huge changes in the health system. Personal health expenses, as a result, soared and the proportion of out-of-pocket health expenditure (which refers to self-paid medical expenses) to the total annual health expenditure rose to 60% in 2001, three times as that in 1978 (which was 20.4%) (Ministry of Health [MoH] of PRC, 2010).

In the 1990s, the Chinese government attempted to offer quality services at a relatively cheap price and put its dedication into controlling the price of healthcare services. Nonetheless, the service fees could not cover the cost and the healthcare institutions had to make profit in the sale of medication and check-ups. The practice of compensating for low medical service charges with high drug prices and drug purchase rebate became increasingly common (Huang *et al.*, 2012; State Council Information Office of PRC, 2012). In addition, the medical security system only served those citizens who worked in the government or state-owned enterprises and there was virtually no protection provided to the rural population. The relationship between medical practitioners and patients has gathered tension, and violence against medical professionals by patients were reported.

Facing public discontent with healthcare services and the associated social instability, the Chinese government has engaged in medical reform since 2003. The system now emphasizes more on the benefits of the public and improving citizens' lives. In 2009, the 'Plan on Deepening the Reform of the Medical and Health Care System' released by the State Council stipulated the objective that every citizen can enjoy basic healthcare services with the healthcare protection system included as a part of the basic healthcare system by 2020 (Central Committee of the Communist Party of China & State Council of PRC, 2009).

At present, a healthcare system which expands both its urban and rural coverage has formed. It encompasses a rural health system and an urban medical service delivery system. The backbone of the rural health system is county-level hospitals, with grassroots being township- and county-level clinics. Meanwhile, in the urban medical service delivery system, community health centres and city hospitals collaborate and coordinate the service delivery. As for the medical security system, the Urban Employee Basic Medical Insurance (UEBMI), Urban Residence Basic Medical Insurance (URBMI), the New Rural Cooperative Medical Scheme (NRCMS), and urban and rural insurance schemes for catastrophic illness provide basic medical security to the urban working population, urban non-working population, rural population, and people who have difficulty affording medical services, respectively. Until 2011, the number of people participating in the insurance system exceeded 1.3 billion, that is, 95% coverage of the population (State Council Information Office of PRC, 2012). The proportion of out-of-pocket health expenditure to total annual health expenditure slumped to 34.8% (MoH of PRC, 2010).

Currently, China's health governance bodies can be divided into four levels. From central to peripheral, they are: (1) the NHFPC; (2) Provincial (municipality's or autonomous region's) Health and Family Planning Commissions; (3) city-level Health and Family Planning Commissions; and (4) county-level Health and Family Planning Commissions. At the village level, there is no independent health governance body (Meng *et al.*, 2015). Like health governance bodies, health institutions were also divided by four levels, namely country level, province level, city level, and county level. Community and village health institutions are usually directly managed by governance departments at the county level.

NHFPC and its affiliated agency, the State Administration of Traditional Chinese Medicine (SATCM), constitute the main health administrative bodies in China. They are the constituting departments of the State Council (NHFPC was originally called the Ministry of Health). In 2013, the first meeting of 12th National People's Congress passed the 'Plan for the Institutional Restructuring of the State Council and Transformation of Functions Thereof' and 'Notice of the State Council on the Setup of Institutions'. Thereafter, the Ministry of Health and National Population and Family Planning Commission were combined, forming the NHFPC, in charge of allocating resources to the management of healthcare planning and services related to fertility policy, organizing the formulation of national drug policy, improving fertility policy, monitoring public health and healthcare services, and the management of population planning and related services (Wang, 2013, March 10). Health governance bodies at the province, city, and county levels follow the principles and directions set by the government and perform the administrative work of the healthcare system within the administrative regions, which includes the supervision of the affiliated healthcare institutions, constructing and executing plans, and decisions and works related to the environment (Fig. 4.2).

4.6.2 General health status

China reported an under-5 mortality rate of 10.7 per 1,000 live births in 2015 (see Table 4.4) and total fertility rate of 1.7 per woman in 2013 (WHO, n.d.). As of 2015, life expectancy for female and male was projected to be 78 and 75 respectively (see Table 4.4). Life expectancy at birth for both sexes increased by 4 years over the period of 2000–2012 when the WHO region average was reported to have an increase of 4 years in the same period. Stroke, accounting for 23.7% of mortality, was the leading cause of death in 2012, while no death was resulted from malaria (WHO, n.d.) and NCDs accounted for 87% of all deaths (WHO, 2014b). In 1981, the life expectancy at birth and infant mortality rate in China were 67.8 and 34.7%, respectively. The maternal mortality rate in 1991 was 80 per 100,000. The health status of Chinese citizens is now one of the highest among developing countries. In 2014, the infant mortality rate dropped to 8.9%, while the maternal mortality rate was 22.2 per 100,000 (National Bureau of Statistics of China, 2015; National Health and Family Planning Commission (NHFPC), 2015). These figures reflect there has been improvement overall, despite the changing health policies.

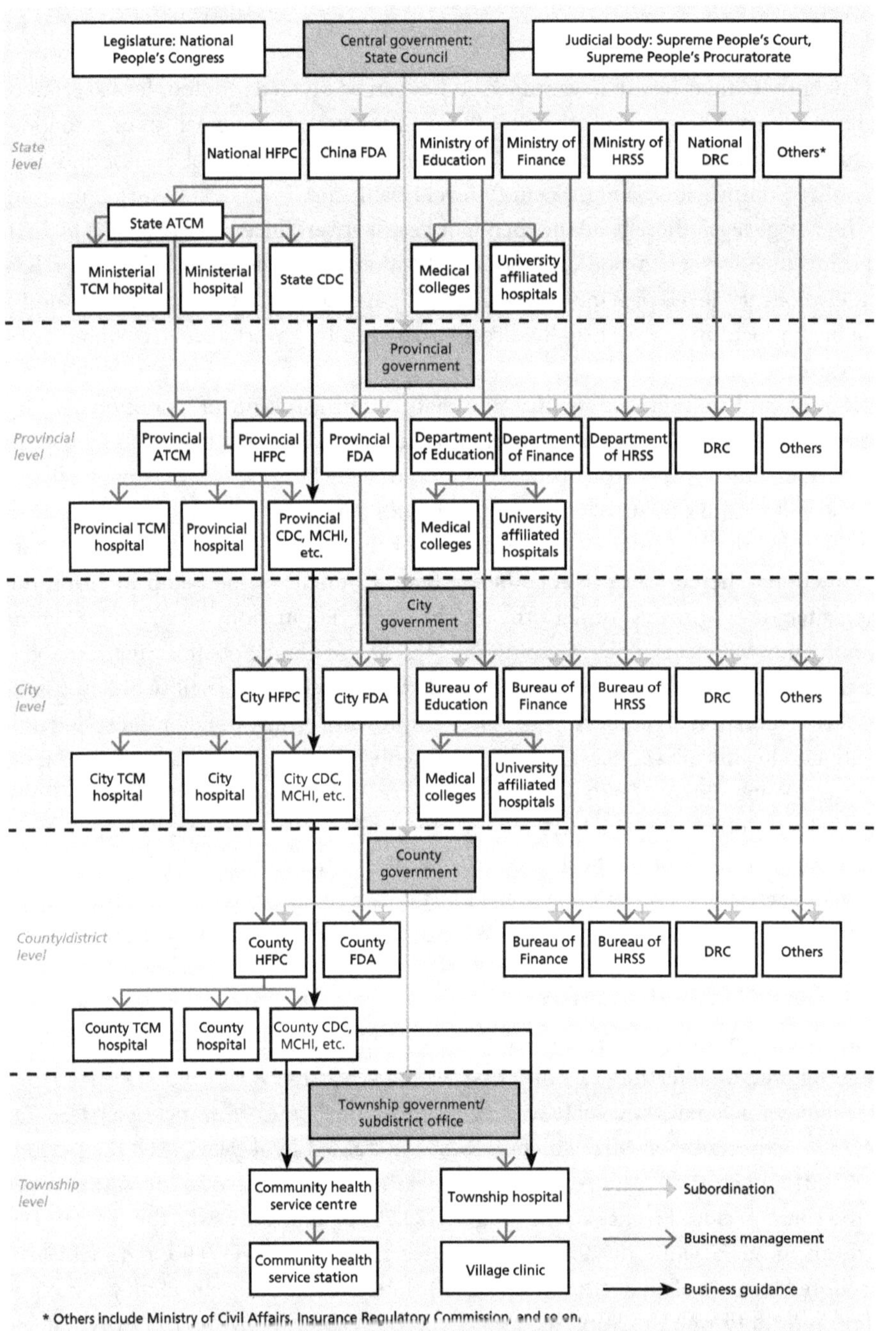

Fig. 4.2 Organizational chart of China's health administration system.

(HFPC = Health and Family Planning Commission; FDA = Food and Drug Administration; HRSS = Human Resource and Social Security; DRC = Development and Reform Commission; ATCM = Administration of Traditional Chinese Medicine; CDC = Center for Disease Control and Prevention; MCHI = Maternal and Children Health Institution.)

Reproduced with permission from Meng Q, Yang H, Chen W, Sun Q, and Liu X. *People's Republic of China health system review (Health Systems in Transition, Vol. 5 No. 7 2015)*. Asia Pacific Observatory on Health Systems and Policies, WHO, Geneva Switzerland, http://www.wpro.who.int/asia_pacific_observatory/hits/series/china_health_systems_review.pdf?ua=1, accessed 13 Feb 2017, Copyright © 2015 World Health Organization.

4.6.3 The rural–urban gap in healthcare

As more people migrated from the rural areas to cities for jobs and education and economic opportunities, 'left-behind children', 'empty nest elderly', and 'grandparents raising grandchildren' have become prevalent phenomena in rural communities. Disease pattern and burden in the rural areas have changed with this shift in demographic pattern. According to the *Floating Population in China Development Report 2015* (NHFPC Department of Floating Population, 2015), the floating population numbered 253 million, with 78% aged between 15 and 59 years. The left-behind elderly and children lacked care due to the migration of the prime working age population, affecting their physical and mental health. The grandparents who raised their grandchildren usually had little health knowledge. The children thus could not receive proper health education. Moreover, the migrated workers moved back due to stress or occupational injuries. Their physical and psychological problems aggravate the heavy burden of the rural healthcare system.

As the rural and urban development polarized, the gap in accessibility to medical services between villages and cities widened. Some 83.5% of urban families resided in locations that were less than 1 km away from their nearest medical care facility, yet, this was the case for only 58% of rural families. It is noteworthy that the conditions of villages in the western regions of the country were worse than that in the eastern and central areas. Some 11% of the rural families in the western provinces were at least 5 km away from their nearest medical care centre while the proportion was much higher than the eastern (2.7%) and central (3.7%) provinces (MoH of PRC, 2008). Quality of healthcare in the rural areas in the western part of the country was worse than that in the eastern and central parts. The ratio of registered medical practitioners (including registered assistant medical practitioners) offering clinical services in village clinics and township clinics, inpatient labour rate, and the rate of main chronic diseases undermanaged were lower in the west. Apart from that, public health facilities such as clean water and sanitation and knowledge on hygiene were lower in the west (Wang *et al.*, 2015). Despite the effort and dedication of the Chinese government, there are still many challenges ahead as evidenced by unequal development among different rural regions.

4.6.4 Public health and primary healthcare system

Health policies in rural China change in accordance with national policies. Before the economic reform, many rural areas implemented the Rural Cooperative Medical Care System. Rural cooperatives were funded by the public, and the medical services provided were almost free. Around five million barefoot doctors who had received basic medical training went to the remote villages and provided simple treatments, referral, vaccination, family planning and infection control (Fang, 2003). In the mid-1970s, the Rural Cooperative Medical Care System covered 90% of the rural population. At that time, the international society agreed the system was successful in improving the health status of low-income regions. The World Health Organization even promoted this system to the developing countries (Huang *et al.*, 2012).

Later, the economic reform caused a breakdown of the system because it was operated by crowd-funding. In 2002, the system coverage was only 9.5%, and 79.1% of the rural population did not have any health insurance, which meant the villagers' medical expenses were mainly out of pocket. In 2003, the Chinese government implemented the NRCMS (Wang *et al.*, 2015). The scheme is a health insurance project targeted at the rural population. The NRCMS is financed by various ways, including governmental organizations, payment by villagers, subsidies from government, and collective support, while enrolment is on a voluntary basis. In the pilot scheme, everyone (the beneficiaries) pays 10 RMB and the central and peripheral government each subsidizes 10 RMB (20 RMB in total); in 2013, the annual personal payment was around 90 RMB and the subsidies from the government became 320 RMB. Although the scheme is not mandatory, the subsidies from the government have increased and the coverage has extended, including subsidies for the expenses of minor illness and inpatient charges due to major illness and chronic NCDs. The system gained the support of the villagers and the number of rural-dwelling people participating in the scheme reached 736 million in 2014. The participation rate was 98.9% (NHFPC, 2015).

Compared to The Rural Cooperative Medical System focusing on minor illness treatment, which aimed to tackle the lack of doctors and drugs in villages before the economic reform, The New Rural Cooperative Medical Scheme, in view of the changing disease burden, focused on the compensation for medical expenses for major illnesses and chronic NCDs. This alleviated the problem of poverty due to medical illness in rural China.

Although the NRCMS enhances the medical security of the rural population, there is a large gap in the medical resources between the rural and urban setting. According to the *2015 China Public Health Statistical Yearbook*, cities had 3.54 registered medical practitioners per 1,000 citizens (including 4.30 registered assistant medical practitioners) and 4.30 registered nurses. However, the figures for the villages were 1.51 and 1.31, respectively. In cities, there were 6.88 beds per 1,000 citizens but only 3.11 in villages. In 2013, the urban health expenditure per capita was 3,234.1 RMB and rural was 1,274.4 RMB. The difference was 2.5 times (NHFPC, 2015).

4.6.5 Disease control and health promotion

In the 1950s, the main disease burden was infectious diseases and pandemics (Liu, 2013). At the end of the 1980s, the main disease-related causes of death were respiratory illness, cerebrovascular diseases, and malignant neoplasm (National Bureau of Statistics of China, 1989), which in 2004 became malignant neoplasm, ischaemic heart diseases, and cerebrovascular diseases (National Bureau of Statistics of China, 2015). From this, the disease burden was found to shift from infectious diseases to chronic NCDs. As older people and children in the villages lacked care, external causes such as injuries and poisoning also showed an increasing trend. The health needs of rural population changed, but this group of people did not have any medical security. This rendered a lot of people unable to receive proper medical treatment or become poor due to high medical expenses.

Disease control and prevention has been one of the key government policies since the establishment of the PRC. Early effort in disease control includes vaccination (e.g. smallpox), environmental hygiene, and sanitation with the great national 'Patriotic Health Campaigns'. Millions of people were immunized and epidemic prevention stations were built in most of the counties (Banister, 1987; Xu, 1994). Sexually transmitted diseases such as syphilis and gonorrhoea declined due to the outlawing of prostitution (Abrams, 2001). Campaigns that eliminated the 'four pests'—sparrows, rats, mosquitoes, and flies (vermin and vectors of disease transmission)—were carried out nationally. While greatly successful in disease control, those efforts mostly benefitted the urban areas and the majority of peasants in rural areas did not have access to formal clinical and public health services in the nascent stage of the PRC. To improve medical access for the rural population, the 'barefoot doctor', a new position for community-level health workers under the cooperative medical scheme was formed shortly after the culture revolution. A barefoot doctor normally received a short period of training (from several months to one year) and served as a primary care 'professional' whose responsibility included basic clinical care, environmental sanitation, and health promotion. Although quality of care was limited, it benefitted that large cohort of population from infectious diseases.

The modern disease control system commenced after the establishment of the Center for Disease Control and Prevention (CDC) System in 2002, which also marks the modernization of public health in China (Walgate, 2002). By the recombination of the Academy of Preventive Medicine, three health research institutes, and the nationwide epidemic prevention stations network, the CDC is the milestone for integration of leadership, resources, and capacity. However, the severe acute respiratory syndrome (SARS) outbreak in 2003 left a tragic lesson learnt by the newly built system. The lack of an early identification, isolation, and coordinated reporting mechanism led to a dreadful epidemic across the county.

In 2004, a new infectious disease surveillance system with a statutory reporting mechanism for 37 notifiable diseases came into force. In rural areas, disease control is now managed by the county-level Health and Family Planning Commission and the CDC with subordinating hospitals and clinics at the county, township, and village levels. For non-communicable diseases, a nationwide disease system with 161 surveillance points was also built in response to this rapidly increased health burden. To deepen health reform in rural areas, the Chinese government launched the 'National Essential Public Health Service' in 2009, providing the establishment of electronic medical records, health education, immunization, health management for children (0–6 years), older people (65 years or above), pregnant women, persons with hypertension, diabetes, and severe mental illness, reporting of communicable disease and emergency public health incidents (NHFPC Department of Primary Health, 2016). Moreover, large-scale government health promotion and disease prevention programmes were implemented in rural China, including subsides for maternal health checks, cervical cancer screening, environmentally friendly toilets, and cataract surgery for persons below the poverty line (State Council Information Office of PRC, 2012).

The population's health literacy is a critical element for disease control and prevention, particularly in rural areas. Health literacy refers to the ability to acquire, process, and understand the health information to make appropriate health decision. In 2008, a Chinese health literacy policy paper, also known as Health 66, was issued and implemented by the national health authority (see Appendix I). It includes 66 essential health messages for basic health knowledge and beliefs, healthy lifestyle and behaviour, and health and safety skills. The results of the first national assessment indicated that only 6.48% of respondents met the standard. Significantly fewer people in the rural areas (3.43%) were health literate compared to their urban counterparts (9.94%), highlighting that the rural communities were in dire need of health education (MoH Department of Maternal and Child Health and Community Health, 2009).

4.6.6 Disaster trends and situations

From 2000 to 2016, droughts (22 times), earthquakes (86 times), riverine floods (133 times), flash floods (16 times), landslides (44 times), tropical cyclones (84 times), and convective storms (61 times) were common types of disaster reported in the country. The deadliest disaster was an earthquake in May 2008, causing 87,476 deaths. The disaster affecting the greatest number of people was a flood in June 2003, affecting 150 million people. The one which caused the greatest economic damage was the earthquake in May 2008, leading to a loss of US$85 billion (CRED, 2017).

4.7 The Republic of India

The Republic of India (India), a low-income country with a large population of 1.3 billion, accounts for 21% of the global disease burden (WHO, 2015). Despite continuous improvements in health indicators, India has very high maternal, infant, and children mortality. With 68% of the population in rural areas (UN, 2015), India has a very high rural–urban disparity in health services provision (Government of India, 2014) (see Table 4.5). According to UNDP (2016), India's HDI value for 2015 was 0.624 in the medium human development category, ranked 131st out of 188 countries and territories.

4.7.1 Development of the health system

India has been actively improving its health system in recent decades. In 2005, the National Rural Health Mission (NRHM) was launched in order to bring all the vertical programmes under one umbrella and to improve federal-state coordination in facing health and health system challenges. In 2008, a health insurance scheme, Rashtriya Swasthya Beema Yojana, was established to target the poor to cover hospitalization costs (WHO, 2015).

The Indian healthcare system comprises both public and private sectors. The public sector has limited infrastructure, technology, drugs, and healthcare workers and the private sector accounted for two-thirds of the healthcare services. In 2010, the government enacted a Clinical Establishment Act to regulate the vast and heterogeneous private sector, despite suboptimal adoption and implementation (WHO, 2015).

Table 4.5 India: Basic facts and key health indicators

Total population (2015)	13.0 billion
Proportion of rural population (2015) (World Bank, n.d.-e)	67%
Life expectancy (years) (2015)	69.9 (female); 66.9 (male); 68.3 (both sexes)
Diphtheria tetanus toxoid and pertussis (DTP3) immunization coverage among one-year-olds (2015)	87%
Measles-containing vaccines (MCV1) immunization coverage for infants (2015) (WHO, 2016, December 1, WHO-UNICEF estimates)	87%
Neonatal mortality rate (per 1,000 live births) (2015)	27.7 [24.0–31.6]
Under-five mortality rate (probability of dying by age five per 1,000 live births) (2015)	47.7 [42.4–53.3]
Maternal mortality rate (per 100,000 live births) (2015)	174 [139–217]
Total expenditure on health as % of GDP (2014)	4.69%
General government expenditure on health as % of total expenditure on health (2014)	30.04%
Private expenditure on health as % of total expenditure on health (2014)	69.96%
Physicians density (per 1,000 population) (2012)	0.702

Source: data from World Health Organization. *Key country indicators—India: key indicators*, http://apps.who.int/gho/data/node.cco.ki-IND?lang=en, accessed 16 Feb 2017, Copyright © 2016 World Health Organization.

The government expenditure on health in India only accounts for 1.2% of gross domestic product (GDP). Out-of-pocket payment is as high as 70% of total health spending, making poor people even poorer because of their healthcare expenses. In 2014, the new Union Government started to pay attention to strengthen the health systems and improve financial protection. The new national health policy for 2015 will focus on primary care in the next five years, with the target of achieving universal health coverage (WHO, 2015). To strengthen the health system, the Ministry of Health and Family Welfare has implemented various e-Health measures including citizen-centric services, information management systems, standardization, and regulation. India's patent law development over the years has shortened the patent protection of pharmaceutical drugs and encouraged the production of low-cost generics (Haley and Hayley, 2012). India also has the expertise in biotechnology which enables it to develop vaccines at a lower cost (Government of India, 2014).

4.7.2 General health status

India reported an under-5 mortality rate of 53 per 1,000 live births in 2015 (see Table 4.5) and total fertility rate of 2.5 per woman in 2013 (WHO, n.d.). As of 2015, life expectancy for female and male was projected to be 70 and 67 respectively (see Table 4.5). Life expectancy at birth for both sexes increased by 5 years over the period of 2000-2012 when the WHO region average was reported to have increased by 5 years in the same period. Ischaemic heart disease, accounting for 12.4% of mortality, was the leading cause of death in 2012, while death due to malaria was reported to be 2.3 per 100,000 population (WHO, n.d.) and NCDs accounted for 60 % of all deaths (WHO, 2014b).

4.7.3 The rural–urban gap in healthcare

India's rural people have poorer health outcomes and less access to healthcare services, when compared to their urban counterparts. There is a 44% difference in total fertility rate between rural areas (2.6) and urban areas (1.8). There is also a difference (63%) in the infant mortality rate between the country's rural population (40 per 1,000 live births) and its urban population (27 per 1,000 live births) (UN, 2015). In 2011–12, the rural population had a higher out-of-pocket healthcare expense as a proportion of total household monthly income per capita (6.9%) than the urban population (5.5%) (Government of India, 2014).

The rural population has less access to healthcare facilities and has lower affordability of treatment, in addition to poorer sanitation. Only 28.5% of the rural population has improved sanitation facilities, much lower than the urban population (62.6%) (WHO, 2016f). Rural residents have access to only one-third of hospital beds while two-thirds are for urban population. The distribution of healthcare workers, including doctors, nurses, and pharmacists, is highly concentrated in urban areas and the private sector. According to a nationwide survey conducted in 2013, to seek outpatient services, nearly one-third (32%) of the rural respondents had to travel over 5 km while only 8% urban citizens had to do the same. The cost of treatment at private healthcare facilities is two to nine times higher than that at public facilities. A more comprehensive health financing should be developed to improve the quality of medical care in India (Aitken *et al.*, 2013).

The National Rural Health Mission (NRHM) was launched in 2005 to provide affordable, accessible, and quality healthcare to the rural population. It introduced almost 900,000 community health volunteers, increased utilization of public services, and improved health behaviours. The NRHM also organized over 18,000 ambulances for free emergency response and patient transport services to over a million patients monthly, added over 178,000 health workers to a public system, provided cash transfers to over 10 million pregnant women annually, empowering and facilitating them to seek free care in the institutions, and began to address infrastructure gaps. An increase in outpatient attendance, bed occupancy, and institutional delivery were recorded. However, only a small proportion of health facilities were fully utilized. Some states had problems such as poor governance and funds are not efficiently utilized. Some service delivery was concentrated on reproductive and child health and disease control instead of a wide range of health services (Government of India, 2014).

4.7.4 Public health and primary healthcare system

India's health system has a mixed ownership. The private sector provides most curative services while the government-funded sector provides publicly financed health promotion as well as preventive and curative health services. The private health sector is further divided into 'not-for-profit' and the 'for-profit': the non-profit ones include health services provided by NGOs and charitable institutions, while the for-profit health sector consists of various types of practitioners and institutions. The private sector takes a major role in all the submarkets including medical education, technology, pharmacy, hospital development, and in the provision of healthcare (India Ministry of Health and Family Welfare, 2011).

The three-tiered primary healthcare system comprises of the subcentre (SC), which is the most peripheral contact point between the primary healthcare system and the community, for a population of 3,000 to 5,000; the primary health centre (PHC), which is the first contact point between the village community and the medical professionals, for 20,000 to 30,000 people; and the community health centre (CHC) which serves as the referral point for every four PHCs, covering 80,000 to 120,000. The district hospitals function as the secondary tier for rural healthcare, and as the primary tier for the urban population (India Ministry of Health and Family Welfare, 2016). In 2016, there were 155,069 subcentres, 25,354 PHCs, and 5,510 CHCs (India Ministry of Health and Family Welfare, 2016).

4.7.5 Disease control and health promotion

Health challenges in India range from infectious diseases to NCDs and the Ministry of Health and Family Welfare is implementing different schemes, programmes, and national initiatives to provide universal access to quality healthcare (India Ministry of Health and Family Welfare, 2011).

India has achieved significant progress in tackling infectious diseases, such as AIDS, tuberculosis, and polio, but continued monitoring is required to secure the gains. People living in poverty are highly vulnerable to health shocks with medical expenses contributing to household poverty and compromising efforts to improve health outcomes. Child malnutrition has been a major concern, notwithstanding economic growth: approximately 40% of the India's children are stunted. Integrated Child Development Services is undergoing restructuring but there are still limitations in terms of technology, capacity, programme, and institution. Access to clean water and sanitation is another pressing health issue. The government has spent US$4 billion annually on improving access to rural water supply and sanitation; however, only one-third of rural households have access to piped water and sanitation (World Bank Group, 2016, October).

Infectious diseases remain a major public .0health challenge. Outbreaks of new emerging and re-emerging infectious diseases also lead to high morbidity, mortality, and negative socioeconomic impact (India Ministry of Health and Family Welfare, 2014). To increase access to the decentralized public health system, the government is building new infrastructure in deprived areas and upgrading the existing infrastructure. Different programmes are put under the umbrella of the National Health Mission (NHM), with the National Rural Health Mission (NRHM) and the National Urban Health Mission (NUHM) as its two Sub-Missions. The major programmes implemented are: Routine Immunization (RI); National Vector Borne Disease Control Programme (NVBDCP); Revised National TB Control Programme (RNTCP); Integrated Diseases Surveillance Programme (IDSP); National Programme for Control of Blindness (NPCB); National Mental Health Programme (NMHP); National Programme for Healthcare of the Elderly (NPHCE); and National Programme for Prevention and Control of Cancer, Diabetes, Cardiovascular Diseases, and Strokes (NPCDCS). Central support is given to strengthen the healthcare management, disaster control, and redevelopment of hospitals and institutions (Aitken *et al.*, 2013). India has made major achievements in tackling infectious diseases such as accomplishing polio-free certification of the WHO South-East Asia Region in March 2014, successful halting and reversal of the spread of HIV/AIDS, significant reduction in the incidence of malaria, tuberculosis, and neglected tropical diseases (WHO, 2015).

Despite these achievements, the emergence of NCDs accounts for 67% of the total morbidity burden and 53% of total deaths in India (WHO, 2015). The change in lifestyle increases the risks factors of NCDs, namely physical inactivity, high intake of salt, sugar, and trans fats, and the use of tobacco and alcohol. To control and prevent chronic diseases, the Ministry of Health and Family Welfare launched a national programme for the prevention of cancer, heart disease, and diabetes, elderly health, and mental health in 100 districts. Training on early detection and referral will be provided to frontline health workers from different health facilities. This decentralization of a comprehensive package of services including prevention, diagnosis, and early treatment will reduce people's out-of-pocket expenditure on health. The country will put more resources into health promotion on behavioural change and healthy lifestyles (India Ministry of Health and Family Welfare, 2011).

4.7.6 **Disaster trends and situations**

From 2000 to 2016, the most common types of natural disaster in India were epidemics (13 viral diseases), extreme temperatures (11 heat waves and 15 cold waves), floods (108 riverine floods and 20 flash floods), landslides (13 times), and storms (14 tropical cyclones and 30 convective storms). The deadliest disaster was an earthquake in January 2001, causing 20,005 deaths. The disasters with the greatest number of affected people were two droughts, one in July 2002 and the other in January 2016, affecting 300 million and 330 million people, respectively. The event causing the greatest economic damage was a flood in September 2014, leading to a loss of US$16 billion (CRED, 2017).

4.8 **The Republic of Indonesia**

In the medium human development category, Indonesia's HDI value in 2015 was 0.689, positioning at 113 out of 188 countries and territories (UNDP, 2016). As the fourth

Table 4.6 Indonesia: Basic facts and key health indicators

Total population (2015)	257.6 million
Proportion of rural population (2015) (World Bank, n.d.-e)	46%
Life expectancy (years) (2015)	71.2 (female); 67.1 (male); 69.1 (both sexes)
Diphtheria tetanus toxoid and pertussis (DTP3) immunization coverage among one-year-olds (2015)	81%
Measles-containing vaccines (MCV1) immunization coverage for infants (2015) (WHO, 2016, December 1, WHO-UNICEF estimates)	69%
Neonatal mortality rate (per 1,000 live births) (2015)	13.5 [10.9–16.8]
Under-five mortality rate (probability of dying by age five per 1,000 live births) (2015)	27.2 [22.5–32.9]
Maternal mortality rate (per 100,000 live births) (2015)	126 [93–179]
Total expenditure on health as % of GDP (2014)	2.85%
General government expenditure on health as % as total expenditure on health (2014)	37.78%
Private expenditure on health as % of total expenditure on health (2014)	62.22%
Physicians density (per 1,000 population) (2012)	0.204

Source: data from World Health Organization. *Key country indicators—Indonesia: key indicators*, http://apps.who.int/gho/data/node.cco.ki-IDN?lang=en, accessed 16 Feb 2017, Copyright © 2016 World Health Organization.

most populous country in the world, the Republic of Indonesia (Indonesia) has been facing challenges to provide universal and accessible healthcare to the entire population. Although improvements have been shown in its health indicators in the last decades (Tandon *et al.*, 2016, October 28), both life expectancy and infant mortality rates are at the average level of a lower-middle-income country (Global Health Workforce Alliance, 2013). Half of the population resides in the rural areas with limited access to healthcare (see Table 4.6).

4.8.1 Development of the health system

In 1999, the MoH released the Health Development Plan Towards Healthy Indonesia 2010, with four missions: to proclaim national development with health concern; to increase the autonomy and awareness of society for healthy living; to maintain and improve health services; and to maintain and enhance individual, family, and public health and the environment (Moeloek, 1999). In 2000, the complex and fragmented interfiscal health system was decentralized to the district level. Based on the national medium-term strategy, each technical unit of MoH, provincial, and district health offices develops its annual operational plans. Region governments gain autonomy and receive substantial financial transfers and increase regional expenditure. Such a completely new intergovernmental fiscal system has reduced the government's effectiveness and its control on corruption (Global Health Workforce Alliance, 2013).

Indonesia launched Jaminan Kesehatan Nasional, a universal health insurance in 2014. Since then, nearly 160 million people have been covered and Indonesia has committed itself to covering the entire population under this social health insurance by 2019 (Tandon *et al.*, 2016, October 28). Under the National Social Security System, the low-income group will be subsidized by the government and the remaining population will be financed through a contributory scheme. The aims are to reduce the prevalence of communicable diseases and to improve maternal and child health (Global Health Workforce Alliance, 2013).

Compared with other countries with a similar income level, Indonesia is among the ones with the lowest proportion of healthcare expenditure, spending at only 2.85% of GDP. Expenditure on healthcare has increased over the last few decades; however, it is still less than optimal to overcome the country's healthcare challenges. Indonesia's health infrastructure is less developed, with fewer hospital beds (per 10,000 people) than its neighbouring countries (Global Health Workforce Alliance, 2013).

4.8.2 General health status

Indonesia reported an under-5 mortality rate of 27.2 per 1,000 live births in 2015 (see Table 4.6) and total fertility rate of 2.3 per woman in 2013 (WHO, n.d.). As of 2015, life expectancy for female and male was projected to be 71 and 67 respectively (see Table 4.6). Life expectancy at birth for both sexes increased by 4 years over the period of 2000-2012 when the WHO region average was reported to have an increase of 5 years in the same period. Stroke, accounting for 21.2% of mortality, was the leading cause of death in 2012, while death due to malaria was reported to be 3.8 per 100,000 population (WHO, n.d.) and NCDs accounted for 71 % of all deaths (WHO, 2014b). Life expectancy at birth has increased from 49 years in 1960, to 63 years in 1990, and to 69 years in 2015. The under-5 mortality rate has declined from 222 per 1,000 live births in 1960 to 85 in 1990 and 27 in 2015; infant mortality has declined sixfold since 1960, down to 23 per 1,000 live births in 2015 (Tandon *et al.*, 2016, October 28; see also Table 4.6).

4.8.3 The rural–urban gap in healthcare

The rural population are disadvantaged as regards healthcare access. The percentage of people without healthcare coverage in rural areas (63.5%) is more than double of that in urban areas (18.4%) (Scheil-Adlung, 2015). Less than half of the rural population (47.5%) has access to improved sanitation, while more than 70% of the urban population are using improved sanitation facilities (WHO, 2016g). Children in rural areas are more likely to be unvaccinated. More than 60% of unvaccinated children live in rural areas (Tandon *et al.*, 2016, October 28).

Despite the implementation of the new unified health insurance programme, people living in remote and rural areas still lack an available and good quality basic benefits package. Geographical unequal distribution of the health workforce and facilities limit the rural population's access to healthcare services (Tandon *et al.*, 2016, October 28).

There is an imbalance in the health workforce distribution across the provinces. Java-Bali, the country's most populated region, has a physician density twice of Kalimantan and three times as Maluku-NTT-Papua. Health workers tend to work in cities due to added financial incentives (Tandon *et al.*, 2016, October 28).

4.8.4 **Public health and primary healthcare system**

Health services in Indonesia are provided by both public and private sectors. The public sector provides the most of care in rural areas and for secondary healthcare. The country has 34 provinces and 514 districts/cities, and some 72,000 villages (Tandon *et al.*, 2016, October 28). From the late 1960s to 1970s, in order to increase primary healthcare access, the Indonesian government started to develop health centres at subdistrict and district level hospitals. The number of health facilities has increased since then. Community services were staffed by doctors, midwives, and nurses under civil service contracts.

Besides public facilities, private services are provided by doctors, nurses, and midwives who are usually employed in public sectors. However, this multiple practice involvement of health workers reduces the efficiency, equity, and overall accessibility of the health system. Faith-based organizations are also active in the healthcare delivery in the country (Global Health Workforce Alliance, 2013).

4.8.5 **Disease control and health promotion**

Indonesia needs to address the community health needs arising from natural disasters, chronic diseases, and infectious diseases. Emerging and re-emerging infectious diseases place burden on the health system and disease control programmes. Accessibility, quality of healthcare, and nutrition are of high public health significance. Morbidity and mortality rates are worsened by food safety and quality issues. Increase in lifestyle and environmental risk factors such as tobacco use, unhealthy diets, physical inactivity, unsafe water, inadequate sanitation, traffic accidents, and use of solid fuels for cooking have also increased the need for more health education promotion (WHO, 2014, May). As the world's fifth-largest tobacco producer, Indonesia's child tobacco workers suffer from occupational diseases (Human Rights Watch, 2016, May 24).

To increase community access to health services, the MoH has launched the Alert Village and Village Health Posts as the community-based health programme since 2006. More than 70,000 villages are covered and that each village must be served by at least one midwife, and each village health post must be served by one midwife and one nurse (Global Health Workforce Alliance, 2013).

The government also enforced compulsory rural and remote service in public sectors to ensure an adequately staffed health workforce (Global Health Workforce Alliance,

2013). As of 2014, at least one community health centre (puskesmas) is available for 30,000 people, with additional subhealth centres accessible at the village level. There were 9,731 health centres as of 2014. Staffed by a doctor or nurses or other qualified healthcare professionals, puskesmases provide basic care services, immunization, antenatal and postnatal care, environmental health, and dental services (Tandon *et al.*, 2016, October 28).

Since the millennium, Indonesia's children have better health outcomes due to the improved access to healthcare services, home care, community care, primary healthcare facilities, and referral facilities. In addition, maternal mortality has declined significantly after the implementation of Mother Class, Maternity Waiting Home, and the family planning programme (Republic of Indonesia, 2012). The government launched a childbirth insurance programme in 2010 to reduce the maternal and neonatal mortality. This childbirth insurance, named the Jampersal Programme, provides insurance in prenatal care, deliveries, postpartum care, and newborn care for all mothers and newborns who do not yet have health insurance.

Indonesia also successfully achieved one of the MDGs by 2015 by halting and beginning to reverse the incidence of tuberculosis (TB) in 2011. The government reduced TB cases by early detection and treatment. The strategies include support in the detection test, development of insurance based payment schemes for patients and expansion of healthcare services for drug-resistant TB patients (Republic of Indonesia, 2012).

4.8.6 Disaster trends and situations

From 2000 to 2016, the most common types of natural disaster in Indonesia were earthquakes (46 ground movements), floods (70 riverine floods and 27 flash floods), landslides (40 times), and volcanic activities (17 ash falls). The deadliest disaster in Indonesia was an earthquake in December 2004, causing 165,708 deaths. The disasters reported with the greatest number of people were two earthquakes occurred in May 2006 and September 2009, where 3.18 million and 2.5 million affected people were affected, respectively. The disaster causing the greatest economic damage was an earthquake in December 2004, leading to a loss of US$4.45 billion (CRED, 2017).

4.9 The Democratic People's Republic of Korea

The Democratic People's Republic of Korea (DPRK) is one of the most isolated regimes in the world. Over the past few years, it has made improvement in some health indicators such as maternal and child health, prevention and control of infectious and non-communicable diseases (WHO Country Office for DPR Korea, 2016). However, it faces challenges in terms of food security, nutrition, and health as well as water, sanitation, and hygiene (WASH). Among the country's population of 25 million, 18 million are in need of humanitarian aid (United Nations DPR Korea Humanitarian Country Team, 2016, April) (see Table 4.7).

4.9.1 Development of the health system

In DPRK, universal and free healthcare is guaranteed in the Constitution of 1960 and Public Health Law of 1980. In 2014, the government allocated 6.4% of its total budget on healthcare. There is no available data on the out-of-pocket private expenditure on health (WHO Country Office for DPR Korea, 2016).

The Ministry of Public Health is the regulatory body of national health programmes. It provides administrative guidance to provincial and county-level health divisions, all hospitals, and hygiene and anti-epidemic stations in order to safeguard supply of drug and equipment. The system consists of the Ministry of Public Health at the central level, health bureaus of the provincial people's committee at provincial level and health department of city/county people's committee at city/county level (WHO Country Office for DPR Korea, 2016).

Over the last two decades, DPRK has encountered acute public health problems caused by geopolitical factors. Before the 1990s, DPRK had established a free universal healthcare system and achieved remarkable health indicators such as life expectancy, infant

Table 4.7 Democratic People's Republic of Korea: Basic facts and key health indicators

Total population (2015)	25.1 million
Proportion of rural population (2015) (World Bank, n.d.-e)	39%
Life expectancy (years) (2015)	74.0 (female); 67.0 (male); 70.6 (both sexes)
Diphtheria tetanus toxoid and pertussis (DTP3) immunization coverage among one-year-olds (2015)	96%
Measles-containing vaccine (MCV1) immunization coverage for infants (2015) (WHO, 2016, December 1, WHO-UNICEF estimates)	98%
Neonatal mortality rate (per 1,000 live births) (2015)	13.5 [7.9–18.6]
Under-five mortality rate (probability of dying by age five per 1,000 live births) (2015)	24.9 [19.5–31.9]
Maternal mortality rate (per 100,000 live births) (2015)	82 [37–190]
Total expenditure on health as % of GDP	No data available
General government expenditure on health as % of total expenditure on health	No data available
Private expenditure on health as % of total expenditure on health	No data available
Physicians density (per 1,000 population) (2014)	3.5

Source: data from World Health Organization. *Key country indicators—Democratic People's Republic of Korea: key indicators*, http://apps.who.int/gho/data/node.cco.ki-PRK?lang=en, accessed 16 Feb 2017, Copyright © 2016 World Health Organization; World Health Organization Country Office for DPR Korea. *WHO country cooperation strategy: Democratic People's Republic of Korea: 2014–2019*. New Delhi: WHO SEARO, New Delhi, India, http://apps.who.int/iris/bitstream/10665/250298/1/9789290224716-eng.pdf, accessed 15 Feb. 2017, Copyright © 2016 World Health Organization.

mortality, access to health services, and water and sanitation. In the early 1990s, the Soviet Union collapsed and hence DPRK suffered from internal economic sanctions with a 50% decrease in per capita income. The economic downturn triggered a decline in healthcare access and resulted in poor nutritional status, outbreaks of infectious diseases, and increases in maternal, child, and infant mortality in the 1990s. To improve people's living standards, the government introduced economic measures to restore the economy (WHO Country Office for DPR Korea, 2016).

As the GDP grew, DPRK's healthcare access and health outcomes have improved gradually. These were indicated by an increase in childhood immunization coverage and access to healthcare services against tuberculosis (TB) and malaria, and women's and children's healthcare access, especially in emergency obstetric care, immunization, and integrated management of childhood illness. There are declines in maternal and child mortality (WHO Country Office for DPR Korea, 2016).

However, with ageing and economic development, DPRK's population is facing the risk of a high prevalence of NCDs, which are the leading cause of the country's morbidity and mortality. DPRK is vulnerable to natural disasters, especially flooding and droughts, which contribute to poorer access to healthcare, outbreaks of infectious diseases, as well as food insecurity (WHO Country Office for DPR Korea, 2016).

According to a report published by UN agencies, more than 75% of the population was under the threat of food insecurity in early 2016 (UN DPR Korea Humanitarian Country Team, 2016, April). The country failed to produce adequate food for its population as food production was limited by available land, quality agricultural products, and frequent dry seasons (UN DPR Korea Humanitarian Country Team, 2016, April). DPRK scored 28.6 in Global Hunger Index score and was classified as 'serious' in 2015. More than 40% of the population was malnourished in 2014–2016 (von Grebmer *et al.*, 2016).

In 2010, Amnesty International released a report, criticizing that the healthcare system in DPRK failed to meet people's basic healthcare needs (Amnesty International, 2010). According to the interviews conducted with the people who already left the country, the hospitals in DPRK were lacking medical supplies and equipment. Many people were unable to afford medical treatment because of the unofficial charges collected by medical staff. However, WHO said the report was unscientific and outdated (Aid agencies row over North Korea healthcare system, 2010, July 16).

4.9.2 General health status

DPRK reported an under-5 mortality rate of 24.9 per 1,000 live births in 2015 (see Table 4.7) and total fertility rate of 2 per woman in 2013 (WHO, n.d.). As of 2015, life expectancy for female and male was projected to be 74 and 67 respectively (see Table 4.7). Life expectancy at birth for both sexes increased by 5 years over the period of 2000-2012 when the WHO region average was reported to have increased by 5 years in the same period. Stroke, accounting for 19.4% of mortality, was the leading cause of death in 2012, while no death was resulted from malaria (WHO, n.d.) and NCDs accounted for 79% of all deaths (WHO, 2014b).

4.9.3 The rural–urban gap in healthcare

The official data shows that DPR Korea has less than 40% rural population. The rural population faces inadequacy in many aspects and is also more vulnerable to natural disasters.

DPRK has inadequate health service delivery in terms of quality of health facilities, equipment, and drugs. While some improvements have been made, the quality of care and services in many health facilities still do not meet international standards. There is a limited availability of essential drugs, medical products, and life-saving equipment at most levels, posing a key constraint for health services (UN DPR Korea Humanitarian Country Team, 2016, April).

There are variations in health outcomes as well as access to care between urban and rural areas.

Urban women have better access to reproductive care. In DPRK, antenatal care services are almost universal, in that all women who were pregnant within the three years prior to the survey received antenatal care from skilled providers. However, more doctors in urban areas provide antenatal care and women in urban areas receive more frequent antenatal check-ups than their rural counterparts. There is also difference in the type of trained personnel assisting in delivery among urban and rural women: 94% of urban women received care from a doctor or assistant doctor, while only around 75% of rural women had the same access (Central Bureau of Statistics of DPRK & UN Population Fund, 2015).

The rural population lacks enough access to clean water, sanitation, and hygiene. Many health facilities do not have functioning water systems and this could result in poor hygiene and, thus, an increase in infection cases and the spread of diseases in hospitals. The lack of access to safe drinking water and sanitation services also lead to higher incidence of diarrhoea, respiratory tract infections, and waterborne diseases. There is an estimated 20% of people in the country who do not have access to clean water and adequate sanitation facilities. These shortages are particularly prominent at the primary level health facilities in the rural areas, where children and women are most vulnerable (UN DPR Korea Humanitarian Country Team, 2016, April).

Children in rural areas are more likely to suffer from malnutrition than their counterparts in urban areas, which is reflected in the weight and stunting rates. Rural children are twice as likely to be underweight (27%) than urban children (13%). Forty-five per cent (45%) of children in rural areas are too short for their age, compared with 23% of their urban counterparts (Central Bureau of Statistics of DPRK, 2010).

4.9.4 Public health and primary healthcare system

DPRK has a centralized healthcare system. It has one of the highest ratios of health workers to population in the region. Across the country, there is an extensive infrastructure of 133 hospitals at central and provincial levels, 1,741 hospitals at county level and RI levels, and 6,263 RI clinics and poly clinics. At all levels, the health programmes are implemented under the guidance of the people's committees (WHO Country Office for DPR Korea, 2016).

The healthcare system is comprised of primary care services by family doctors; secondary healthcare services at districts/country hospitals; and tertiary healthcare services at central and provincial people's hospitals, medical school hospitals, paediatric and maternity hospitals, and medical specialty institutes located in cities (WHO Country Office for DPR Korea, 2016).

The 'family doctor system' is the basis of DPRK's health system. It ensures universal healthcare access by providing integrated first-contact preventive and curative services through assigning one family doctor for every 130 households. Household doctors deliver primary healthcare services to the community at the polyclinic or clinic in urban areas, and at the RI hospital or RI clinic in rural areas. These hospitals are also responsible for reporting of disease and outbreak response. However, there have been reports on insufficient monitoring of facility equipment and poor management at county hospitals and RI clinics (WHO Country Office for DPR Korea, 2016).

The health referral system is limited by transportation and communication constraints, and is sometimes affected by extreme weather in winter. In an attempt to overcome these barriers, the government initiated a telemedicine programme in 2007 with the support of WHO to improve access to clinical advice and diagnostic services for remote areas. The telemedicine network today is run across the country, connecting hospitals at central, provincial, and county levels (WHO Country Office for DPR Korea, 2016).

4.9.5 Disease control and health promotion

The high immunization coverage in DPRK has been recognized as an achievement. Since 1997, WHO and United Nations Children's Fund (UNICEF) have been providing technical and operational support in terms of vaccination, logistics, cold chain equipment, transportation, and training for the local human workforce. DPRK has achieved polio-free status since 2006 and is at the status of eliminating measles. In 2012, Hib-containing pentavalent vaccine was also introduced in routine immunization (WHO Country Office for DPR Korea, 2016).

However, some health issues remain major concerns, including maternal mortality, high prevalence of low birth weight and childhood malnutrition, as well as tuberculosis (TB), malaria, and hepatitis B (WHO Country Office for DPR Korea, 2016). For example, an estimated 2,500 people in the country die from TB annually. The lack of treatment for approximately 3,900 multidrug-resistant TB patients leads to many avoidable deaths and continued high transmission in the community (DPRK United Nations Country Team, 2015). According to an UN report released in July 2015, the number of North Korean children being treated for severe acute malnutrition increased by 38% in 2014 compared to the previous year. The increase was considered to coincide with the beginning of a drought period (UN Office for the Coordination of Humanitarian Affairs, 2015, July).

4.9.6 Disaster trends and situations

From 2000 to 2016, the DPRK experienced 26 natural disasters (13 and 7 out of 27 were riverine floods and tropical cyclones, respectively). The deadliest natural disasters were two floods in August 2007 and August 2016, causing 610 and 538 deaths, respectively. The disaster reported to have the greatest number of affected people was a drought in June 2015, where 18 million people were affected. The disaster with the greatest economic damage was a storm in August 2000, leading to a loss of US$6 billion (CRED, 2017).

4.10 Lao People's Democratic Republic

The Lao People's Democratic Republic (Lao PDR) is a landlocked country comprised of mountainous landscape. With a population of 6.8 million people living in its 18 provinces, 61% of the population are currently living in rural settings and in the most extreme cases, some even live in areas with no roads. Lao PDR has made remarkable progress in the past three decades. Its HDI value significantly increased from 0.345 in 1980 to 0.586 in 2015, putting it in the medium human development category and ranking 138th out of 188 countries and territories (UNDP, 2016). In fact, the life expectancy rate at birth extended by 19 years from 1985 to 2012 (see Table 4.8).

4.10.1 Development of the health system

Since the establishment of Lao People's Democratic Republic in 1975, the country has undergone multiple governance phases, from centralized to decentralized. Now, the healthcare system in Lao PDR is delivered in three levels: the central (Ministry of Health [MoH]), provincial, and district levels. Developed by the MoH, the system is composed of two national health plans including the medium-term five-year health sector development plan and the annual operational plan, aimed at improving the health status of the population (Akkhavong *et al.*, 2014)

In 1975, when the administrations were all centralized, the central government was organized and responsible for developing national plans, managing budget, and allocating resources for the population. However, while the government had implemented a series of initiations to improve the productivity of all public sectors, the lack of human and financial resources in the central government pressured the central level to decentralize and disseminate all their sectors and authority to the provincial levels (Akkhavong *et al.*, 2014).

As the central government handed over its responsibilities of planning, budgeting, and delivering healthcare services to the provincial governments, multiple issues emerged, one of which was disparity. The lack of regulations among the decisions of each province generated inequalities, including the disparity of revenues and expenditures across the 17 provinces. As a result, in the 2000s, regulations were established to reform coordination and management in a horizontal perspective among the provinces. While the levels from the provincial to the district were responsible for financial management and delivering all types of services including transportation, education, health, and rural development directly to the general population, the central government played a major role in allocating budget for central hospitals and national-planned projects (Akkhavong *et al.*, 2014).

Table 4.8 Lao PDR: Basic facts and key health indicators

Total population (2015)	6.8 million
Proportion of rural population (2015) (World Bank, n.d.-e)	61%
Life expectancy (years) (2015)	67.2 (female), 64.1 (male), 65.7 (both sexes)
Diphtheria tetanus toxoid and pertussis (DTP3) immunization coverage among one-year-olds (2015)	89%
Measles-containing vaccine (MCV1) immunization coverage for infants (2015) (WHO, 2016, December 1, WHO-UNICEF estimates)	88%
Neonatal mortality rate (per 1,000 live births) (2015)	30.1 [20.7–42.7]
Under-five mortality rate (probability of dying by age five per 1,000 live births) (2015)	66.7 [48.8–89.7]
Maternal mortality rate (per 100,000 live births) (2015)	197 [136–307]
Total expenditure on health as % of GDP (2014)	1.87%
General government expenditure on health as % of total expenditure on health (2014)	50.53%
Private expenditure on health as % of total expenditure on health (2014)	49.47%
Physicians density (per 1,000 population) (2012)	0.182

Source: data from World Health Organization. *Key country indicators—Laos: key indicators*, http://apps.who.int/gho/data/node.cco.ki-LAO?lang=en, accessed 16 Feb 2017, Copyright © 2016 World Health Organization.

4.10.2 **General health status**

Laos reported an under-5 mortality rate of 66.7 per 1,000 live births in 2015 (see Table 4.8) and total fertility rate of 3 per woman in 2013 (WHO, n.d.). As of 2015, life expectancy for female and male was projected to be 67 and 64 respectively (see Table 4.8). Life expectancy at birth for both sexes increased by 7 years over the period of 2000-2012 when the WHO region average was reported to have an increase of 4 years in the same period. Lower respiratory infections, accounting for 11.3% of mortality, were the leading cause of death in 2012, while death due to malaria was reported to be 4.4 per 100,000 population (WHO, n.d.) and NCDs accounted for 48 % of all deaths (WHO, 2014b).

Despite the enhancements made, disparity remains a major issue that has hindered the country from its development. Geographical disparity has consequently generated a limitation for the poor from accessing distant services. As public transportations are inadequate and unsuitable for its mountainous landscape, only 33.3% of the rural areas have access to roads (Akkhavong *et al.*, 2014). Some 93% of the population require an average of a 90- minute walk to access to the nearby healthcare facility (WHO & MoH of Lao PDR, 2012). Moreover other examples of inequalities that have increased the level of disparity include differences in ability to access food, education, and healthcare, not only between the rich and the poor but also males and females (WHO & MoH of Lao PDR, 2012).

Rapid increase in medical costs as well as the weak healthcare financial system cause further inequalities to accessing healthcare services. Although the undeveloped healthcare structure has successfully introduced user fees and out-of-pocket payment, these concepts have negatively affected the rural population through delayed care, as many who are poor cannot afford these services. In addition, due to the high costs and low-quality of these services, utilizations of services are low and inefficient. Among the poor, only 25% of this population lives in a village with a medical practitioner, whereas 50% of the better-off live near a doctor (WHO & MoH of Lao PDR, 2012).

4.10.3 The rural–urban gap in healthcare

Poverty has been a prominent issue in Lao PDR as 27.6% of the population are still living below the poverty line. The mountainous landscape of the country impedes its population's access to basic needs such as sanitation and electricity, and the inability to retain healthcare workers in a rural setting has been a major issue among the rural populations (Akkhavong *et al.*, 2014).

In response to the rural community and its poverty status, the government has developed multiple services to tackle the issues, such as offering cash crop replacements. The government also encourages villagers to relocate to lowland areas to increase access to roads and community services. However, this resettlement idea is rather challenging for the villagers as they may not adapt well with the new environment where traditional cultivation methods may not be applicable (Akkhavong *et al.*, 2014).

To address the lack of access in the rural community, the government has enacted an initiation entitled MoH regulation No. 103. Aiming to evenly distribute healthcare professionals across the country, this regulation requires all healthcare graduates to work in a rural setting for their first three years after graduation. With adequate incentives, the government attempts to retain healthcare professionals in the rural communities to improve the quality of deliverance and the system as a whole. In addition, the government has initiated strengthening of this development in different directions such as establishing programmes for drugs and for maternal, neonatal, and child health, while renovating and upgrading healthcare facilities to improve quality (Akkhavong *et al.*, 2014).

As the rural and urban gap widened, the government has also introduced and attempted to implement multiple policies and programmes for the poor and those living in the rural communities. However, due to weak governance and monitoring, many of these initiations were ineffective to benefit the poor. For example, the government introduced a policy named Prime Ministerial Decree No. 52/PM to exempt the poor, other disadvantaged groups, and civil servants from healthcare expenses. However, due to the underdeveloped healthcare financial system and the poorly defined eligibility criteria, this exemption is often not applied for the poor with regards to accessibility of healthcare facilities (Akkhavong *et al.*, 2014).

4.10.4 Public health and primary healthcare system

Public health in Lao PDR is promoted through many services including district health centres, and provincial and central hospitals. It focuses and prioritizes on communicable diseases such as vector-, water-, and food-borne diseases. More significantly, the outbreak of SARS in 2003 has allowed the government to develop a National Coordination Committee on Communicable Diseases aiming to lower the impacts of future emerging epidemics (Akkhavong *et al.*, 2014).

In Lao PDR, primary healthcare is provided through district hospitals and health centres and village drug kits. Provision of health education in Lao has successfully developed a large primary healthcare network while nurturing a good number of village healthcare workers and qualified volunteers. However, mainly due to the limited availability of paid posts offered for healthcare graduates, many qualified healthcare workers are left waiting for approval and retention of healthcare workers in rural communities has been difficult within the country (Akkhavong *et al.*, 2014).

District health centres are often the first level of healthcare facility in Lao PDR. These centres offer primary healthcare services such as prevention, health promotion, diagnosis, and treatments that are limited to their ability and capacity. However, the inability to monitor the healthcare service in the rural communities has consequently led to poor quality healthcare services for the poor which in return has decreased the general population's acceptance towards these offered services (Akkhavong *et al.*, 2014).

4.10.5 Disease control and health promotion

Since 2003, a variety of programmes has been established to monitor the levels of communicable diseases within the country. After reviewing the Expanded Programme on Immunization in 2012, it has offered protection against eight antigens including BCG, diphtheria, tetanus and pertussis, poliomyelitis, Haemophilus influenzae type B, measles, and hepatitis B. This program aims to fully immunize 85% of the infants. However, recent studies done by the Lao Social Indicator Survey in 2012 reveal the necessity to implement further promotion of this programme, as only 39% of the population are fully vaccinated (Akkhavong *et al.*, 2014). Contributing to the MDGs, Lao PDR demonstrated progress in reducing hunger and provision of education. However, issues regarding nutrition and maternal mortality remain unchanged and are still severely prevalent in the country.

4.10.6 Disaster trends and situations

From 2000 to 2016, floods and epidemics were considered as the most common types of natural disaster in Laos. The deadliest disaster was an epidemic in January 2013, causing 77 deaths and the disaster with the greatest number of affected people was a flood in August 2001, affecting 453,000 people. The disaster causing the greatest economic damage was a storm in September 2009, leading to a loss of US$100 million (CRED, 2017).

References

Abrams, H. K. (2001). The resurgence of sexually transmitted disease in China. *J Public Health Policy*, **22**, 429–40.

Afghanistan Central Statistics Organization (2014). *National Risk and Vulnerability Assessment 2011–12: Afghanistan Living Condition Survey*. Afghanistan Central Statistics Organization, Ministry of Public Health, Kabul, Afghanistan, and ICF International, Rockville, MD.

Afghanistan Central Statistics Organization, Afghanistan Ministry of Public Health, ICF International (2016). *Afghanistan Demographic and Health Survey 2015: Key Indicators*. Afghanistan Central Statistics Organization, Ministry of Public Health, Kabul, Afghanistan, and ICF International, Rockville, MD.

Afghanistan Ministry of Public Health (2015). *Ministry of Public Health National Health Strategy 2015–2020*. Kabul, Afghanistan: Ministry of Public Health.

Afghanistan Ministry of Public Health (2016). *Ministry of Public Health National Health Strategy 2016–2020*. Kabul, Afghanistan: Ministry of Public Health.

Aid agencies row over North Korea health care system (2010, July 16) *BBC News*. Available at: https://www.bbc.com/news/world-asia-pacific-10665964 (accessed 25 January 2017) [Online].

Aitken, M., Backliwal, A., Chang, M., & Udeshi, A. (2013). Understanding healthcare access in India. What is the current state? Parsippany, NJ: IMS Institute for Healthcare Informatics. Available at: http://www.esocialsciences.org/Download/Download.aspx?fname=A20141224155255_33.pdf&fcategory=Articles&aid=6366 (accessed 15 February 2017) [Online].

Akkhavong, K., Paphassarang, C., Phoxay, C., Vonglokham, M., Phommavong, C., & Pholsena, S. (2014). *Lao People's Democratic Republic: Health System Review* (Health Systems in Transition Vol. 4 No. 1 2014). Geneva Switzerland: Asia Pacific Observatory on Health Systems and Policies, WHO. Available at: http://www.wpro.who.int/asia_pacific_observatory/hits/series/Lao_Health_System_Review.pdf (accessed 15 February 2017) [Online].

Amnesty International (2010). *The Crumbling State of Health Care in North Korea*. London, UK: Amnesty International. Available at: https://www.amnesty.org/en/documents/asa24/001/2010/en/ (accessed 15 February 2017) [Online].

Banister, J. (1987). *China's Changing Population*. Stanford, CA: Stanford University Press.

Bhutan Ministry of Health (2014a). *2012 National Health Survey*. Thimphu, Bhutan: Ministry of Health.

Bhutan Ministry of Health (2014b). *Human Resources for Health: Country Profile Bhutan*. Bhutan, Thimphu: Ministry of Health.

Bhutan Ministry of Health (2016). *Annual Health Bulletin 2016*. Thimphu, Bhutan: Ministry of Health.

Bhutan National Statistics Bureau (2011). *Bhutan Multiple Indicator Survey 2010*. Thimphu, Bhutan: National Statistics Bureau. Available at: https://mics-surveys-prod.s3.amazonaws.com/MICS4/South%20Asia/Bhutan/2010/Final/Bhutan%202010%20MICS_English.pdf (accessed 17 February 2017) [Online].

Boyd, C. P., Hayes, L., Wilson, R. L., & Bearsley-Smith, C. (2008). Harnessing the social capital of rural communities for youth mental health: An asset-based community development framework. *Aust J Rural Heal*, **16**, 189–93.

Bragg, F., Holmes, M. V., Iona, A., *et al.* (2017). Association between diabetes and cause-specific mortality in rural and urban areas of China. *JAMA*, **317**, 280–9.

Cambodia National Institute of Statistics, Cambodia Directorate General for Health, ICF International (2015, September). *Cambodia Demographic and Health Survey 2014*. Available at: https://dhsprogram.com/pubs/pdf/FR312/FR312.pdf (accessed 13 February 2017) [Online].

Central Bureau of Statistics of Democratic People's Republic of Korea (2010). *Democratic People's Republic of Korea Multiple Indicator Cluster Survey 2009: Final Report.* Central Bureau of Statistics, Pyongyang, DPR Korea. Available at: http://catalog.ihsn.org/index.php/catalog/2878/download/43765 (accessed 15 February 2017) [Online].

Central Bureau of Statistics of Democratic People's Republic of Korea & United Nations (UN) Population Fund (2015). *Democratic People's Republic of Korea: socio-economic, demographic and health survey 2014.* Central Bureau of Statistics, Pyongyang, DPR Korea. Available at: http://kp.one.un.org/content/dam/unct/dprk/docs/2014%20SDHS%20Report_E_final.pdf (accessed 15 February 2017) [Online].

Central Committee of the Communist Party of China, State Council of the People's Republic of China (2009). [On deepening the medical and healthcare system reform]. Available at: http://www.gov.cn/jrzg/2009-04/06/content_1278721.htm (accessed 23 January 2017) (Chinese) [Online].

Centre for Research on the Epidemiology of Disasters (CRED) (2017). EM-DAT: The Emergency Events Database. Available at: http://.emdat.be/emdat_db/ (accessed 14 July 2017) [Online].

DPRK United Nations Country Team (2015). DPR Korea 2015: Needs and Priorities. Available at: https://www.humanitarianresponse.info/system/files/documents/files/20150401%20DPR_Korea_NP_FINAL.pdf (accessed 15 February 2017)

Fang, X. (2003). [The barefoot doctors and Rural Cooperative Medical Scheme: the case of Fuyang County, Zhejiang Province]. *21st Century*, (10), 87–97 (Chinese).

Global Health Workforce Alliance (2013). *Mid-level Health Workers for Delivery of Essential Health Services: A Global Systematic Review and Country Experiences.* Available at: http://www.who.int/workforcealliance/knowledge/resources/ghwa_mid_level_report_2013.pdf (accessed 15 February 2017) [Online].

Gong, P., Liang, S., Carlton, E. J., *et al.* (2012). Urbanisation and health in China. *Lancet*, **379**(9818), 843–52.

Government of India (2014). *National Health Policy 2015.* New Delhi, India: Ministry of Health and Family Welfare.

Haley, G. T. & Hayley, U. C. V. (2012). The effects on patent-law changes on innovation: the case of India's pharmaceutical industry. *Technological Forecasting & Social Change*, **79**, 607–19.

Huang, Y., Zeng, L., Li, Y., Zhou, X., & Liu, P. (2012). Performance evaluation on healthcare reform policy in rural China: a systematic review. *CJEBM*, **12**, 293–304.

Human Rights Watch (2016, May 24). 'The Harvest is in My Blood': Hazardous Child Labor in Tobacco Farming in Indonesia. Available at: https://www.hrw.org/report/2016/05/24/harvest-my-blood/hazardous-child-labor-tobacco-farming-indonesia (accessed 10 February 2017) [Online].

India Ministry of Health and Family Welfare (2011). *Annual Report to the People on Health.* New Delhi, India: Ministry of Health and Family Welfare.

India Ministry of Health and Family Welfare (2014). *Annual Report of Department of Health & Family Welfare for 2013–14.* New Delhi, India: Ministry of Health and Family Welfare.

India Ministry of Health and Family Welfare (2016). *Rural Health Statistics.* New Delhi, India: Ministry of Health and Family Welfare.

Liu, J. (2013). [Development of Chinese medical and health system reform and policy connotation of new health care system]. *Social Security Studies*, (1), 125–34. Available at: http://mall.cnki.net/onlineread/Mall/MallIndex?sourceid=10&fName=SHBB201301*1* (accessed 14 February 2017) (Chinese) [Online].

Médecins Sans Frontières (2014). Between rhetoric and reality: The ongoing struggle to access healthcare in Afghanistan. Available at: http://www.msf.org/en/article/between-rhetoric-and-reality-ongoing-struggle-access-healthcare-afghanistan [Online].

Meng, Q., Yang, H., Chen, W., Sun, Q., & Liu, X. (2015). People's Republic of China Health System Review (Health Systems in Transition Vol. 5 No. 7 2015). Geneva Switzerland: Asia Pacific

Observatory on Health Systems and Policies, WHO. Available at: http://www.wpro.who.int/asia_pacific_observatory/hits/series/china_health_systems_review.pdf?ua=1 (accessed 13 February 2017) [Online].

Ministry of Health of the People's Republic of China, Department of Maternal and Child Health and Community Health (2009). Report of the First Chinese Residents' Health Literacy Survey. Available at: http://wenku.baidu.com/view/651453a5f524ccbff121840a.html (accessed 14 February 2017) [Online].

Ministry of Health of the People's Republic of China, Center for Health Statistics and Information (2008). [*An Analysis Report of National Health Services Survey in China, 2008*]. Available at: http://www.nhfpc.gov.cn/cmsresources/mohwsbwstjxxzx/cmsrsdocument/doc9911.pdf (accessed 23 January 2017) (Chinese) [Online].

Ministry of Health of the People's Republic of China (2010). *2010 China Public Health Statistical Yearbook*. Beijing, China: Peking Union Medical College Press.

Moeloek, F. A. (1999). *Health Development Plan Towards Healthy Indonesia 2010*. Jakarta, Indonesia: Ministry of Health.

National Bureau of Statistics of China (1989). *China Statistical Yearbook 1989*. Beijing, China: China Statistics Press.

National Bureau of Statistics of China (2015). *2015 China Public Health Statistical Yearbook*. Beijing, China: China Statistics Press. Available at: http://www.stats.gov.cn/tjsj/ndsj/2015/indexeh.htm (accessed 23 January 2017) [Online].

National Health and Family Planning Commission (NHFPC) of the People's Republic of China (2015). *2015 China health and family planning statistical yearbook*. Beijing, China: Peking Union Medical College Press.

National Health and Family Planning Commission (NHFPC) of the People's Republic of China Department of Floating Population (2015). [*Floating Population in China Development Report 2015*]. Beijing, China: China Population Publishing House. (Chinese).

National Health and Family Planning Commission (NHFPC) of the People's Republic of China Department of Primary Health (2016). [*Notice on the effective implementation of National Basic Public Health Services Project 2016*]. Available at: http://www.nhfpc.gov.cn/jws/s3577/201606/f29a4659c7f4455ca6f62f8d14eb4b02.shtml (accessed 24 January 2017) (Chinese) [Online].

Population pyramids of the world from 1950 to 2100: Cambodia 2015 (n.d.). Available at: https://populationpyramid.net/cambodia/2015/ (accessed 26 January 2017) [Online].

Republic of Indonesia & Ministry of National Development Planning/National Development Planning Agency (BAPPENAS) (2012). *Report on the Achievement of the Millennium Development Goals in Indonesia 2011*. Indonesia: Ministry of National Development Planning/National Development Planning Agency, Jakarta, Indonesia

Scheil-Adlung, X. (2015). *Global Evidence on Inequities in Rural Health Protection: New Data on Rural Deficits in Health Coverage for 174 Countries*. Geneva, Switzerland: International Labour Office.

Schelzig, K. (2014). Cambodia: Country Poverty Analysis 2014. Mandaluyong City, Philippines: Asian Development Bank. Available at: https://www.adb.org/sites/default/files/institutional-document/151706/cambodia-country-poverty-analysis-2014.pdf (accessed 26 January 2017) [Online].

Singh, P. N., Arthur, K. N., Orlich, M. J., *et al.* (2014). Global epidemiology of obesity, vegetarian dietary patterns, and noncommunicable disease in Asian Indians. *Am J Clin Nutr*, **100**(suppl), 359S–64S.

Smith, K. B., Humphreys, J. S., & Wilson, M. G. (2008). Addressing the health disadvantage of rural populations: How does epidemiological evidence inform rural health policies and research? *Aust J Rural* Heal, **16**, 56–66.

State Council Information Office of the People's Republic of China (PRC) (2012). *White paper on medical and health services in China.* Available at: http://www.scio.gov.cn/zfbps/ndhf/2012/Document/1262402/1262402.htm (accessed 23 January 2017) [Online].

Tandon, A., Pambudi, E. S., Harimuti, P., *et al.* (2016, October 28). *Indonesia—Health Financing System Assessment: Spend More, Right and Better* (Policy Brief). World Bank Group, Washington, DC. Available at: http://documents.worldbank.org/curated/en/453091479269158106/pdf/110298-REVISED-PUBLIC-HFSA-Nov17-LowRes.pdf (accessed 15 February 2017) [Online].

United Nations Development Programme (2016). *Human Development Report 2016.* New York, NY: United Nations Development Programme.

United Nations (UN) DPR Korea Humanitarian Country Team (2016, April). *DPR Korea Needs and Priorities 2016.* New York, NY: United Nations Office for the Coordination of Humanitarian Affairs. Available at: https://www.humanitarianresponse.info/system/files/documents/files/2016_dprk_needs_and_priorities_final_draft_140416.pdf (accessed 15 February 2017) [Online].

United Nations (UN) Office for the Coordination of Humanitarian Affairs (2016). *Afghanistan 2017 Humanitarian Needs Overview.* New York, NY: United Nations. Available at: https://www.humanitarianresponse.info/en/operations/afghanistan/document/afghanistan-2017-humanitarian-needs-overview [Online].

United Nations (UN) Office for the Coordination of Humanitarian Affairs (2015, July). *Democratic People's Republic of Korea: Drought (as of Jul 2015).* New York, NY: United Nations. Available at: https://www.reliefweb.int/sites/reliefweb.int/files/resources/PRK_drought_150701.v3.pdf (accessed 15 February 2017) [Online].

United Nations (UN) Department of Economic and Social Affairs, Population Division (2014). *Our urbanizing world* (Population Facts No.2014/3). New York, NY: United Nations. Available at: http://www.un.org/en/development/desa/population/publications/pdf/popfacts/PopFacts_2014-3.pdf (accessed 20 January 2017) [Online].

United Nations (UN) Department of Economic and Social Affairs, Population Division (2015). *World Urbanization Prospects: The 2014 Revision* (ST/ESA/SER.A/366). New York, NY: United Nations. Available at: https://esa.un.org/Unpd/Wup/Publications/Files/WUP2014-Report.pdf (accessed 15 February 2017) [Online].

von Grebmer, K., Bernstein, J., Nabarro, D., *et al.* (2016). *2016 Global Hunger Index: Getting to Zero Hunger.* Washington, DC, Dublin, Ireland, Bonn, Switzerland: International Food Policy Research Institute, Concern Worldwide, Welthungerhilfe, United Nations. Available at: http://ebrary.ifpri.org/utils/getfile/collection/p15738coll2/id/130707/filename/130918.pdf (accessed 15 February 2017) [Online].

Walgate, R. (2002). China sets up Centre for Disease Control and Prevention. *Bull World Health Organ,* **80**(4), 335.

Wang, M., Fang, H., Bishwajit, G., Xiang, Y., Fu, H., & Feng, Z. (2015). Evaluation of rural primary health care in western China: a cross-sectional study. *Int J Envion Res Public Health,* **12**, 13843–60.

Wang, Z. (2013, March 10). The plan for institutional reform and functional transformation of the State Council. *Xinhua News Agency.* Available at: http://news.xinhuanet.com/2013lh/2013-03/10/c_114968104.htm (accessed 23 January 2017). (Chinese) [Online].

World Bank (n.d.-a). Maternal mortality ratio (modeled estimate, per 100,000 live births). Available at: http://data.worldbank.org/indicator/SH.STA.MMRT (accessed 26 January 2017) [Online].

World Bank (n.d.-b). Mortality rate, neonatal (per 1,000 live births). Available at: http://data.worldbank.org/indicator/SH.DYN.NMRT (accessed 26 January 2017) [Online].

World Bank (n.d.-c). Mortality rate, under-5 (per 1,000 live births). Available at: http://data.worldbank.org/indicator/SH.DYN.MORT (accessed 26 January 2017) [Online].

World Bank (n.d.-d). Out-of-pocket health expenditure (% of private expenditure on health). Available at: http://data.worldbank.org/indicator/SH.XPD.OOPC.ZS (accessed 26 January 2017) [Online].

World Bank (n.d.-e). Rural population (% of total population). Available at: http://data.worldbank.org/indicator/SP.RUR.TOTL.ZS (accessed 26 January 2017) [Online].

World Bank Group (2016, October). *India: Country Snapshot*. Available at: http://documents.worldbank.org/curated/en/341851476782719063/pdf/109249-WP-IndiaCountrySnapshots-highres-PUBLIC.pdf (accessed 15 February 2017) [Online].

World Health Organization (WHO) (n.d.). Country statistics. Available at: http://www.who.int/gho/countries/en/ (accessed 4 October 2017) [Online].

World Health Organization (WHO) (2014a). *Country Cooperation Strategy 2014–2018: Bhutan*. New Delhi, India: WHO.

World Health Organization (WHO) (2014b). *Noncommunicable Diseases Country Profiles 2014*. Geneva, Switzerland: WHO.

World Health Organization (WHO) (2014, May). *WHO Country Cooperation Strategy at a Glance: Indonesia*. Available at: http://apps.who.int/iris/bitstream/10665/136896/1/ccsbrief_idn_en.pdf?ua=1 (accessed 15 February 2017) [Online].

World Health Organization (WHO) (2015). *WHO Country Cooperation Strategy at a Glance: India*. Available at: http://apps.who.int/iris/bitstream/10665/136895/1/ccsbrief_ind_en.pdf (accessed 14 February 2017) [Online].

World Health Organization (WHO) (2015, January). *Democratic People's Republic of Korea: WHO statistical profile*. Available at: http://www.who.int/gho/countries/prk.pdf?ua=1 (accessed 23 January 2017) [Online].

World Health Organization (WHO) (2016, May). WHO Country Cooperation Strategy at a Glance: Afghanistan. Available at: http://apps.who.int/iris/bitstream/10665/136852/1/ccsbrief_afg_en.pdf?ua=1 (accessed 20 January 2017) [Online].

World Health Organization (WHO) (2016a). *Afghanistan Health Profile 2015*. Cairo, Egypt: WHO.

World Health Organization (WHO) (2016b). Afghanistan: key indicators. Available at: http://apps.who.int/gho/data/node.cco.ki-AFG?lang=en (accessed 16 February 2017) [Online].

World Health Organization (WHO) (2016c). Bhutan: key indicators. Available at: http://apps.who.int/gho/data/node.cco.ki-BTN?lang=en (accessed 16 February 2017) [Online].

World Health Organization (WHO) (2016d). Cambodia: key indicators. Available at: http://apps.who.int/gho/data/node.cco.ki KHM?lang=en (accessed 16 February 2017) [Online].

World Health Organization (WHO) (2016e). China: key indicators. Available at: http://apps.who.int/gho/data/node.cco.ki-CHN?lang=en (accessed 16 February 2017) [Online].

World Health Organization (WHO) (2016f). India: key indicators. Available at: http://apps.who.int/gho/data/node.cco.ki-IND?lang=en (accessed 16 February 2017) [Online].

World Health Organization (WHO) (2016g). Indonesia: key indicators. Available at: http://apps.who.int/gho/data/node.cco.ki-IDN?lang=en (accessed 16 February 2017) [Online].

World Health Organization (WHO) (2016h). Democratic People's Republic of Korea: key indicators. Available at: http://apps.who.int/gho/data/node.cco.ki-PRK?lang=en (accessed 16 February 2017) [Online].

World Health Organization (WHO) (2016i). Laos: key indicators. Available at: http://apps.who.int/gho/data/node.cco.ki-LAO?lang=en (accessed 16 February 2017) [Online].

World Health Organization (WHO) (2016, December 1). WHO vaccine-preventable diseases: monitoring system: 2016 global summary. Available at: http://apps.who.int/immunization_monitoring/globalsummary/ (accessed 16 February) [Online].

World Health Organization (WHO) Country Office for DPR Korea (2016). *WHO Country Cooperation Strategy: Democratic People's Republic of Korea: 2014–2019*. New Delhi, India: WHO SEARO. Available at: http://apps.who.int/iris/bitstream/10665/250298/1/9789290224716-eng.pdf (accessed 15 February 2017) [Online].

World Health Organization (WHO) Regional Office for Western Pacific & Cambodia Ministry of Health (2012). *Health Service Delivery Profile: Cambodia 2012*. Available at: http://www.wpro.who.int/health_services/service_delivery_profile_cambodia.pdf (accessed 26 January 2017) [Online].

World Health Organization (WHO) & Ministry of Health of Lao People's Democratic Republic (2012). *Health Service Delivery Profile: Lao PDR*. Available at: http://www.wpro.who.int/health_services/service_delivery_profile_laopdr.pdf (accessed 15 February 2017) [Online].

World Health Organization (WHO) & United Nations Children's Fund (2016, July 6a). *Afghanistan: WHO and UNICEF Estimates of Immunization Coverage: 2015 revision*. Available at: https://www.who.int/immunization/monitoring_surveillance/data/afg.pdf (accessed 13 February 2017) [Online].

World Health Organization & United Nations Children's Fund (2016, July 6b). *China: WHO and UNICEF estimates of immunization coverage: 2015 revision*. Available at: http://www.who.int/immunization/monitoring_surveillance/data/chn.pdf (accessed 14 February 2017) [Online].

World Heart Foundation (2012). Urbanization and Cardiovascular Disease (Fact Sheet). Available at: http://www.world-heart-federation.org/fileadmin/user_upload/documents/Fact_sheets/2012/Urbanization_and_CVD.pdf (accessed 20 January 2017) [Online].

Xu, X. (1994). Control of communicable diseases in the People's Republic of China. *Asia Pac J Public Health*, 7, 123–31.

Chapter 5

Public health in rural Asia II

This chapter highlights another eight countries in the Asia-Pacific region, namely: Mongolia Uls (Republic of Mongolia/Mongolia); Republic of the Union of Myanmar (Myanmar); the Federal Democratic Republic of Nepal (Nepal); Islamic Republic of Pakistan (Pakistan); the Independent State of Papua New Guinea (PNG); Republic of the Philippines (the Philippines); Kingdom of Thailand (Thailand); and Socialist Republic of Vietnam (Vietnam) (see Fig. 5.1).

5.1 Mongolia Uls (Republic of Mongolia)

Situated in East Asia and sandwiched between China and Russia, Mongolia Uls (Mongolia) is the second largest landlocked country in the world. It is also one of the most sparsely populated countries, with a population of around three million people scattered in a territory which is mostly covered by grassy steppes. With mountains to the west and north, and the Gobi Desert to the south in the country's terrain, healthcare delivery has always been a major challenge, particularly for those who live in remote areas and have a nomadic lifestyle (see Table 5.1). According to UNDP (2016), its HDI value for 2015 was 0.735 in the high human development category, ranked 92nd out of 188 countries and territories.

5.1.1 Development of a health system

Administratively the country is divided into two segments: aimags and capital city. Aimags are further divided into soums, and soums into baghs. The capital city is divided into districts, and districts into khoroos.

The modern Mongolian health service was developed under the strong influence of the Soviet Union in the twentieth century and modelled on a highly centralized Semashko healthcare system which was financed by the government. Mongolia's healthcare system is based on a two-tier system which provides primary and specialized care (WHO, 2013). In the early 1990s, with the collapse of the Soviet Union and the democratic reforms in Mongolia, it was getting difficult for the system to continue to be self-sustained. Since then, international aid has started to play an important role in the healthcare provision in Mongolia (WHO, 2013).

Mongolia's healthcare system transited from a centralized Semashko model to a market-oriented system in the 1990s. Reform was emphasized in its decentralization, which was

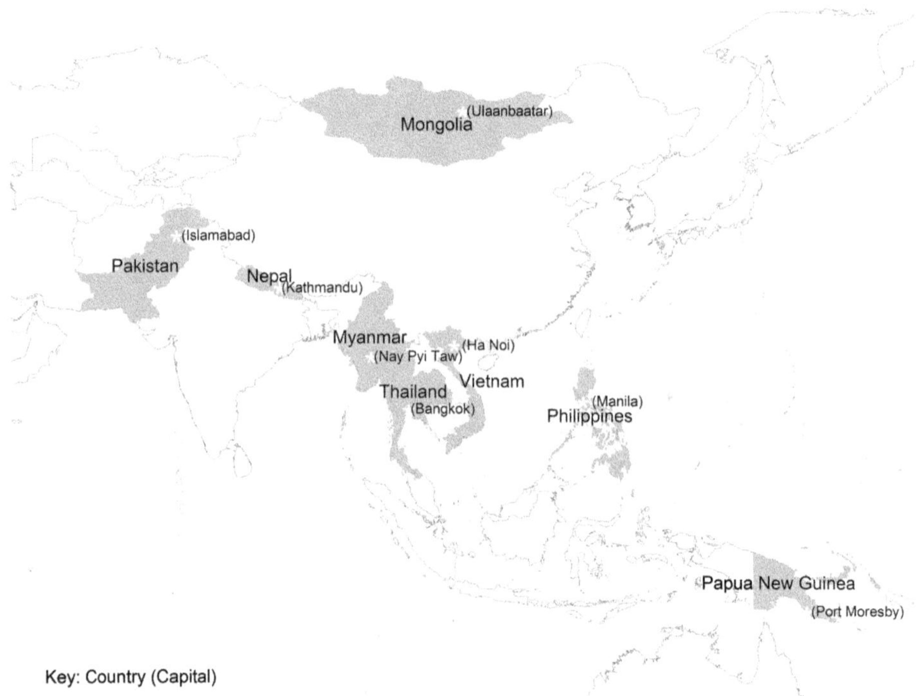

Fig. 5.1 Locations of countries discussed in Chapter 5, including Mongolia, Myanmar, Nepal, Pakistan, Papua New Guinea, the Philippines, Thailand, and Vietnam in the Asia–Pacific.

Table 5.1 Mongolia: Basic facts and key health indicators (WHO, 2016a)

Total population (2015)	3 million
Proportion of rural population (2015) (World Bank, n.d.-b)	28%
Life expectancy (years) (2015)	73.2 (female), 64.7 (male), 68.8 (both sexes)
Diphtheria tetanus toxoid and pertussis (DTP3) immunization coverage among one-year-olds (2015)	99%
Measles containing vaccines (MCV1) immunization coverage for infants (2015) (WHO, 2016, December 1, WHO-UNICEF estimates)	98%
Neonatal mortality rate (per 1,000 live births) (2015)	11.1 [6.7–16.8]
Under-five mortality rate (probability of dying by age five per 1,000 live births) (2015)	22.4 [16.3–30.0]
Maternal mortality rate (per 100,000 live births) (2015)	44 [35–55]
Total expenditure on health as % of GDP (2014)	4.73%
General government expenditure on health as % of total expenditure on health (2014)	55.40%
Private expenditure on health as % of total expenditure on health (2014)	44.60%
Physicians density (per 1,000 population) (2011)	2.837

Source: data from World Health Organization. *Key Country Indicators—Mongolia: key indicators*, http://apps.who.int/gho/data/node.cco.ki-MNG?lang=en, accessed 16 Feb 2017, Copyright © 2016 World Health Organization.

based on the transfer of the financial responsibility for local level health facilities to the local governments. However, due to a lack of clear guidelines, the decentralization process is as yet incomplete (WHO, 2013).

5.1.2 General health status

Mongolia reported an under-5 mortality rate of 22.4 per 1,000 live births in 2015 (see Table 5.1) and total fertility rate of 2.4 per woman in 2013 (WHO, n.d.). As of 2015, life expectancy for female and male was projected to be 73 and 65 respectively (see Table 5.1). Life expectancy at birth for both sexes increased by 5 years over the period of 2000-2012 when the WHO region average was reported to have an increase of 4 years in the same period. Ischaemic heart disease, accounting for 20.9% of mortality, was the leading cause of death in 2012, while no death was resulted from malaria (WHO, n.d.) and NCDs accounted for 79 % of all deaths (WHO, 2014).

5.1.3 The rural–urban gap in healthcare

The extreme low population density in Mongolia is a major challenge to the delivery of health services. In the capital city of Ulaanbaataar, primary healthcare services are mainly provided through family group practices (FGPs). In suburban areas, three village health centres support the services to the communities. In the aimag or provincial level, primary healthcare is delivered by FGPs (one per aimag), and soum hospitals (one per soum). In addition, there are also intersoum hospitals that serve multiple soums (WHO, 2013).

Bagh feldshers, who undergo a four-year medical training, deliver healthcare services in remote areas. They report to the soum health centre and refer people to the soum doctors. FGPs provide general professional care and focus on health promotion and preventive care. An intersoum hospital located in a suitable location is used for primary referral services for the neighbouring soums. Soum health centres and intersoum hospitals also have a limited number of beds to provide rehabilitation and emergency health services (WHO, 2013).

Wide disparities are reported in infant mortality and especially in the neonatal and maternal mortality between rural and urban areas. The sparse distribution of the rural population makes it extremely difficult to deliver healthcare to the rural population in the remote areas, especially the herders who lead a nomadic life (Ministry of Health [MoH] Mongolia & WHO Western Pacific Region [WHO WPRO], 2010).

While Mongolia has made steady improvement in its control of communicable diseases, the country's disease burden has shifted to NCDs. As of 2010, the leading causes of morbidity were diseases of the respiratory, digestive, genitourinary and circulatory systems, and injuries and poisoning. Overall morbidity for respiratory, digestive, and genitourinary diseases is higher in rural areas, while incidence rates for injuries and cardiovascular diseases are higher in urban areas (MoH Mongolia, 2010). Disparity exists in the provision of the healthcare workforce between rural and urban settings. In 2008, there were 18.8 physicians per 10,000 people in rural areas, while there were 43.4 physicians per 10,000 people in the capital city of Ulaanbaatar (MoH Mongolia & WHO WPRO, 2010).

5.1.4 Public health and primary healthcare system

As mentioned above, primary healthcare services are provided mostly by soum healthcare workers at soum hospitals, bagh feldshers at bagh clinics, and practitioners at FGPs in urban family clinics in the capital and aimag cities. Six districts in the capital city also provide primary and secondary health services (MoH Mongolia & WHO WPRO, 2010).

5.1.5 Disease control and health promotion

In Mongolia, liver cancer is one of the most common causes of mortality, with hepatitis B and C as the main causes of chronic liver disease and hepatocellular carcinoma in the country. The high intake of alcohol among the Mongolians accelerates the course of processes caused by these viruses, leading to the development of chronic hepatitis and liver cancer at a much younger age than in other countries (MoH Mongolia & WHO WPRO, 2010). Respiratory and gastrointestinal diseases dominate the non-communicable morbidity pattern, though the incidence of infectious diseases associated with behaviour and lifestyle, as well as living conditions remain significant. These diseases include HIV/AIDS, sexually transmitted infections (STIs), tuberculosis (TB), viral hepatitis, and zoonotic diseases (WHO, 2013). Although the HIV/AIDS prevalence is low in Mongolia, the risk is still high due to the relatively young population and the increase in STI cases in recent years. There is a high prevalence of STIs, which accounted for 35% of all registered infectious diseases as of 2010, indicating a high risk of HIV/AIDS. The increasing migratory trend and the growing HIV/AIDS epidemics in neighbouring countries are also considered as risk factors (WHO, 2013).

Mongolia's large herder-based population has a greater chance of contracting zoonotic diseases. In 2009, the livestock population in Mongolia was estimated at 43 million. Several anthrax and plague cases have been recorded yearly (MoH Mongolia & WHO WPRO, 2010). In addition, Mongolia is one of the countries with the highest prevalence of Brucellosis (Pappas *et al.*, 2006).

In recent years, the country has seen great internal migration from rural to urban areas. This migration has resulted in the creation and expansion of slum areas in the periphery of the cities. Migrants in general lack safe water supplies and live in poor conditions. They also have limited access to healthcare (MoH Mongolia & WHO WPRO, 2010).

5.1.6 Disaster trends and situations

From 2000 to 2016, meterological disaster (i.e. storms) was the most common type of natural disaster in Mongolia. The deadliest disaster in Mongolia during this period was a storm in May 2008, causing 52 deaths. The disaster with the greatest number of affected people was an extreme temperature in November 2015, affecting 965,000 people. The event causing the greatest economic damage was a storm in January 2000, leading to a loss of US$80 million (Centre for Research on the Epidemiology of Disasters [CRED], 2017).

5.2 Republic of the Union of Myanmar

The Republic of the Union of Myanmar (Myanmar) has been experiencing changes in the political system and administrative structures since the 2010 national elections. The government has undertaken reforms in different dimensions, including in the health sector. Healthcare expenditure has been increased to expand the health coverage for the poor. However, challenges remain for improving health equity for the rural and border populations. Ongoing conflicts and natural disasters in Myanmar have further affected disease pattern healthcare access. The ethnic clashes and fighting in Kachin and the northern Shan States, and the persecution on the Muslim ethnic minority Rohingyas have been escalating over the last two decades. Myanmar is prone to natural disasters, with its coastal regions being exposed to cyclones and tropical storms, and the whole country is at risk from earthquakes (see Table 5.2). The country was ranked 145th out of 188 countries and territories in terms of HDI in 2015, with a HDI value of 0.556 in the medium human development category (UNDP, 2016).

Table 5.2 Myanmar: Basic facts and key health indicators (WHO, 2016b)

Total population (2015)	53.9 million
Proportion of rural population (2015) (World Bank, n.d.-b)	66%
Life expectancy (years) (2015)	68.5 (female); 64.6 (male); 66.6 (both sexes)
Diphtheria tetanus toxoid and pertussis (DTP3) immunization coverage among one-year-olds (2015)	75%
Measles containing vaccines (MCV1) immunization coverage for infants (2015)	86%
Neonatal mortality rate (per 1,000 live births) (2015) (WHO, 2016, December 1, WHO-UNICEF estimates)	26.4 [17.0–38.1]
Under-five mortality rate (probability of dying by age five per 1,000 live births) (2015)	50.0 [37.9–65.4]
Maternal mortality rate (per 100,000 live births) (2015)	178 [121–284]
Total expenditure on health as % of GDP (2014)	2.28%
General government expenditure on health as % of total expenditure on health (2014)	45.91%
Private expenditure on health as % of total expenditure on health (2014)	54.09%
Physicians density (per 1,000 population) (2012)	0.612

Source: data from World Health Organization. *Key Country Indicators—Myanmar: key indicators*, http://apps.who.int/gho/data/node.cco.ki-MMR?lang=en, accessed 16 Feb 2017, Copyright © 2016 World Health Organization.

5.2.1 Development of a health system

Myanmar's healthcare system has been affected by the evolution of the political system over the last century. The Ministry of Health (MoH) is the major healthcare provider, governing body, administrator, and regulator of the health sector. The government used to be the main source of financing, with provision of services being virtually free until user charges were introduced in the form of cost sharing in 1993. Household out-of-pocket expenses have become the main source of finance since then (WHO, 1997).

Led by one minister and two deputies, the MoH is split into seven separate departments, each responsible for separate functions. The Department of Health is the main service provider in the public sector, providing curative services (primary, secondary, and tertiary care) through a network of facilities. Regional administrative teams provide technical support to local facilities and manage referrals to tertiary care. While the general structure of the system seems to be functional, better coordination between departments is required to meet mutual goals (Than *et al.*, 2014).

The National Health Committee, chaired by the Minister of Health, sets the country's health policy, which is then implemented by the Department for Healthcare Planning through formulation of a National Health Plan (NHP).

The private sector has been the major source of service provision since the establishment of Myanmar's health system and it remains predominant in urban settings and principally in the form of primary and ambulatory care. Recent years have seen some expansion to private inpatient care in major cities, but the majority of secondary care remains public (Than *et al.*, 2014). The non-profit organizations provide social-franchising approaches to strengthen the capacity of private services to improve healthcare access for low-income and vulnerable populations.

5.2.2 General health status

Myanmar reported an under-5 mortality rate of 50.0 per 1,000 live births in 2015 (see Table 5.2) and total fertility rate of 1.9 per woman in 2013 (WHO, n.d.). As of 2015, life expectancy for female and male was projected to be 69 and 65 respectively (see Table 5.2). Life expectancy at birth for both sexes increased by 3 years over the period of 2000-2012 when the WHO region average was reported to have an average increase of 5 years in the same period. Stroke, accounting for 12.7% of mortality, was the leading cause of death in 2012, while death due to malaria was reported to be 5.4 per 100,000 population (WHO, n.d.) and NCDs accounted for 59 % of all deaths (WHO, 2014).

5.2.3 The rural–urban gap in healthcare

Despite the policy to expand services to rural and border areas, disparities were found in access to and utilization of health services. In 2011, access to and utilization of services such as delivery in healthcare facility (25% for rural and 65% for urban) and childbirth attended by skilled personnel (63% for rural and 90% for urban) and children under five with diarrhoea treated with oral rehydration (62% for rural and 85% for urban) were more common in urban than in rural areas (Ministry of National Planning and Economic Development Myanmar [MNPED] & MoH Myanmar, 2011).

In terms of region/state, while Yangon Region has the highest (69%) availability of healthcare facilities, Chin State, a mountainous region which borders with Bangladesh and India, has the lowest rate (6%). Shan State borders with China, Laos, and Thailand. It is largely rural and inhabited mainly by ethnic minority Shan people. Shan State has the lowest rate in children under five with diarrhoea treated with oral rehydration (28%), while Tanintharyi Region has the highest (90%) (MNPED & MoH Myanmar, 2011). A major reform is needed to address the inequality and inequities to ensure healthcare reaches the poor and the disadvantaged groups, particularly the minority groups, hard-to-reach population, and people in the conflict affected areas (Than *et al.*, 2014).

5.2.4 **Public health and primary healthcare system**

Based on geographical location, health facilities in Myanmar range from subrural health centres to tertiary hospitals. The last 20 years have seen the development of an extra 140 public hospitals, in addition to increases in the numbers of rural and subrural health centres, through funding from central government (Smith and Chan, 2016).

The country's 'National Health Policy' was developed to reduce health inequality in Myanmar, particularly in rural and border areas (Than *et al.*, 2014). While point-of-use healthcare fees were introduced in 1993, it was envisaged that the charges for the poorest members of society would be waived. The government suggested that public hospital formed trust funds in order to generate interest to account for this lack of revenue. Subsequent efforts were also made by international partners to establish community-based schemes (Than *et al.*, 2014). The township health system is regarded as the backbone of the health system of Myanmar and is a network of basic healthcare infrastructure in 330 townships across the country, covering both rural and urban areas. The township health system is governed by the Township Health Department and provides comprehensive health services through facilities and individuals (fixed and mobile; public and private). It has reached into the remote rural areas through a network of volunteer health workforce and local community-based social organizations. A typical system each includes a 25-bed township hospital, an urban unit/maternal health centre, one to two station hospitals, 4–5 rural health centres, and 20–25 subrural health centres. The facilities are staffed by trained medical personnel, and volunteer health workers are involved (Than *et al.*, 2014).

Myanmar's total health workforce increased by 20% between the financial years 2006/07 and 2010/11, to 1.49 health workers per 1,000 population (Than *et al.*, 2014), but this is still significantly lower than the global standard of 2.28 health workers per 1,000 (WHO, 2006). Efforts have been made to address health workforce planning for the next 20–30 years in the government's 'Human Resources for Health Master Plan' (2012) (Than *et al.*, 2014). In addition to doctors, nurses, and midwives, voluntary health workers have been providing rural health services since 1980. Community health workers (CHWs) and auxiliary midwives (AMVs) act as a bridge between healthcare professionals and the community. Commonly trained by international organizations for one and six months, respectively, CHWs and AMVs have been involved in supportive roles, for example environmental sanitation and health education. Recent years have seen voluntary health workers performing more clinical duties, such as nutrition surveillance, identification of cases of malaria, and treatment of diarrhoea in children (Than *et al.*, 2014).

There is minimal private healthcare insurance available in Myanmar and government spending on social security is low (1.3% of the government's health expenditure), resulting in only 1% of the population being covered by the existing programme (Than *et al.*, 2014). The 'Social Security Law' (Republic of the Union of Myanmar, 2012) proposed in 2012 aims to expand the programme's coverage, while the MoH's township health system initiative targets primary care services access, and provides free, essential medicines to the entire population (Than *et al.*, 2014).

5.2.5 **Disease control and health promotion**

The country's top three national priority diseases are tuberculosis (TB), malaria, and HIV/AIDS (MoH Myanmar, 2013).

Malaria remains a leading cause of mortality and morbidity and is responsible for 8.1% of the total mortality, although there has been a large reduction of cases in recent years. Malaria is re-emerging due to climatic and ecological changes, migration, and natural-extraction industries, artemisinin resistance, and changes in behaviour of disease vectors. High-risk groups also include labourers in extraction industries (such as dams, mining, logging, rubber plantation, subsistence farmers in the forest, and other forest workers) female sex workers and their clients, men who have sex with men, and people who inject drugs (MoH Myanmar, 2005, 2011). HIV prevalence in adults was estimated at 0.6% in 2011 (World Bank, 2011). Despite the persisting burden of infectious disease, studies of Myanmar's population have shown that between 1990 and 2010, overall disability-adjusted living years (DALYs) due to communicable, maternal, and neonatal causes are declining, while NCDs are increasing (University of Washington, 2010).

Cardiovascular diseases, cancers, and chronic respiratory diseases are the leading causes of the NCD burden in Myanmar (Than *et al.*, 2014), which currently accounts for 40% of the country's deaths (Than *et al.*, 2014). The top five risk factors for NCD-associated DALYs have been identified as dietary risks, tobacco smoking, domestic air pollution from solid fuels, high blood pressure, and high fasting blood sugar (University of Washington, 2010).

Myanmar's government has several behavioural initiatives focused at reducing smoking and consumption of alcohol (Than *et al.*, 2014), including the implementation of all the recommendations from the WHO 'Framework Convention on Tobacco Control' and restriction on outdoor advertising or corporate sponsorship by companies selling alcohol (Than *et al.*, 2014). As with most countries, Myanmar's healthcare system needs to acknowledge the need to reduce NCD risk factors through improving access to, and investing in, primary care as well health promotion.

5.2.6 Disaster trends and situations

From 2000 to 2016, floods were the most common type of natural disaster was floods. The deadliest among these disasters was a storm in May 2008, causing 138,366 deaths. The disaster with the greatest number of affected people was a flood in July 2015, affecting nine million people. The disaster causing the greatest economic damage was a storm in May 2008, leading to a loss of US$4 billion (CRED, 2017).

5.3 Federal Democratic Republic of Nepal

The Federal Democratic Republic of Nepal (Nepal) is a small, landlocked South Asian country situated between China and India, sharing almost 3,000 km of land borders with these two countries. There are five major regions and 75 districts in the country, with an area of 147,181 sq km. The terrain in Nepal varies from the flat river plains of the Ganges in the south, to the rugged mountain setting in the north at an elevation of 8,850 m. Despite rapid urbanization, Nepal remains a predominant rural country with an 81% rural population in 2015. Politically, Nepal was an absolute monarchy until 1990, when there were large-scale political reforms after mounting pressure and political movement among the people. The reforms established a multiparty democracy within the framework of a constitutional monarchy (Central Intelligence Agency, 2017). Nepal had a HDI value of 0.558 in 2015, positioning it at 144 out of 188 countries and territories in the medium human development category (UNDP, 2016). Its healthcare system faces challenges from emerging infectious diseases, increasing burden from NCDs, and also natural disasters (WHO, 2016, May, -a) (see Table 5.3).

5.3.1 Development of a health system

Ministry of Health and Population (MoHP) plays a leading role in improving people's health. The private sector and non-government organizations are increasingly engaged in the implementation of health programmes (WHO, 2016, May, -a) and in developing a comprehensive framework of health plans, strategy, and policy.

The Nepal National Health Policy (1991) is the foundation of the health sector's developmental framework, with the aim to expand the primary healthcare system to rural people and increase their access to quality health services. The country's Second Long-Term Health Plan 1997–2017 defines a cost-effective package of Essential Health Care Services (EHCS) and focuses on improving the health status of the most vulnerable groups, including women and children, the rural population, the poor, and the underprivileged, and the marginalized (WHO Country Office for Nepal, 2007). The government provides emergency and inpatient services free of charge to poor, destitute, disabled, senior citizens, and female community health volunteers (MoHP Nepal, 2011). 'The Health Sector Strategy: An Agenda for Reform 2004' is being implemented through the Nepal Health Sector Programme to improve the health of the poor and those living in remote areas (WHO Country Office for Nepal, 2013). The implementation plan adopted a sector-wide approach to enhance development assistance effectiveness (MoHP Nepal, 2011). The

Table 5.3 Nepal: Basic facts and key health indicators (WHO, 2016c)

Total population (2015)	28.5 million
Proportion of rural population (2015) (World Bank, n.d.-b)	81%
Life expectancy (years) (2015)	70.8 (female); 67.7 (male); 69.2 (both sexes)
Diphtheria tetanus toxoid and pertussis (DTP3) immunization coverage among one-year-olds (2015)	91%
Measles containing vaccines (MCV1) immunization coverage for infants (2015) (WHO, 2016, December 1, WHO-UNICEF estimates)	85%
Neonatal mortality rate (per 1,000 live births) (2015)	22.2 [17.1–28.8]
Under-five mortality rate (probability of dying by age five per 1,000 live births) (2015)	35.8 [28.1–45.5]
Maternal mortality rate (per 100,000 live births) (2015)	258 [176–425]
Total expenditure on health as % of GDP (2014)	5.80%
General government expenditure on health as % of total expenditure on health (2014)	40.33%
Private expenditure on health as % of total expenditure on health (2014)	59.67%
Physicians density (per 1,000 population) (2004)	0.209

Source: data from World Health Organization. *Key Country Indicators—Nepal: key indicators*, http://apps.who.int/gho/data/node.cco.ki-NPL?lang=en, accessed 16 Feb 2017, Copyright © 2016 World Health Organization.

Nepal Health Sector Programme—II (NHSP-II) 2010–2015, based on the experiences and improvement in health indicators in NHSP-I, focuses on enhancement in health standards with a stronger healthcare system and equitable healthcare access to the whole population (WHO Country Office for Nepal, 2013).

Nepal's government has developed policies to protect its citizens' constitutional right to access free basic care. With an emphasis on universal health coverage and quality equitable access to healthcare, the national health strategy has prioritized improvement for the health workforce, public financial management, infrastructure, procurement, and health governance. The results framework of the Nepal Health Sector Strategy 2015–2020 not only monitors United Nations' Millennium Development Goals (MDG)-related indicators, but also focuses on mental health, injuries, financial burden of healthcare, and different components of health systems like the human workforce and health infrastructure (WHO, 2016, May, -a).

Nepal decided to minimize the equity gaps and increase the accessibility of health services for the population in need. The introduction of free healthcare programmes, targeted health package schemes, and a safe delivery incentive scheme, has limited effects due to other health challenges. Given the out-of-pocket health expenditure at 49%, the country faces challenges in providing quality health services, retaining adequate skilled health workers, and securing regular availability of essential medical supplies to deliver basic healthcare. As Nepal is moving towards universal health coverage, the MoHP has defined a basic healthcare package and started to introduce social insurance schemes to plug equity gaps (WHO, 2016, May, -a).

5.3.2 General health status

Nepal reported an under-5 mortality rate of 35.8 per 1,000 live births in 2015 (see Table 5.3) and total fertility rate of 2.3 per woman in 2013 (WHO, n.d.). As of 2015, life expectancy for female and male was projected to be 71 and 68 respectively (see Table 5.3). Life expectancy at birth for both sexes increased by 6 years over the period of 2000-2012 when the WHO region average was reported to have an increase of 5 years in the same period. Chronic obstructive pulmonary disease, accounting for 9.2% of mortality, was the leading cause of death in 2012, while death due to malaria was reported to be 0.1 per 100,000 population (WHO, n.d.) and NCDs accounted for 60% of all deaths (WHO, 2014).

5.3.3 The rural–urban gap in healthcare

Despite the expansion of health services in the public sector, people living in rural and remote areas still have limited access to health facilities. About 40% people in mountainous areas and 30% people in hilly regions have to travel one to four hours to access a health or subhealth post (World Health Organization Country Office for Nepal, 2013). On average, rural women give birth to 2.8 children, when urban women give birth to 1.6 children (MoHP Nepal, 2012). Rural children are more likely to be underweight (30%) than urban children (17%) (MoHP Nepal, 2011).

The shortage of health workers is more acute in remote and rural areas. Understaffing and absenteeism become more serious. MoHP is unable to attract and retain adequate qualified health workers in government facilities. Private hospitals, mostly used by the rich, are concentrated in the urban areas. In 2008, a third of primary healthcare centres did not have any doctors. Doctors may prefer to join the private sector in urban areas or migrate to developed countries, rather than serving in rural areas (MoHP Nepal, 2012).

5.3.4 Public health and primary healthcare system

The Department of Health Services is responsible for providing preventive, diagnostic, and curative health services. The government health service operates at national, regional, zonal, district levels and below, as well as at the community level. Ayurveda services are available at each level of the health system, as Ayurveda is the traditional medicine in Nepal (MoHP Nepal, 2012).

At the regional level, five Regional Health Directorates provide technical support and programme monitoring to the districts. The formation of Hospital Development Boards has brought decentralized authority to regional, subregional, and zonal hospitals.

Meanwhile, tsraining centres, laboratories, TB centres, and medical stores are available at the regional level (MoHP Nepal, 2016).

At the district level, districts managed by the District Health Office (DHO) and District Public Health Office (DPHO) have different structures. The DPHOs and DHOs are responsible for implementing EHCS and monitoring the activities and outputs of district hospitals, primary healthcare centres (PHCCs), and health posts (HPs). The public service delivery outlets in the country include HPs, PHCCs/HCs, district/other hospitals, zonal hospitals, subregional hospitals, regional hospitals, and central level hospitals (MoHP Nepal, 2016).

The health post, as the first institutional contact point for basic health services, monitors the activities of the female community health volunteer (FCHV) as well as community-based activities by primary healthcare outreach clinics and Expanded Program on Immunization (EPI) clinics. In addition, HP also functions as the referral centre of FCHVs as well as a venue for community-based initiatives, such as Primary health care outreach clinics and EPI clinics. The referral hierarchy is from health posts to PHCCs, to district, zonal subregional, and regional hospitals, and finally to tertiary care hospitals. This referral system is designed to ensure that accessible and affordable public health and minor treatment is available for most people. It also acts as a supporting mechanism that the lower levels will receive logistical, financial, supervisory, and technical support from the centre to the periphery (MoHP Nepal, 2016).

5.3.5 Disease control and health promotion

Nepal has a triple health burden in terms of infectious diseases, NCDs, and disasters. The immunization coverage for DPT3 and polio has consistently remained above 90% since 2011 and it has increased to approximately 88% for measles. Polio eradication has been achieved, leprosy is at the elimination stage, and malaria is in the pre-elimination phase. Nepal's government has put substantial efforts into halting and reversing the trends of tuberculosis (TB) and HIV. With a decreasing incidence of HIV infection, the treatment coverage rate is low at 27% due to the difference between the estimated and identified HIV cases. Despite the high treatment success rate for drug- susceptible TB (91%) and multidrug-resistant TB (76.6%), the treatment success rate of extensively drug- resistant TB is low at 11%. NCDs contribute to 60% of mortality. The major NCDs in Nepal are cardiovascular diseases, diabetes, cancer, chronic respiratory diseases, oral diseases, and mental disorders. Lifestyle-related chronic diseases are on a rising trend. Moreover, Nepal is also vulnerable to natural hazards; the 2015 earthquake damaged Nepal's health structures and facilities (WHO, 2016, May, -a). Migrants in Nepal are vulnerable to health risks as well (Amnullah *et al.*, 2015).

Nepal has been exemplary in the management of drug-resistant tuberculosis by operating Directly Observed Treatment Short-Course (DOTS) services throughout all health institutions of the healthcare system as a public–private partnership. The fully ambulatory and supervised multidrug-resistant TB services increases the cure rates up to international standards. Even with minimal hospitalization, countrywide programme coverage for multidrug-resistant and extensively drug-resistant TB can be achieved. Socioeconomic support is provided to drug-resistant TB patients so that they can stay with their family while receiving treatment, health education, infection control instructions, and moral support. The public–private partnership enables a much wider range of expertise, infrastructure, and human resources (WHO Country Office for Nepal, 2013).

Nepal has made significant progress in reducing the maternal mortality due to the promotion of delivery at health facilities, delivery by skilled birth attendants, the expansion of birthing units and basic and comprehensive emergency obstetrical care sites, the safe delivery incentive programme, a free maternity programme, birth preparedness, and expansion of safe abortion services. To address the increase in the older population and high dependency ratio, the Ministry of Public Health (MoPH) has implemented health promotion programmes for older people. They distribute health-related essential appliances and equipment, provide health check-ups, and offer treatment support to cardiovascular diseases patients aged 75 or above through a social security programme. However, much still needs to be done to create an age-friendly environment, and to foster the health and participation of old people in society (WHO Country Office for Nepal, 2013).

5.3.6 Disaster trends and situations

From 2000 to 2016, the most common types of natural disaster in Nepal were floods (18 riverine floods) and landslides (10 times). The deadliest among these disasters was the dual earthquakes occurred in April and May 2015, causing 8,831 deaths. The disaster with the greatest number of affected people was the same earthquakes, affecting 5.64 million people, which also caused the greatest economic loss of US$5.174 billion (CRED, 2017).

5.4 Islamic Republic of Pakistan

The Islamic Republic of Pakistan (Pakistan) is the fifth most populous country in the world. In the past 25 years, the population growth has been as high as 40% and this growth rate has led to Pakistan being a relatively young nation with over a third of its population aged under 14 years. According to UNDP (2016), Pakistan's HDI value for 2015 was 0.550 in the medium human development category, positioning it at 147 out of 188 countries and territories. With the socioeconomic, political, and cross-border challenges together with natural disasters in the past decades, Pakistanis' health status has improved at a much slower pace when compared to its neighbouring countries (Government of Pakistan, 2014) (see Table 5.4).

5.4.1 Development of a health system

The country is divided into eight federal units with provinces and administrative territories through the Eighteenth Constitutional Amendment of 2010. The Federal Ministry of Health was dissolved and the provinces gained the responsibility for health services policy direction and planning. In 2010, a draft of the National Health Policy introducing an Essential Health Services Package was developed but could not be approved. The provinces then developed their own health strategic planning such as improving access

Table 5.4 Pakistan: Basic facts and key health indicators (WHO, 2016d)

Total population (2015)	188.9 million
Proportion of rural population (2015) (World Bank, n.d.-b)	61%
Life expectancy (years) (2015)	67.5 (female); 65.5 (male); 66.4 (both sexes)
Diphtheria tetanus toxoid and pertussis (DTP3) immunization coverage among one-year-olds (2015)	72%
Measles containing vaccines (MCV1) immunization coverage for infants (2015) (WHO, 2016, December 1, WHO-UNICEF estimates)	61%
Neonatal mortality rate (per 1,000 live births) (2015)	45.5 [33.4–60.1]
Under-five mortality rate (probability of dying by age five per 1,000 live births) (2015)	81.1 [64.7–102.2]
Maternal mortality rate (per 100 000 live births) (2015)	178 [111–283]
Total expenditure on health as % of GDP (2014)	2.61%
General government expenditure on health as % of total expenditure on health (2014)	35.15%
Private expenditure on health as % of total expenditure on health (2014)	64.85%
Physicians density (per 1,000 population) (2010)	0.827

Source: data from World Health Organization. *Key Country Indicators—Pakistan: key indicators*, http://apps.who.int/gho/data/node.cco.ki-PAK?lang=en, accessed 16 Feb 2017, Copyright © 2016 World Health Organization.

to healthcare, increasing health workers, strengthening governance in health sector, and optimizing health financing (WHO, 2016, May, -b).

The provincial and regional Departments of Health have major responsibilities for health, whereas the Federal Ministry of National Health Services, Regulation, and Coordination is responsible for certain critical national health functions. The provinces have different degree of capacity, infrastructure, and level of governance, which is often worsened by security issues or natural disasters (WHO, 2016, May, -b). The provincial departments encountered challenges in fragmented structure, lack of resources, limited management capacity in devolved structure, insufficient specific functions, and gender insensitivity (WHO Regional Office for the Eastern Mediterranean [EMRO], 2016).

Pakistan has a very low per capita expenditure on health, which has not increased significantly in the last decade. In 2011, public health spending was as low as less than 0.5% of the GDP (Government of Pakistan, 2014). In 2013, the newly established Ministry of Health Services, Regulations, and Coordination consolidated the scattered federating units. The Ministry and the provinces need to redefine their roles and responsibilities. In regard to the high out-of-pocket expenses on healthcare, the government has introduced a social health insurance scheme to reduce the spending and safeguard against catastrophic expenditure (WHO EMRO, 2016). In 2016, the government launched National Health Vision 2016–2025.

5.4.2 General health status

Pakistan reported an under-5 mortality rate of 81.1 per 1,000 live births in 2015 (see Table 5.4) and total fertility rate of 3.2 per woman in 2013 (WHO, n.d.). As of 2015, life expectancy for female and male was projected to be is 68 and 66 respectively (see Table 5.4). Life expectancy at birth for both sexes increased by 3 years over the period of 2000-2012 and the WHO region average was reported to have an increase of 3 years in the same period. Ischaemic heart disease, accounting for 8.4% of mortality, was the leading cause of death in 2012, while death due to malaria was reported to be 1.1 per 100,000 population (WHO, n.d.) and NCDs accounted for 50% of all deaths (WHO, 2014).

5.4.3 The rural–urban gap in healthcare

According to the 2012–13 Pakistan Demographic and Health Survey, rural areas have higher mortality rates in all categories than urban areas, especially infant and under-five mortality rates (National Institute of Population Studies Pakistan & ICF International, 2013). Infant mortality in rural areas is 88 deaths per 1,000 live births, as compared with 63 deaths per 1,000 live births in urban areas. The under-five mortality is 106 per 1,000 live births in rural areas, compared to 74 per 1,000 live births in urban areas.

Rural households have limited access to clean water and sanitation. Eighty-six per cent (86%) of urban households have access to improved sanitation compared to less than half (45%) of households in rural areas. About 10% of rural households do not have access to clean water, soap, or any cleansing agent for handwashing compared to 1% among urban households. Women residing in urban areas have 3.2 children on average, compared with 4.2 children per woman in rural areas. Around one-third of married women in urban areas use modern family planning methods, compared to 23% in rural areas. Home births are more common in rural areas (60%) than urban areas (32%). Rural women are more likely to mention problems in healthcare access than urban women, particularly in Sindh (46% in urban areas and 86% in rural areas).

Children in rural areas are more likely to suffer from chronic malnutrition which is indicated by a higher stunting rate (48%) than in urban areas (37%). Less than half of rural children aged 12–23 months have received all recommended vaccines: Bacillus Calmette–Guérin (BCG), measles, DPT, and polio, when compared to two-thirds of children in urban areas. Urban citizens are more knowledgeable than rural counterparts about AIDS and tuberculosis (TB).

5.4.4 Public health and primary healthcare system

Primary healthcare services are provided through over 7,500 primary care facilities and outreach services in the public sector (WHO EMRO, 2016). All vertical primary healthcare programmes were also devolved successive to the Eighteenth Constitutional Amendment. Two provinces (Punjab and Khyber Pakhtunkhwa) have recently developed and approved an integrated package of services including maternal, newborn, and child health, immunization, nutrition, and population welfare programmes.

Besides more than 100,000 female health workers serving rural and slum urban areas, community midwives and other community-based workers who have gained success and trust in the communities provide outreach primary care services (Government of Pakistan, 2014). Hospital and curative care is the major healthcare service in terms of access by the people and financial allocation by the government. The health system has low utilization rates and a lack of institutional frameworks for outsourcing health services. Healthcare providers at primary care and hospital levels face challenges in healthcare quality and safety. The global health initiative supports health system strengthening as a national health strategy and plan, and promotes integrated service delivery. Without any federal or national human resources for a health development policy, human resources have been compiled by three provinces and this will help in the development of the respective provincial human resources for health strategies.

5.4.5 Disease control and health promotion

The country has a high maternal mortality rate, infant mortality rate, and under-five child mortality. Pakistan has double disease burdens on both communicable (such as TB, malaria, and hepatitis B and C) and NCDs (WHO, 2016, May, -b).

The government provides funding for various health programmes. All four provinces have developed their own provincial hepatitis control programmes. Pakistan established 16 sentinel sites to manage patients with TB and HIV co-infection for those most affected, including injecting drug users and transgender sex workers in concentrated epidemic areas in the joint efforts of the national TB programme and the national HIV/AIDS and sexually transmitted infections control programme. The country has a low routine immunization coverage rate and the government has responded by expanding the immunization programme and bearing the full cost of all routine traditional vaccines (WHO EMRO, 2016).

Although NCDs constitute more than half of the preventable mortality and morbidity, there are very limited integrated programmes available for prevention and control (WHO EMRO, 2013). To combat diseases like cancers, diabetes, and mental illnesses, the Non-Communicable Diseases Unit was established under the Ministry of National Health Services, Regulation, and Coordination. To address the growing mental health problems, 15 districts have integrated mental health services into primary care at the Institute of Psychiatry (WHO EMRO, 2016).

Tobacco use is common in Pakistan, with more than 10% of adolescents of age 13–15 years using tobacco product and 21% of young people aged 15–24 being exposed to tobacco smoke at home. The implementation of the Framework Convention on Tobacco Control is ongoing despite many challenges. Pakistan introduced 40% pictorial health warning on cigarette packs in 2010 and increased it to 85% in 2015. The government has also provided 100 indoor, smoke-free environments; however, tobacco taxation is still too low (WHO EMRO, 2016).

5.4.6 Disaster trends and situations

Pakistan is a natural disaster- prone country, threatened by natural hazards such as avalanches, cyclones and storms, droughts, earthquakes, epidemics, floods, glacial lake outbursts, and landslides. Its human hazards are associated with transport, industry, oil spills, forest fires, civil conflicts, and internal displacements of communities as a result of multiple factors (WHO EMRO, 2013). In response, the government has adopted the risk management approach for emergency preparedness (WHO EMRO, 2016). National disaster risk reduction policy in 2013 focused on risk assessment, prevention, mitigation, and preparedness (Government of Pakistan, 2013).

From 2000 to 2016, the most common types of natural disaster in Pakistan were earthquakes (14 times) and floods (31 riverine floods and 15 flash floods). The deadliest among these disasters was an earthquake in October 2005, causing 73,338 deaths. The disaster with the greatest number of affected people was a flood in July 2010, affecting 20.34 million people, which caused the greatest economic loss of US$ 9.5 billion (CRED, 2017).

5.5 Independent State of Papua New Guinea

The Independent State of Papua New Guinea (PNG), after 30 years of political independence and economic development, remains a poor country with a low life expectancy and high infant mortality rate. In the low human development category, the country had a HDI value of 0.516 in 2015, ranked 154th out of 188 countries and territories (UNDP, 2016). The majority of the population (almost 90%) are living in rural areas, including remote highlands and far-flung islands that are often inaccessible with any road transport. PNG is a vastly diverse country, with hundreds of ethnic groups speaking more than 800 languages. All of these pose great challenges to the healthcare provision. People generally identify the failure of the health system as a major cause of the very poor health status of the people in PNG (WHO, 2016, May, -c) (see Table 5.5).

5.5.1 Development of a health system

Health system in PNG is largely decentralized. In 2007, its Provincial Health Authorities (PHAs) combined the management of hospital and rural health services into one authority. In the provinces with PHA, hospitals and rural health services are accountable to the Chief Executive Officer of the PHA. In non-PHA provinces, National Department of Health manages hospitals, and the provincial government manages the rural health services. In 2015, the government established the District Development Authority (DDA) (WHO, 2016, May, -c). In 2011, the National Health Services Standards defined seven levels of the PNG health service delivery model, with a package of health services and set standards, types, and mix of staff at each level and an accreditation system for hospitals and health centres (WHO, 2016, May, -c). By 2014, the 'Free Primary Healthcare and Subsidized Specialist Services Policy' was implemented as a step towards universal health coverage. In 2016, the government developed a partnership framework with Christian churches to provide primary healthcare in PNG (WHO, 2016, May, -c).

Table 5.5 Papua New Guinea: Basic facts and key health indicators (WHO, 2016e)

Total population (2015)	7.6 million
Proportion of rural population (2015) (World Bank, n.d.-b)	87%
Life expectancy (years) (2015)	65.4 (female); 60.6 (male); 62.9 (both sexes)
Diphtheria tetanus toxoid and pertussis (DTP3) immunization coverage among one-year-olds (2015)	62%
Measles containing vaccines (MCV1) immunization coverage for infants (2015) (WHO, 2016, December 1, WHO-UNICEF estimates)	60%
Neonatal mortality rate (per 1,000 live births) (2015)	24.5 [13.5–43.7]
Under-five mortality rate (probability of dying by age five per 1,000 live births) (2015)	57.3 [35.0–95.7]
Maternal mortality rate (per 100,000 live births) (2015)	215 [98–457]
Total expenditure on health as % of GDP (2014)	4.26%
General government expenditure on health as % of total expenditure on health (2014)	81.28%
Private expenditure on health as % of total expenditure on health (2014)	18.72%
Physicians density (per 1,000 population) (2012)	0.058

Source: data from World Health Organization. *Key Country Indicators—Papua New Guinea: key indicators*, http://apps.who.int/gho/data/node.cco.ki-PNG?lang=en, accessed 16 Feb 2017, Copyright © 2016 World Health Organization.

The National Health Plan (NHP, 2011–2020) focuses on primary care services and set key objectives related to the MDGs (Government of Papua New Guinea, 2010). The goal is to increase universal health coverage and equity for the rural majority and the urban poor (WHO, 2016, May, -c). After the World Bank released a report on PNG's health worker crisis in 2011, the government developed a manpower policy (Government of Papua New Guinea, 2015a) and a Workforce Enhancement Plan (2013–2018) to improve the health of the workforce (WHO, 2016, May, -c).

The healthcare system has suffered ongoing difficulties including a severe shortage of health workers, frequent shortages of medications, and poor governance (WHO, 2016, May, -c). Although the decentralization policy allows the provinces and districts to deliver rural health services, the lack of financial resources and management capacity hampers health services delivery (WHO WPRO, 2010).

5.5.2 General health status

Papua New Guinea reported an under-5 mortality rate of 57.3 per 1,000 live births in 2015 (see Table 5.5) and total fertility rate of 3.8 per woman in 2013 (WHO, n.d.). As of

2015, life expectancy for female and male was projected to be 65 and 61 respectively (see Table 5.5). Life expectancy at birth for both sexes increased by 3 years over the period of 2000-2012 when the WHO region average was reported to have an average increase of 4 years in the same period. Lower respiratory infections, accounting for 16% of mortality, were the leading cause of death in 2012, while death due to malaria was reported to be 38.5 per 100,000 population (WHO, n.d.) and NCDs accounted for 42% of all deaths (WHO, 2014).

5.5.3 The rural–urban gap in healthcare

The NHP (2011–2020) puts increasing equity in access to rural health services as its top priority. However, inadequate access to and poor quality of healthcare services, and low medical expenditure have worsened the health equity. Rural areas even face geographical limitations leading to expensive service costs with lower access to health resources (WHO & Papua New Guinea National Department of Health, 2012).

Of note, maternal mortality is one of the highest in the world. Maternal deaths are high, but especially in rural areas and particularly in the Highlands Region. Neonatal deaths are also a concern in rural areas. Infants have twice the chance of dying before their first birthday in rural areas than in urban areas (Government of Papua New Guinea, 2015a). Only one-third (32.8%) of the rural population have access to improved drinking water, a much lower rate than the urban population (88%). While only half (56.4%) of the urban population have improved sanitation services, the situation in rural areas (13.3%) is even worse (WHO & Papua New Guinea National Department of Health, 2012).

5.5.4 Public health and primary healthcare system

Health services are mainly provided by the government and facilities run by churches, with a mix of funding from government tax revenues, out-of-pocket payments, and donations. The central government is responsible for the national referral hospital, the specialist hospital, and 4 regional and 16 provincial public hospitals. Provincial and local governments provide most of the rural health services, including rural hospitals, health centres, health subcentres, and aid posts. The government plans to build the health system in a hierarchical structure of seven levels by 2050. Level 1 is the basic health service delivered by aid posts and community HPs, whereas level 7 is the most complex health services provided at the national referral hospital (Government of Papua New Guinea, 2016).

Government-subsidized health services run by churches are important in the system. In rural areas, churches provide almost half of the outpatient services. Regulated under the Churches Medical Council, these services are non-profit making. The government grants over 80% of the service costs without any formal contract. In practice, these services are coordinated by local authorities and the churches have limited participation in the healthcare decision-making (Government of Papua New Guinea, 2016).

Private enterprises, for example farms, factories, and mines, provide health services for their employees and families, and such services often also extend to the surrounding communities. International and national non-governmental organizations provide services for underprivileged groups, including as women and children (Government of Papua New Guinea, 2016).

5.5.5 Disease control and health promotion

The NHP (2011–2020) describes the policies and strategies to improve rural health. To increase access to health services, the government has planned to provide more outreach services and increased medical supplies. It provides more funding for operations and referral transport of patients to health facilities. To improve child survival, the government increased the coverage of childhood immunization and introduced the Integrated Management of Childhood Illness (IMCI) (Government of Papua New Guinea, 2010). IMCI is a strategy composed of improvement in health providers' skills, enhancement of health system, and the promotion of quality child care to family and community (Costello and Dalglish, 2016). To reduce maternal mortality, the government has enhanced the promotion of family planning, and increased access to safe delivery services and emergency obstetric care. Improving maternal health can reduce neonatal deaths as well (Government of Papua New Guinea, 2010).

Infectious diseases are the main cause of morbidity and mortality, especially malaria, tuberculosis (TB), diarrhoeal diseases, and acute respiratory infections. Although PNG has sustained its polio-free status since 2000, there were measles outbreaks in 2005 and in 2013–2014 (WHO, 2016e). Similar to the neighbouring countries in the Western Pacific Region, PNG has an increasing burden from NCDs (Government of Papua New Guinea, 2016).

HIV/AIDS has remained below 1% over the last decade. PNG had an HIV epidemic mostly due to heterosexual transmission. Care and treatment for people living with HIV have improved significantly since 2006 (WHO WPRO, 2010). As of 2014, the coverage of HIV/AIDS counselling, testing, and treatment services has achieved almost 90%. The HIV prevalence among pregnant women has stabilized at 0.56%. The provision of antiretroviral therapy (ART) at national levels started from 2000, and the coverage increased significantly to 86% of all eligible adults and children living with HIV in 2014 (Government of Papua New Guinea, 2015b).

The mortality and incidence of malaria have both reduced to achieve the MDGs. The partnership between governments, donors, technical partners, civil society, and local communities has contributed to the reduction of malaria, a leading cause of infant and maternal mortality. Malaria is a significant public health issue with 1.5–1.8 million suspected cases every year, and more than 50% of the population residing in areas with potentially higher risks. National household surveys recorded a decrease in parasite prevalence (Government of Papua New Guinea, 2015b).

DOTS for TB were expanded from two provinces in 2008 to 22 provinces in 2012 and contributed to an increase in case reporting. Incidence of TB increased from 308 in 1990 to 348 in 2012 (per 100,000 people) and the prevalence declined from 715 in 1990 to 437 in2013. TB with drug resistance is more prevalent, with extremely drug-resistant (XDR) TB reported in some areas. Drug-resistant TB and TB/HIV co-infection are on a rising trend (Government of Papua New Guinea, 2015b).

5.5.6 Disaster trends and situations

From 2000 to 2016, floods (seven riverine floods and two coastal floods), epidemics (four viral diseases and two bacterial diseases), landslides (seven times), volcanic activities (six ash falls), and earthquakes (five ground movements) were the most common types of natural disaster in Papua New Guinea. The natural disaster affecting the greatest number of people was a drought in May 2015, where 2.52 million people were affected. This event also caused the greatest economic damage, leading to a loss of US$60 million (CRED, 2017).

5.6 Republic of the Philippines

The Republic of the Philippines (the Philippines) is an archipelago-based country composed of more than 7,000 islands. Historically, with its geographic location of being in the centre of Asia's ocean, the Philippines was a transitive point in East Asia during the time of the Spanish Colonial Era. In the 1950s, with the rapid development of national industries, the country had once been one of the richest countries in Asia. Nowadays, the Philippines is regarded as of the most dynamic economies in the East Asia region, with sound economic fundamentals and a globally recognized competitive workforce (World Bank, n.d.-a) (see Table 5.6). Its HDI values for 2015 was 0.682 in the medium human development category, positioning it at 116 out of 188 countries and territories (UNDP, 2016).

5.6.1 Development of a health system

Healthcare reform in the Philippines started in the 1970s. After the country has established a republican government in 1987, a series of health polices were implemented from 1988. Health services were devolved to local government units in 1991 and the universal coverage with financial access to quality and affordable medical care for all Filipinos was expected by 2010. The financing sources of the healthcare system in the country include national and local governments, insurance (government and private), user fees/ out-of-pocket and donors. Among the total health expenditure, out-of-pocket expenditure takes up the largest share, increased from 47% in 1997 to 57% in 2007. Social health insurance programmes were also developed to include the poor in 1995 (Herrera *et al.*, 2010; Republic of Philippines, 2012; Romualdez *et al.*, 2011). In 1999, the Department of Health launched the Health Sector Reform Agenda (HSRA) to improve the way healthcare is delivered, regulated, and financed (e.g. corporatization of government hospitals) (Romualdez *et al.*, 2011). The Reproductive Health and Population Development Act 2008 was also introduced to improve people's quality of life and guarantee universal access to reproductive healthcare (Herrera *et al.*, 2010).

The Philippines has a mixed public–private healthcare system. Forty per cent (40%) of its hospitals are managed by the public (Republic of Philippines, 2012). However, private

Table 5.6 The Philippines: Basic facts and key health indicators (WHO, 2016f)

Total population (2015)	100.7 million
Proportion of rural population (2015) (World Bank, n.d.-b)	46%
Life expectancy (years) (2015)	72.0 (female); 65.3 (male); 68.5 (both sexes)
Diphtheria tetanus toxoid and pertussis (DTP3) immunization coverage among one-year-olds (2015)	60%
Measles containing vaccines (MCV1) immunization coverage for infants (2015) (WHO, 2016, December 1, WHO-UNICEF estimates)	82%
Neonatal mortality rate (per 1,000 live births) (2015)	12.6 [9.0–17.1]
Under-five mortality rate (probability of dying by age five per 1,000 live births) (2015)	28.0 [21.2–36.7]
Maternal mortality rate (per 100 000 live births) (2015)	114 [87–175]
Total expenditure on health as % of GDP (2014)	4.71%
General government expenditure on health as % of total expenditure on health (2014)	34.28%
Private expenditure on health as % of total expenditure on health (2014)	65.72%
Physicians density (per 1,000 population) (2004)	1.153

Source: data from World Health Organization. *Key Country Indicators—Philippines: key indicators*, http://apps.who.int/gho/data/node.cco.ki-PHL?lang=en, accessed 16 Feb 2017, Copyright © 2016 World Health Organization.

healthcare, which is based on the user's fee and caters for 30% of the population, is considered to be of better quality in human and financial terms, and more advanced in technological resources (Allianz Worldwide Care, n.d.; Romualdez *et al.*, 2011).

5.6.2 General health status

Philippines reported an under-5 mortality rate of 28.0 per 1,000 live births in 2015 (see Table 5.6) and total fertility rate of 3 per woman in 2013 (WHO, n.d.). As of 2015, life expectancy for female and male was projected to be 72 and 65 respectively (see Table 5.6). Life expectancy at birth for both sexes increased by 1 year over the period of 2000-2012 when the WHO region average was reported to have an increase of 4 years in the same period. Ischaemic heart disease, accounting for was 15.4 % of mortality, was the leading cause of death in 2012, while death due to malaria was reported to be 0.1 per 100,000 population (WHO, n.d.) and NCDs accounted for 67% of all deaths (WHO, 2014).

5.6.3 The rural–urban gap in healthcare

Although there is ongoing efforts of upgrading rural health facilities, the rural–urban gap in healthcare still exists. Brain drain of health professionals from rural to urban areas is one of the major barriers to upgrade rural healthcare provision (Lorenzo *et al.*, 2007). Average travel time to a health facility is longer in rural areas (45 minutes) than in urban areas (32 minutes) (Republic of Philippines, 2012). People in urban areas are more likely to use regional hospitals than those in rural areas, and the use of private facilities is higher in urban areas than in rural areas (National Statistics Office Philippines & ICF Macro, 2009). Last but not least, health insurance coverage is higher in urban areas (49%) than in rural areas (35%) (National Statistics Office Philippines & ICF Macro, 2009).

In the 1950s, rural health units were set up all over the country to ensure better access to healthcare. By early 1990s, health service provision was decentralized to local government units by Republic Act No. 7160 'Local Government Code', resulting in fragmentation of administrative control of health services and the quality of healthcare being substantially subject to the local governments (Republic of Philippines, 2012). From 2007 to 2010, for rehabilitating and upgrading rural health units, investments in infrastructure and equipment were expanded to support health sector reforms and the MDGs (Romualdez *et al.*, 2011).

Although reforms were launched to provide financial protection, with priority given to the poor and improve health insurance coverage, inadequate health facilities, health personnel, and medicines available remain prevalent in many rural areas. Child mortality is significantly higher in rural areas, especially among women who have no education and among the poorest of the poor (Republic of Philippines, 2012).

5.6.4 **Public health and primary healthcare system**

Primary healthcare in Philippines is provided by both public and private sectors. Barangay health stations, rural health units, clinics, and other small facilities of the public sectors serve as the first point of contact with health workers, and are key areas for disseminating health information on a community level. Reports have indicated that 63% of services provided by government primary care facilities are preventive in nature (i.e. immunization and the like); 30% are for the treatment of minor illnesses and accidents and other services (e.g. pre/postnatal care and deliveries), and the remainder are for laboratory services (Herrera *et al.*, 2010). The private sector, as just mentioned, generally caters for the more wealthy. People of lower income are more likely to use primary care facilities such as rural health units and village health stations than those of higher income, and these facilities are generally perceived to provide low-quality health services (Asian Development Bank, 2007). Aside from the price and service quality, rural communities also lack pharmacies (Republic of the Philippines, 2012).

5.6.5 **Disease control and health promotion**

People in the rural areas are in great need of healthcare because of limited access to healthcare facilities (Republic of the Philippines, 2012). Endemic diseases areas are usually rural, hilly, or mountainous, and difficult to reach. While overnutrition is an emerging issue in the country, undernutrition remains a pressing problem, especially in rural and poor areas (Republic of the Philippines, 2012). Toilets that flush into a septic tank are much more common in urban areas than in rural areas, while pit latrines are just the opposite; 15% of households in rural areas have no toilet facility, compared with only 4% in urban areas (National Statistics Office Philippines & ICF Macro, 2009).

5.6.6 Disaster trends and situations

From 2000 to 2016, floods (47 riverine floods and 28 flash floods), landslides (11 times), and storms (128 tropical cyclones) were the most common types of natural disaster in the Philippines. The deadliest among these disasters was a storm in November 2013, causing 7,354 deaths, 16.11 million people were affected, and leading to the greatest economic damage of a reported loss of US$10 billion (CRED, 2017).

5.7 Kingdom of Thailand

The Kingdom of Thailand (Thailand) is a middle-income country with a population of almost 70 million (WHO, 2016g). Over the last decade, the proportion of people living in poverty has decreased while life expectancy has increased (Wibulpolprasert, 2011). According to UNDP (2016), Thailand was in the high human development category with an HDI value of 0.740 for 2015, positioning it at 87 out of 188 countries and territories. The country's healthcare reform in 2002 aimed to improve health equity and contributed to its overall health improvement, helping make Thailand one of the first developing countries to achieve universal health coverage. (Health Insurance System Research Office, 2012) (see Table 5.7).

5.7.1 Development of a health system

Thailand took 30 years to achieve universal health security (Jongudomsuk *et al.*, 2015). After developing health infrastructure and increasing the healthcare manpower by 2000, the Thai government launched the Universal Coverage Scheme (UCS) as an evolution of the health insurance schemes, which included the Civil Servant Medical Benefit Scheme (CSMBS), the Social Security Scheme (SSS), the Medical Welfare Scheme (MWS), and the Voluntary Health Card Scheme (VHCS). The UCS provides a comprehensive benefits package for preventive care, curative, and rehabilitation services and it is important for improving health equity in Thailand, as most of the registered are poor rural residents (Health Insurance System Research Office, 2012). Use of healthcare has also increased with better access, while incidence of catastrophic health expenditure and impoverishment from medical payments has decreased. The infant mortality decreased from 37 per 1,000 live births in 1990 to 13 per 1,000 live births in 2013 (WHO, 2016g).

The CSMBS provided health insurance to government sector employees, their dependents, and retirees. The SSS was a compulsory health insurance programme for private sector employees, and dependents and retirees were not covered by the scheme. The MWS

Table 5.7 Thailand: Basic facts and key health indicators (WHO, 2016g)

Total population (2015)	68.0 million
Proportion of rural population (2015) (World Bank, n.d.-b)	50%
Life expectancy (years) (2015)	78.0 (female); 71.9 (male); 74.9 (both sexes)
Diphtheria tetanus toxoid and pertussis (DTP3) immunization coverage among one-year-olds (2015)	99%
Measles containing vaccines (MCV1) immunization coverage for infants (2015) (WHO, 2016, December 1, WHO-UNICEF estimates)	99%
Neonatal mortality rate (per 1,000 live births) (2015)	6.7 [3.5–12.3]
Under-five mortality rate (probability of dying by age five per 1,000 live births) (2015)	12.3 [7.7–19.9]
Maternal mortality rate (per 100,000 live births) (2015)	20 [14–32]
Total expenditure on health as % of GDP (2014)	6.53%
General government expenditure on health as % of total expenditure on health (2014)	86%
Private expenditure on health as % of total expenditure on health (2014)	14%
Physicians density (per 1,000 population) (2010)	0.393

Source: data from World Health Organization. *Key Country Indicators—Thailand: key indicators*, http://apps.who.int/gho/data/node.cco.ki-THA?lang=en, accessed 16 Feb 2017, Copyright © 2016 World Health Organization.

was a government-subsidized programme, with the target population expanded from the poor in 1975 to older people in 1992 and children in 1994. The VHCS included the people not eligible for the other three programmes. The government further integrated the MWS and VHCS and established the UCS programme in 2002. Currently, three health insurance programmes are implemented for the entire population, which are the CSMBS (9%), the SSS (16%), and the UCS (75%) (Wibulpolprasert, 2011).

The UCS accounts for approximately 17% of the country's total health expenditure (Jongudomsuk *et al.*, 2015). The universal health coverage, funded by tax revenue, increased public spending on health from 63% in 2002 to 77% in 2011 and decreased out-of-pocket payments from 27.2% to 12.4% in this period (WHO, 2016g).

5.7.2 General health status

Thailand reported an under-5 mortality rate of 12.3 per 1,000 live births in 2015 (see Table 5.7) and total fertility rate of 1.4 per woman in 2013 (WHO, n.d.). As of 2015, life expectancy for female and male was projected to be 78 and 72 respectively (see Table 5.7). Life expectancy at birth for both sexes increased by 4 years over the period of 2000-2012 when the WHO region average was reported to have an increase of 5 years in the same period. Ischaemic heart disease, accounting for 13.7% of mortality, was the leading cause of death in 2012, while death due to malaria was reported to be 0.2 per 100,000 population (WHO, n.d.) and NCDs accounted for 71% of all deaths (WHO, 2014).

5.7.3 The rural–urban gap in healthcare

As aforesaid, one key concern is the distribution of health services across regions. When compared to other regions, urban residents in Bangkok have much greater access to healthcare services, in terms of number of doctors and the number of medical appliances per person (Wibulpolprasert, 2011). Only around 20% of doctors and dentists serve the rural areas, with the health workforce density being five times lower than that of the urban areas. Urban areas have a nurse density two times higher than that of rural areas (Wibulpolprasert, 2011). There is an uneven distribution between rural and urban areas and the rural health system is worsened due to the failure in retention of health workers. Since the 1970s, the government has introduced a range of strategies to address unequal distribution and rural turnover. For example, the government recruits more students from rural areas to public medical and nursing schools, making rural service compulsory for three years upon medical, dental, and pharmaceutical students' graduation, and provides special quotas for nursing graduates from public schools to work in the public sector. The government has also increased financial allowances for healthcare personnel working in remote areas according to the proximity of the region. Healthcare workers in remote areas can obtain better opportunities for professional training and career prospects (Jongudomsuk *et al.*, 2015). Since the introduction of the UCS, the situation has improved as the difference in medical personnel between the most urbanized area and the most isolated area has become narrowed (Tangkitvanich and Sasiwuttiwat, 2012). However, this improvement has not provided the entire population with adequate healthcare.

5.7.4 Public health and primary healthcare system

The Thai health system is complex, dominated by the public sector, especially in the rural areas. It is a three-tier system composed of subdistrict health centres, district hospitals, and general/regional hospitals (Health Insurance System Research Office, 2012). The rural health system primarily comprises district hospitals and subdistrict health centres. Under the strong network of MoPH, all villages and subdistricts are covered by primary healthcare providers in Thailand. There are about 50,000 community HPs covering all villages with community health volunteers and at least one health centre per subdistrict that provides public health services and outpatient primary healthcare services. Most private facilities were situated in urban areas. At the subdistrict level, the health centre staff use population household lists to monitor and implement programmes such as vaccinations and chronic disease screening. The health centres have adequate supplies of medication and effective health workers. At the village level, the village health volunteers have information on the households with children, disabled, and chronic disease patients in their geographic area of responsibility.

In Thailand, community healthcare services were provided at homes, communities, or villages where people live. The services include health promotion and disease prevention for healthy people, and long-term care for elders and chronic disease patients in communities or villages. The service providers are trained village health volunteers, elderly groups, trained caregivers, and mainstream health workers including primary healthcare workers, public health physicians, and nurses (WHO Regional Office for South-East Asia & Ministry of Health Thailand, 2010).

Another challenge is the ageing population which will create a burden on the healthcare system, especially in poor rural regions. Despite the UCS, older people aged 80 or above in rural areas have difficulty in using the available services as they rely on carers or relatives to access the healthcare services (World Bank Group, 2016). In light of the increasing number of dependent elderly, long-term care policies are needed for health and social welfare systems (Health Insurance System Research Office, 2012).

To further enhance the primary healthcare system, the government provides funding on diabetes and hypertension screening and treatment, and offers financial incentives to providers upon the completion of prenatal care services. The local government and UCS provide funding for health-promoting activities at subdistricts as well.

5.7.5 Disease control and health promotion

Malaria remains a concern, particularly at the border areas with Cambodia and Myanmar, due to the movement and activities of the mobile and migrant populations around the areas. Thailand is prioritizing malaria elimination and is working together with other countries in the Greater Mekong Subregion to tackle multidrug-resistant malaria, in particular.

Incidence of HIV/AIDS in Thailand has continued to decline. New infections among adults have reduced 65% during 2000–2010. There were an estimated 7,700 infections in 2014, a decline of 23% from 2010. Progress in eliminating HIV infections among children has been dramatic. In 2014, an estimated 121 children were newly infected with HIV, representing about 41% reduction compared with 2010. The mother-to-child transmission rate was 2.1% in 2014, meaning Thailand is very close to eliminating new HIV infections among children (National AIDS Committee, 2015). The Thai Health Promotion Foundation, established in 2001, serves as a funding catalyst to support health promotion programmes and activities held by state and non-state actors, especially the civil society. This independent agent, funded by a tobacco and alcohol excise tax, has made progress in tackling health issues such as smoking, alcohol, and road accidents. However, the recent review suggests the importance of policy development complementing the programmes for further success (Jongudomsuk *et al.*, 2015).

5.7.6 Disaster trends and situations

From 2000 to 2016, floods (24 riverine floods and 16 flash floods) were the most common type of natural disaster in Thailand. The deadliest among these disasters was an earthquake in December 2004, causing 8,345 deaths. The disaster reported to have affected the greatest number of people was a drought in April 2008, where 10 million people were affected. The one causing the greatest economic damage was a flood occurred in August 2011, leading to a loss of US$40 billion (CRED, 2017).

5.8 Socialist Republic of Vietnam

The Socialist Republic of Vietnam (Vietnam) is located on the eastern coast of the Indochina Peninsula in Southeast Asia. The former French colony gained independence in 1954 but was divided into two rival states which entered into a prolonged conflict known as the Vietnam War. As a result of this war, which ended in 1975, Vietnam has suffered from a severe economic crisis throughout the 1970s and 1980s. To improve the critical state, Vietnam has established multiple initiations such as the *Doi Moi* process, Socio-economic Development Strategy (SEDS), and Vietnam's Development Goals (VDGs) (United Nations in VietNam, n.d.-b). Focusing on the ideas of reconstruction and development, Vietnam has successfully reformed the nation as a 'middle-income country', as described by the World Bank, since 2010 (UNDP, 2015). Vietnam's HDI was 0.683 in the medium human development category in 2015, ranked 115th out of 188 countries and territories (UNDP, 2015).

5.8.1 Development of a health system

Since the Vietnam War (1954–1975), Vietnam has made remarkable improvements among different areas of health even before it earned its status as a middle-income country (Tran *et al.*, 2011). Before the war, similar to many historical socialist countries, Vietnam's healthcare system was built and highly dependent on the revenue of its general government. This system successfully delivered free primary healthcare services to all citizens. However, due to the consequences of the war, Vietnam underwent a major economic crisis. With the primary intention to relieve the critical state of its economy, the Vietnamese government introduced a reforming initiation entitled *Doi Moi* in 1986. Under the health sector of this initiation, Vietnam successfully introduced the private healthcare sector, with concepts such as out-of-pocket payment, health insurance, and delivering a pharmaceutical market (United Nations in VietNam, n.d.-b).

The healthcare system in Vietnam is levelled into four layers: national, provincial, district, and communal. The national level is also entitled as the Ministry of Health [MoH]. This level bears the main authority of the healthcare system, as it bears responsibility for formulating and disseminating health policies into different provinces of the country. The provincial level is composed of 63 provincial health bureaus altogether. This level aims to practice the given health policy by the MoH. The primary level consists of district and commune levels and it provides a general basic health network for the public population (Tran *et al.*, 2011).

Since the 1980s, there has been a $2,000 increase on the GDP per capita. This improvement has significantly lowered the number of people living in extreme poverty by 47%, from 50% in early 1990s to 3% in 2012. Moreover, the introduction of the MDGs by the United Nations in the year 2000 has inspired Vietnam to compose a set of its own, entitled Vietnam's Development Goals (VDGs), generating strategies for the country's own specific issues, such as poverty. By implementing these values through its development, Vietnam has successfully tackled the major issues, reaching multiple goals of the MDGs. While the maternal mortality rate has been reduced below the expected average for upper-middle-income countries, the under-five mortality has also decreased by 50% (World Bank, n.d.-c).

To further enhance the situations for the country, Vietnam has pledged to continue its development in the 10-year SEDS for 2011–2020. While SEDS 1990–2000 and SEDS 2000–2010 focused on helping the poor while developing a structured market, SEDS 2011–2020 aims to industrialize and modernize the country (United Nations in VietNam, n.d.-b).

5.8.2 General health status

Vietnam reported an under-5 mortality rate of 21.7 per 1,000 live births in 2015 (see Table 5.8) and total fertility rate of 1.7 per woman in 2013 (WHO, n.d.). As of 2015, life expectancy for female and male was projected to be 81 and 71 respectively (see Table 5.8). Life expectancy at birth for both sexes increased by 2 years over the period of

Table 5.8 Vietnam: Basic facts and key health indicators (WHO, 2016h)

Total population (2015)	93.4 million
Proportion of rural population (2015) (World Bank, n.d.-b)	66%
Life expectancy (years) (2015)	80.7 (female); 71.3 (male); 76.0 (both sexes)
Diphtheria tetanus toxoid and pertussis (DTP3) immunization coverage among 1-year-olds (2015)	97%
Measles containing vaccines (MCV1) immunization coverage for infants (2015) (WHO, 2016, December 1, WHO-UNICEF estimates)	97%
Neonatal mortality rate (per 1,000 live births) (2015)	11.4 [9.4–13.4]
Under-five mortality rate (probability of dying by age five per 1,000 live births) (2015)	21.7 [20.8–22.7]
Maternal mortality rate (per 100,000 live births) (2015)	54 [41–74]
Total expenditure on health as % of GDP (2014)	7.07%
General government expenditure on health as % of total expenditure on health (2014)	54.06%
Private expenditure on health as % of total expenditure on health (2014)	45.94%
Physicians density (per 1,000 population) (2013)	1.19

Source: data from World Health Organization. *Key Country Indicators—Viet Nam: key indicators*, http://apps.who.int/gho/data/node.cco.ki-VNM?lang=en, accessed 16 Feb 2017, Copyright © 2016 World Health Organization.

2000-2012 when the WHO region average was reported to have an increase of 4 years in the same period. Stroke, which accounted for 21.7% of mortality, was the leading cause of death in 2012, while death due to malaria was reported to be 0.1 per 100,000 population (WHO, n.d.) and NCDs accounted for 73% of all deaths (WHO, 2014).

5.8.3 The rural–urban gap in healthcare

Since the post-war era, Vietnam has made substantial improvements in many areas of health. One major development is the access to basic infrastructure. Today, access to electricity is available to almost all and access to clean water has increased by at least 25% since 1993 (World Bank, n.d.-c). Although significant improvements have been made, up to one-third of the population, approximately 30 million people, is still living near the poverty line and falls into the state of being 'poor'. As the 54 ethnic minority groups contribute up to 15% of the population, those who are considered 'extremely poor' are mainly found within these groups (World Bank, n.d.-c). While roughly 30% of the population resides in an urban area, more than 60% of the population lives in a rural setting (WHO, n.d.).

Although Vietnam has been acknowledged for its remarkable improvements, the issue on disparity has been watered down. Masked by the compliments of the country's development, the statistics between different regions of the country reveal a gap between the urban and rural areas. According to the United Nations, while the infant mortality in areas such as Central Highlands and the north of Vietnam is significantly higher than the stated average, the maternal mortality is higher among the ethnic minority population as well (United Nations in VietNam, n.d.-b).

Comparing the wealthiest 20% with the poorest 20%, the issue on disparity can be easily identified. For example, in 2011 while only 60% of the poor had been given the DPT3 vaccine, more than 85% of the wealthiest were vaccinated. In a more extreme case, one of the greatest inequalities lies among reproductive health, where there is a 60% difference between the poor and the rich having access to antenatal care services (Countdown to 2015, 2013, May).

5.8.4 Public health and primary healthcare system

There are four levels of the healthcare system in Vietnam; the district and community levels, also regarded as part of the basic health network, are the levels that provide primary healthcare services for the general population.

In 2010, there were approximately 11,000 community health stations. The community health stations are mainly responsible in delivering primary care and national health programmes to populations who reside in the rural and mountainous areas. These services include education, diagnosis, and intervention. Some examples of these include vaccinations, antenatal care, and safe delivery, screening examinations, and referrals for outpatients. Community health workers tend to collaborate with village health workers in disseminating outreach activities within the rural residents. Within the community level, 99% have their own community health station and 70% of these stations have a doctor. As the community level is in close contact with the rural community, 79.3% of these health stations will provide traditional medical services. In fact, those who face difficulties in accessing healthcare services due to distance will access primary care services through traditional medical practice (WHO & MoH Viet Nam, 2012).

5.8.5 Disease control and health promotion

In Vietnam, public health services which include prevention and promotion are offered by the public sector. More specifically, the district and provincial levels are mainly responsible for disease control. The district level provides preventive medicine centres which act as some of the public health facilities for prevention purposes, while the provincial level provides specific centres, such as AIDS Centres and Reproductive Health Centres for specific diseases and or populations (WHO & MoH Viet Nam, 2012). As a member of the United Nations, Vietnam has also been proactively collaborating with the UN in developing policies to provide protection and services such as education and governance for all and especially the vulnerable, including migrants and ethnic minorities. One proposed framework entitled the One Plan Management Plan aims to implement the idea of having one common service to increase efficiency and to lower costs. This plan also aligns with the SEDS 2011–2020 (United Nations in VietNam, n.d.-a).

5.8.6 Disaster trends and situations

From 2000 to 2016, floods (37 riverine floods) and storms (41 tropical cyclones) were the most common types of natural disaster in Vietnam. The deadliest among these disasters was a flood in July 2000, causing 460 deaths, which also affected the greatest number of people of five million. The disasters reported of the greatest economic damage were two storms in September 2009 and November 2013, leading to losses of US$785 million and US$734 million, respectively (CRED, 2017).

5.9 Conclusion

While Asia hosts a number of countries with large population size, major health disparities exist alongside with the mosaic patterns of socioeconomic development. It remains as operational and policy challenges to address the multiple health needs and health promotion in the rural contexts. Additional country case examples will be presented and discussed in Chapters 8, 9, and 10 which will discuss various contemporary rural health challenges.

References

Allianz Worldwide Care (n.d.). Healthcare in the Philippines. Available at: https://www.allianzworldwidecare.com/en/support/view/national-healthcare-systems/healthcare-in-philippines/ (accessed 16 February 2017) [Online].

Amnullah, A. S. M., Baral, S. C., Khatri, R., Uprety, S., & Dulal, B. (2015). *Health Vulnerabilities of Migrants from Nepal: Baseline Assessment.* Geneva, Switzerland: International Organization for Migration. Available at: https://www.researchgate.net/publication/290437618_Health_Vulnerabilities_of_Migrants_from_Nepal (accessed 17 February 2017) [Online].

Asian Development Bank (2007). *Philippines: Critical Development Constraint* (Country Diagnostic Studies). Manila, the Philippines: Asian Development Bank.

Central Intelligence Agency. (2017). The world factbook: South Asia - Nepal. Available at: https://www.cia.gov/library/publications/the-world-factbook/geos/np.html (accessed 14 July 2017) [Online].

Costello, A. M. & Dalglish, S. L. (on behalf of the Strategic Review Study Team) (2016). *Towards a Grand Convergence for Child Survival and Health: A Strategic Review of Options for the Future Building on Lessons Learnt from IMNCI*. Geneva, Switzerland: WHO. Available at: http://apps.who.int/iris/bitstream/10665/251855/1/WHO-MCA-16.04-eng.pdf?ua=1 (accessed 17 February 2017) [Online].

Countdown to 2015 (2013, May). Vietnam health data—2013 accountability profile. Available at: http://countdown2015.org/documents/2013Report/Vietnam_Accountability_profile_2013.pdf (accessed 18 February 2017) [Online].

Centre for Research on the Epidemiology of Disasters (CRED) (2017). EM-DAT: The Emergency Events Database. Available at: http://emdat.be/emdat_db/ (accessed 14 July 2017) [Online].

Government of Pakistan. Ministry of Climate Change. National Disaster Management Authority (2013). *National Disaster Risk Reduction Policy*. Islamabad, Pakistan: National Disaster Management Authority. Available at: http://www.ndma.gov.pk/Documents/drrpolicy2013.pdf (accessed 17 February 2017) [Online].

Government of Pakistan. Ministry of Planning, Development & Reform. Planning Commission (2014). *Pakistan 2025: One Nation—One Vision*. Islamabad, Pakistan: Pakistan Vision 2025 Secretariat. Available at: http://www.pakbj.org/statics/css/pakbj/pdf/Pakistan-Vision-2025.pdf (accessed 17 February 2017) [Online].

Government of Papua New Guinea. Department of National Planning and Monitoring (2015a). *Papua New Guinea Medium Term Development Plan 2: 2016–2017*. Waigani, Papua New Guinea: Department of National Planning and Monitoring. Available at: http://www.planning.gov.pg/images/dnpm/pdf/MTDP2.pdf (accessed 17 February 2017) [Online].

Government of Papua New Guinea. Department of National Planning and Monitoring (2015b). *Papua New Guinea: Millennium Development Goals final summary report 2015*. Waigani, Papua New Guinea: Department of National Planning and Monitoring. Available at: http://www.pg.undp.org/content/papua_new_guinea/en/home/library/millennium-development-goals-final-summary-report-2015.html (accessed 17 February 2017) [Online].

Government of Papua New Guinea. National Department of Health (2010). *National Health Plan 2011–2020* (Volume 1: Policies and Strategies). Waigani, Papua New Guinea: National Department of Health. Available at: http://www.wpro.who.int/health_services/papua_new_guinea_nationalhealthplan.pdf (accessed 17 February 2017) [Online].

Government of Papua New Guinea. National Department of Health (2016). *2015 Sector Performance Annual Review*. Waigani, Papua New Guinea: National Department of Health.

Health Insurance System Research Office (2012). *Thailand's Universal Coverage Scheme: Achievements and Challenges: An Independent Assessment of the First 10 Years (2001–2010)*. Nonthaburi, Thailand: HISRO.

Herrera, M. E. B., Roman, F. L., & Alarilla, M. C. I. (2010). *Overview of Health Sector Reform in the Philippines and Possible Opportunities for Public–Private Partnerships* (AIM Working Paper No. 10–002). Available at: http://ps4h.org/docs17_PHSA/ppp.Philippines.20101124.final.pdf (accessed 14 July 2017) [Online].

Jongudomsuk, P., Srithamrongsawat, S., Patcharanarumol, W., *et al.* (2015). *The Kingdom of Thailand Health System Review* (Health Systems in Transition Vol. 5 No. 5 2015). Available at: http://www.

wpro.who.int/asia_pacific_observatory/hits/series/thailand_health_systems_review.pdf?ua=1 (accessed 17 February 2017) [Online].

Lorenzo, F. M. E., Galvez-Tan, J., Icamina, K., & Javier, L. (2007). Nurse migration from a source country perspective: Philippine country case study. *Health Serv Res*, **42**(3p2), 1406–18.

Ministry of Health and Population Nepal (2011). *Department of Health Services Annual Report 2009–2010.* Kathmandu, Nepal: Ministry of Health and Population.

Ministry of Health and Population Nepal (2012). *Human Resources for Health Strategic Plan 2011–2015* (draft). Available at: http://www.nhssp.org.np/human_resources/HRH%20Strategic%20Plan%20 Final.pdf (accessed 17 February 2017) [Online].

Ministry of Health and Population Nepal (2016). *Department of Health Services Annual Report 2014–2015.* Kathmandu, Nepal: Ministry of Health and Population.

Ministry of Health Mongolia (2010). *Evaluation of the Soum Hospital Development Programme.* Ulaabaatar, Mongolia: Ministry of Health Mongolia.

Ministry of Health Mongolia, World Health Organization Western Pacific Region (2010). *WHO Country Cooperation Strategy for Mongolia 2010–2015.* Available at: http://www.wpro.who.int/mongolia/publications/who_ccs_for_mongolia.pdf?ua=1 (accessed 16 February 2017) [Online].

Ministry of Health Myanmar (2005). *Malaria Situation in Myanmar (1976–2004)* (Vector Borne Disease Control Programme). Available at: http://actmalaria.net/downloads/pdf/info/2005/ Myanmar.pdf (accessed 15 June 2013) [Online].

Ministry of Health Myanmar (2011). *Myanmar national strategic plan and operational plan on HIV and AIDS 2011–2015: concise version.* Available at: http://www.ilo.org/wcmsp5/groups/public/---ed_protect/---protrav/---ilo_aids/documents/legaldocument/wcms_174886.pdf (accessed 17 February 2017)

Ministry of Health Myanmar (2013). *Health in Myanmar 2013.* Nay Pyi Taw, Myanmar: Ministry of Health.

Ministry of National Planning and Economic Development Myanmar, Ministry of Health Myanmar (2011). *Myanmar Multiple Indicator Cluster Survey 2009–2010: Final Report.* Nay Pyi Taw, Myanmar: Ministry of National Planning and Economic Development and Ministry of Health. Available at: https://www.unicef.org/myanmar/MICS_Myanmar_Report_2009-10.pdf (accessed 18 February 2017) [Online].

National AIDS Committee (2015). *Thailand Ending AIDS: Thailand AIDS Response Progress Report 2015.* Available at: www.unaids.org/sites/default/files/country/documents/THA_narrative_report_2015.pdf (accessed 17 February 2017) [Online].

National Institute of Population Studies Pakistan, ICF International (2013). *Pakistan Demographic and Health Survey 2012–13.* Pakistan, Calverton, MD: National Institute of Population Studies Pakistan, ICF International, Islamabad. Available at: http://www.nips.org.pk/abstract_files/ PDHS%20Final%20Report%20as%20of%20Jan%2022-2014.pdf (accessed 17 February 2017) [Online].

National Statistics Office Philippines, ICF Macro (2009). *National Demographic and Health Survey 2008.* Available at: https://dhsprogram.com/pubs/pdf/FR224/FR224.pdf (accessed 2 March 2017) [Online].

Pappas, G., Papadimitriou, P., Akritidis, N., Christou, L., & Tsianos, E. V. (2006). The new global map of human brucellosis. *Lancet Infect Dis*, **6**, 91–9.

Republic of the Philippines, Department of Health (2012). *2011–2016 National Objectives for Health* (Health Sector Reform Agenda Monograph No. 12). Manila, Republic of the Philippines: Department of Health. Available at: http://www.doh.gov.ph/sites/default/files/basic-page/toc-foreword-preface.pdf (accessed 2 March 2017) [Online].

Republic of the Union of Myanmar, The Pyidaungsu Hluttaw (2012). *The Social Security Law, 2012.* Available at: http://www.burmalibrary.org/docs15/2012-Social_Security_Bill-ocr-en.pdf (accessed 17 February 2017) [Online].

Romualdez, A. G. Jr., de la Rosa, J. F. E., Flavier, J. D. A., *et al.* (2011). *The Philippines Health System Review* (Health Systems in Transition Vol. 1 No. 2 2011). Available at: http://www.wpro.who.int/asia_pacific_observatory/Philippines_Health_System_Review.pdf (accessed 16 February 2017) [Online].

Smith, A. D. & Chan, E. Y. Y. (2016). *Health Challenges & Disaster Risk Reduction in Myanmar* (Policy Brief). Hong Kong, China: Collaborating Centre for Oxford University and CUHK for Disaster and Medical Humanitarian Response (CCOUC), The Chinese University of Hong Kong.

Tangkitvanich, S. & Sasiwuttiwat, S. (2012). Revamping the Thai education system: quality for all. *TDRI Quarterly Review*, **27**(2), 3–14.

Than, T. S., Phone, M., Nilar, T., Htay, W., San, S. A., & Than, S. (2014). *The Republic of the Union of Myanmar: Health System Review* (Health Systems in Transition Vol.4 No. 3 2014). Geneva Switzerland: Asia Pacific Observatory on Health Systems and Policies, WHO. Available at: http://www.wpro.who.int/asia_pacific_observatory/hits/series/myanmar_health_systems_review.pdf (accessed 17 February 2017) [Online].

Tran, V. T., Hoang, T. P., Mathauer, I., Nguyen, T. K. P. (2011). *A Health Financing Review of Vietnam with a Focus on Social Health Insurance.* Geneva, Switzerland: WHO. Available at: http://www.who.int/health_financing/documents/oasis_f_11-vietnam.pdf (accessed 17 February 2017) [Online].

United Nations Development Programme (2015). Briefing Note for Countries on the 2015 Human Development Report: Viet Nam. Available at: http://hdr.undp.org/sites/all/themes/hdr_theme/country-notes/VNM.pdf (accessed 24 January 2017) [Online].

United Nations Development Programme (2016). *Human Development Report 2016.* New York, NY: United Nations Development Programme.

United Nations in VietNam (n.d.-a). One Plan. Available at: http://www.un.org.vn/en/the-one-un-initiative-in-viet-nam-mainmenu-265/one-plan/1064-one-plan.html (accessed 24 January 2017) [Online].

United Nations in VietNam (n.d.-b). Viet Nam at a glance. Available at: http://www.un.org.vn/en/about-viet-nam/overview.html (accessed 24 January 2017) [Online].

University of Washington. Institute for Health Metrics and Evaluation (2010). *GBD Profile: Myanmar.* Available at: https://www.healthdata.org/sites/default/files/files/country_profiles/GBD/ihme_gbd_country_report_myanmar.pdf (accessed 17 February 2017) [Online].

Wibulpolprasert, S. (2011). *Thailand Health Profile 2008–2010.* Nonthaburi, Thailand: Ministry of Public Health.

World Bank (n.d.-a). Philippines: Overview. Available at: http://www.worldbank.org/en/country/philippines/overview (accessed 16 February 2017) [Online].

World Bank (n.d.-b). Rural population (% of total population). Available at: http://data.worldbank.org/indicator/SP.RUR.TOTL.ZS (accessed 26 January 2017) [Online].

World Bank (n.d.-c). Vietnam: Overview. Available at: http://www.worldbank.org/en/country/vietnam/overview (accessed 24 January 2017) [Online].

World Bank (2011). *World Development Indicators 2011.* Available at: http://siteresources.worldbank.org/DATASTATISTICS/Resources/wdi_ebook.pdf (accessed 17 February 2017)

World Bank Group (2016). *Closing the Health Gaps for the Elderly: Promoting Health Equity and Social Inclusion in Thailand.* Available at: http://documents.worldbank.org/curated/en/148431468299339382/pdf/AUS13326-REVISED-TITLE-HAS-CHANGED-PUBLIC-Closing-the-Health-Gaps-for-the-Elderly-English-final-for-IDU.pdf [Online].

World Health Organization (WHO) (n.d.). Country statistics. Available at: http://www.who.int/gho/countries/en/ (accessed 4 October 2017) [Online].

World Health Organization (WHO) (1997). *Financing Drugs in South-East Asia: Report of the first meeting of the WHO/SEARO Working Group on Drug Financing, Korat, Thailand, 26–28 November 1996*. Geneva, Switzerland, New Delhi, India: Action Programme on Essential Drugs, WHO Regional Office for South-East Asia.

World Health Organization (WHO) (2006). *The World Health Report 2006: Working Together For Health*. Available at: http://www.who.int/whr/2006/whr06_en.pdf (accessed 17 January 2017) [Online].

World Health Organization (WHO) (2013). *Mongolia Health System Review* (Health Systems in Transition Vol. 3 No. 2 2013). Geneva, Switzerland: WHO.

World Health Organization (WHO) (2014). *Noncommunicable Diseases Country Profiles 2014*. Geneva, Switzerland: WHO.

World Health Organization (WHO) (2016a). Mongolia: key indicators. Available at: http://apps.who.int/gho/data/node.cco.ki-MNG?lang=en (accessed 16 February 2017) [Online].

World Health Organization (WHO) (2016b). Myanmar: key indicators. Available at: http://apps.who.int/gho/data/node.cco.ki-MMR?lang=en (accessed 16 February 2017) [Online].

World Health Organization (WHO) (2016c). Nepal: key indicators. Available at: http://apps.who.int/gho/data/node.cco.ki-NPL?lang=en (accessed 16 February 2017) [Online].

World Health Organization (WHO) (2016d). Pakistan: key indicators. Available at: http://apps.who.int/gho/data/node.cco.ki-PAK?lang=en (accessed 16 February 2017) [Online].

World Health Organization (WHO) (2016e). Papua New Guinea: key indicators. Available at: http://apps.who.int/gho/data/node.cco.ki-PNG?lang=en (accessed 16 February 2017) [Online].

World Health Organization (WHO) (2016f). Philippines: key indicators. Available at: http://apps.who.int/gho/data/node.cco.ki-PHL?lang=en (accessed 16 February 2017) [Online].

World Health Organization (WHO) (2016g). Thailand: key indicators. Available at: http://apps.who.int/gho/data/node.cco.ki-THA?lang=en (accessed 16 February 2017) [Online].

World Health Organization (WHO) (2016h). Viet Nam: key indicators. Available at: http://apps.who.int/gho/data/node.cco.ki-VNM?lang=en (accessed 16 February 2017) [Online].

World Health Organization (WHO) (2016, May, -a). *WHO Country Cooperation Strategy at a Glance: Nepal*. Available at: http://apps.who.int/iris/bitstream/10665/136955/1/ccsbrief_npl_en.pdf?ua=1 (accessed 17 February 2017) [Online].

World Health Organization (WHO) (2016, May, -b). *WHO Country Cooperation Strategy at a Glance: Pakistan*. Available at: http://apps.who.int/iris/bitstream/10665/136607/1/ccsbrief_pak_en.pdf?ua=1 (accessed 17 February 2017) [Online].

World Health Organization (WHO) (2016, May, -c). *WHO Country Cooperation Strategy at a Glance: Papua New Guinea*. Available at: http://apps.who.int/iris/bitstream/10665/136819/1/ccsbrief_png_en.pdf?ua=1 (accessed 17 February 2017) [Online].

World Health Organization (WHO) (2016, December 1). WHO vaccine-preventable diseases: monitoring system: 2016 global summary. Available at: http://apps.who.int/immunization_monitoring/globalsummary/ (accessed 16 February) [Online].

World Health Organization (WHO) Country Office for Nepal (2007). *Policy papers on health, Nepal*. Kathmandu, Nepal: WHO.

World Health Organization (WHO) Country Office for Nepal (2013). *WHO country cooperation strategy Nepal, 2013–2017*. WHO, New Delhi, India. Available at: http://apps.who.int/iris/bitstream/10665/161133/1/B4946.pdf (accessed 17 February 2017) [Online].

World Health Organization (WHO) Regional Office for South-East Asia, Ministry of Health Thailand (2010). *Human Resources for Health: Country Profile: Thailand.* Available at: http://www.searo.who.int/entity/human_resources/data/tha_profile.pdf (accessed 17 February 2017) [Online].

World Health Organization (WHO) Regional Office for the Eastern Mediterranean (EMRO) (2013). *Country Cooperation Strategy for WHO and Pakistan: 2011–2017* (WHO-EM/PME/001/E). World Health Organization Regional Office for the Eastern Mediterranean, Cairo, Egypt. Available at: http://apps.who.int/iris/bitstream/10665/113228/1/CCS_Pakistan_2013_EN_14946.pdf (accessed 17 February 2017) [Online].

World Health Organization (WHO) Regional Office for the Eastern Mediterranean (2016). *Pakistan Health Profile 2015.* Cairo, Egypt: World Health Organization Regional Office for the Eastern Mediterranean. Available at: http://applications.emro.who.int/dsaf/EMROPUB_2016_EN_19266.pdf?u (accessed 17 February 2017) [Online].

World Health Organization (WHO) Western Pacific Regional Office (2010). *WHO Country Cooperation Strategy: Papua New Guinea 2010–2015.* World Health Organization Western Pacific Regional Office, Manila, Philippines. Available at: http://www.wpro.who.int/countries/png/ccs_png_en.pdf (accessed 17 February 2017) [Online].

World Health Organization (WHO), Ministry of Health Viet Nam (2012). Health services delivery profile: Viet Nam: 2012. Available at: http://www.wpro.who.int/health_services/service_delivery_profile_vietnam.pdf (accessed 24 January 2017) [Online].

World Health Organization (WHO), Papua New Guinea National Department of Health (2012). *Papua New Guinea Health Service Delivery Profile.* Available at: http://www.wpro.who.int/health_services/service_delivery_profile_papua_new_guinea.pdf (accessed 17 February 2017) [Online].

Chapter 6

From theory to practice

This chapter examines how theories may be applied in field practices for promoting health risk awareness, disaster preparedness, and bottom-up health resilience in rural communities. Practical challenges and problems encountered when designing field-based interventions in rural Asian settings, the field-policy nexus, international policy frameworks (such as the Sustainable Development Goals (SDGs), the Sendai Framework for Disaster Risk Reduction (2015–2030) (UN, 2015), and the Paris Agreement for Climate Change) to improve health resilience and emergency and disaster risk reductions in field contexts are discussed. Throughout the chapter, the CCOUC Ethnic Minority Health Project model (as described in Chapter 1: Introduction) will be used as an example to illustrate how to bridge theory and practical.

6.1 Introduction: Health needs in remote rural areas

In general, population health outcomes fare worse in rural contexts when compared with urban settings (Khosh-Chashm, 1995). Issues with water, sanitation facilities, electricity systems, housing constructions, solid waste collection and disposal, animal, waste, and stagnant water management, indoor air quality, vector control, food safety, and fuel poverty are common contributing factors to rural vulnerability towards health risks (Khosh-Chashm, 1995; World Health Organization Regional Office for the Eastern Mediterranean [WHO EMRO], 1994).

6.2 Healthy Settings: The Healthy Village programme

The Healthy Settings movement came out of the World Health Organization (WHO) strategy of 'Health for All' in 1980 (Mahler, 1981).

The Healthy Village is a holistic approach to address the critical environmental health problems in rural areas and was a concept first proposed by WHO/EMRO in 1989 in a Technical Consultation on Urban Environmental Health at the WHO Regional Office for the Eastern Mediterranean (1990, 1994) in Alexandria, Egypt. The basis of the Healthy Village programme (Howard *et al.*, 2002) is similar to the Healthy City programme, but applied in rural areas as opposed to urban areas. Achievement of better health is again defined by the area's residents; however, the generally accepted definition of a Healthy Village includes a community with low rates of infectious diseases, access to basic healthcare services, and a stable, peaceful social environment. According to Howard *et al.* (2002), environment, awareness of individuals, personal hygiene, healthcare, and faecal–oral and vector-borne diseases are the five main health-affecting components that might need to be addressed to develop a 'Healthy Village'.

6.3 Project planning

6.3.1 Methods and planning strategy: The Health Settings approach

A project cycle describes the entire project process and is usually divided into four or five stages to allow a project team to monitor progress and to evaluate project efforts. For example, the EMHP project (see Chapter 1) adopted the project cycle suggested by the International Federation of Red Cross and Red Crescent Societies and had encompassed four project stages, namely needs assessment, planning, implementation, and monitoring and evaluation, in its cycle (see Fig. 6.1 and Fig. 6.2).

The planning of the 'Healthy Village' project for EMHP (see Chapter 1) was based on the MAP-IT approach described by United States Department of Health and Human Services in 2001 in its planning guide titled *Healthy People in Healthy Communities* (Guidry *et al.*, 2001). MAP-IT is the acronym for Mobile, Assess, Plan, Implement, and Track. (See Table 3.1).

6.3.2 Needs assessment

Needs assessment aims to collect information to inform project planning and development. Different assessment tools and methods may be used to identify and understand the health problems of the target community. The main objective is to examine the epidemiological health profile and beliefs of patients and stakeholders, and to analyse the determinants of health behaviour. Results will also help identify interventions and review priorities when multiple concurrent needs (e.g. alcohol abuse, smoking, and high-salt diet) are identified.

Collecting background information about the project site

Technology advancement has enabled information access beyond physical boundaries. Yet, information accuracy may vary with its sources, information collection methods, and timing of data collection. To obtain a holistic view of the context and to prevent a mismatch between the project design and the actual needs, information triangulation from

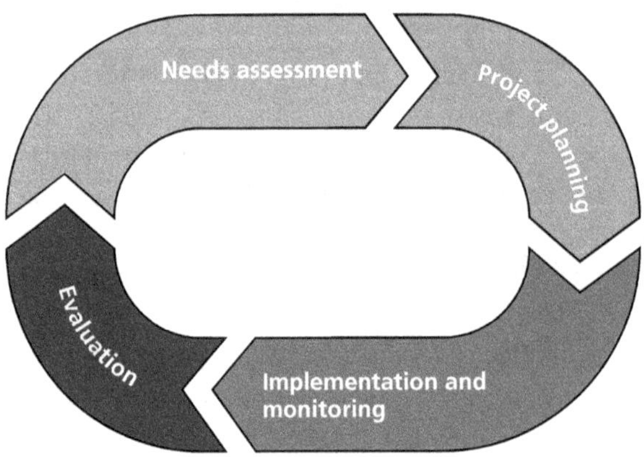

Fig. 6.1 A Project cycle.

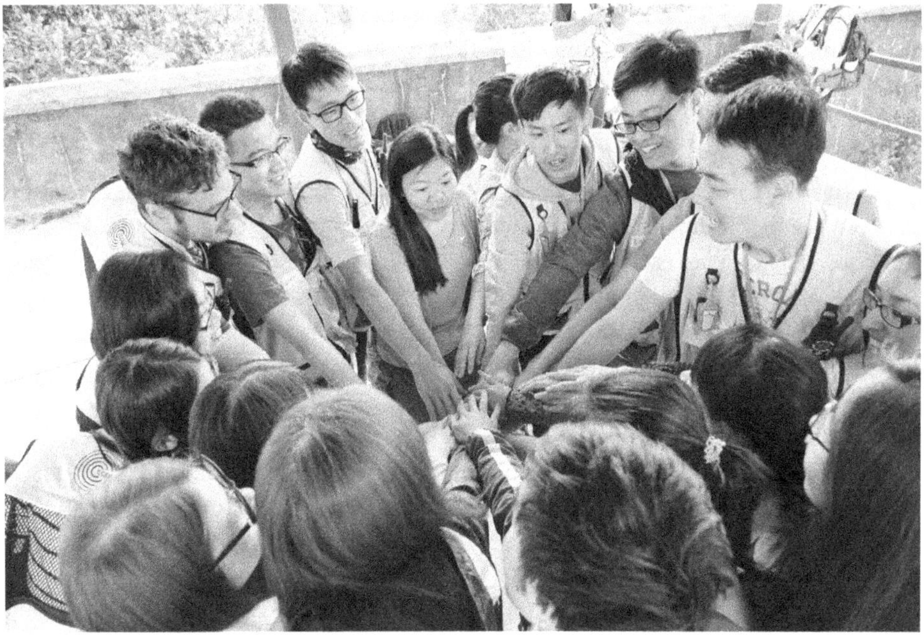

Fig. 6.2 A project team will go through the project cycle.

various sources, supplemented with direct field assessments, is always preferable. Official information sources such as local government statistics, newspapers, reports from volunteer organizations, and publications in different disciplines should be consulted and verification of the field situation with the local co-organizers and field data collection should be attempted whenever possible.

Reviewing existing databases/reports is usually the first step in understanding the patterns and trends of the relevant health outcomes for the intended interventions. Nevertheless, for many Asian countries, regular data collection and surveillance processes might be limited by a lack of the relevant capacity, system, or simply even the policy to support such an attempt. Moreover, most data collection efforts might attempt to provide a generalized view through cluster sampling and neglect certain secluded communities or population subgroups that might be traditionally hard to reach. Thus, general patterns might not reveal real health outcome patterns of the intended audience if target audience are minority groups. Most practitioners or researchers who target specific underserved communities are often likely to have to collect their own baseline data in order to understand the potential health impacts and needs of a condition or situation.

In addition, for some rural contexts, simple extrapolation of the provincial statistics may not reflect the actual health needs in the activity area, as the available information might either be out of date (much of it was published more than five years ago, even before the 2008 earthquake) or not relevant (provincial statistics that were collected from rural/

suburban communities rather than from remote ethnic minority areas). Specifically, for rural ethnic minority-based communities, their health and behaviour patterns might not be represented in the general statistical reports.

To collect information for health needs assessment, appropriate tools, specified target group, and sampling frame, as well as sufficient resources (such as time, manpower, and facilitation from or by stakeholders) are all crucial determinants to assess the real needs of a community. Data collection methods may be quantitative or qualitative. In some locations, language or certain cultural practices (e.g. a community in which the discussion of death or illness might be taboo) might also present additional barriers for simple data collection efforts. Regardless of the tools and methods used for the data collection, it is essential to enquire and consider environmental (physical—such as rivers and earthquake-prone areas) and socioeconomical factors, as well as the existing health burden and service availability.

Needs priorities might be ranked by health impacts on the community (e.g. incidence, prevalence), but implementation depends on feasibility assessment of the underlying circumstance, resource availability, individual and community perceptions of the severity and importance of the programme.

Before conducting household-based field needs assessment in a village, the team might wish to consider first conducting in-depth stakeholder interviews with key village members (e.g. village chief, the village committee, and village doctors) to understand the general context and health situation in the village (see Appendix 2). Additional focus groups and household-based surveys will be valuable to provide insights for activities relevancy and programme planning. Of note, when conducting focus group studies, whenever possible, gender and age stratified focus groups might allow better discussion of the issues specific to gender and age needs. Some important questions to be explored and agreed before the needs assessment include:

- Determining the priority population groups for internventions;
- Determining the health needs and groups to be addressed; and
- The priority of resources allocation.

During the assessment, the availability of existing database (government local office report) or reports of other organizations' current health projects should be explored. This not only prevents duplications, but also helps identify potential working partners on the site. Appendices 3 to 5 show the focus group questions devised by CCOUC, the questionnaire on the basic demographics of interviewees, and also the questionnaire for the household survey (see Chapter 1: Introduction). Study tools should be adjusted according to the targets and projects. Ethnics approval should be sought from the research committee of the team's affiliated organization and related local organizations or personnel before the start of the project.

In rural communities, the senior male in a family may not always be the main decision-makers when it comes to family issues. Actual decision-makers need to be identified to prevent a bias in the assessment.

6.3.3 Field programme planning

Field programme planning and implementation is a complex process. Four key principles should be considered (Hadridge, 2001): (1) evidence-based information should be used to plan the programme, to ensure its appropriateness and relevance to the local needs and to various stakeholders' interests. Stakeholder interviews, focus groups, as well as local epidemiological and health knowledge studies should be conducted; (2) multidisciplinary actors and stakeholders should be involved in the planning process and be engaged in the programme implementation. With the aim of maintaining sustainability at the field level, local and community-based collaborators/champions will need to be identified; (3) a continuous feedback mechanism should be built into the programme; and (4) resources (both internal and external) mapping must be conducted before designing the programme, in order to maximize the local involvement and programme cost-effectiveness.

Community partner

Effective planning of rural community-based interventions requires community facilitation, local participation, and political endorsement. To maximize the impact, multidisciplinary collaborative teams should always be attempted to maximize synergy and project outcomes.

6.3.4 Setting the objectives

Objectives should be mapped with expected intervention outcomes. They should be built on specific, measurable, achievable, relevant, and time-bound (SMART), principles. Table 6.1 described the SMART principles.

Due to resource constraints (such as time, manpower, and money), programme objectives should consider local incentives, political interests, and resources availability.

A statement of intent which clarify programme aims and objectives will help bring related stakeholders to agree on the purpose of a project or programme. The three most important strategic programme planning questions to be discussed between stakeholders and programme team will be: (1) Where we are now (i.e. baseline)?; (2) What do we want to do (i.e. objectives)?; and (3) How do we plan to get there (i.e. strategy)? Once the

Table 6.1 The SMART principles

Principle	Definition
Specific	Project objectives should be specific and unambiguous
Measurable	The objectives should be quantifiable and may be tracked throughout the project
Achievable	The objectives should be feasible under field constraints
Relevant	The objectives should be relevant to the identified issue(s)
Time-bound	The objectives should be achievable within a specific time frame

objectives have been specified, the 'target' measures, which are more specific and often measurable, might then be developed (see SMART criteria previously described).

Project planning

The success of a programme often depends on content design and development. The project organizers need to consider the following points:

- The characteristics of the target audience.
- The scope of the project.
- The approach (methods and resources) used to achieve the project goals.
- Key project messages.
- Methods of communication.
- Project outcome indicators.
- Evaluation of project effectiveness.
- Level of community participation.
- Availability of contingency plans.

For a more detailed discussion of designing project content, refer to the theories and models in Chapter 3.

6.3.5 **Resources consideration**

Funding/financial budget, logistics, and human resources (technical capacity and skills, experiences, personality, and availability), legal and system requirements, as well as the availability of materials (drugs, equipment) are all key components for building programmes and enabling implementation success. Scale and the size of programme, staff commitment, and relevance of proposed initiatives to existing programme/policy directions are also important factors.

Budgeting

Resources for programme implementation will need to be translated to a budget for management purposes. Typical programme costs that must be considered and budgeted (if applicable) include: capital expenditures (constructions, facilities, commodities, equipment, vehicles, and furniture); personnel (staff and administrative costs—part-time or full-time); training; travel; supplies; and running and maintenance (utilities, communications, and insurance). Potential pitfalls may include a lack of funds, relevant resources, and manpower, input timing, local resistance to change, neglect of institutional or legal requirements, unexpected results, poor coordination, and unforeseen circumstances.

Cost of the intervention

A health promotion campaign should include a budget plan which stipulates the required items, their respective uses, and the expenses. It usually includes several types of expenses:

1. Equipment expenses: appliances (such as walkie-talkies, amplifiers, and batteries), teaching materials (such as posters, items for demonstration, and stationery), souvenirs for the villagers or the local representative, first aid kits and medication, and team uniform/clothing.
2. Logistics and transportation fees: budget should carefully balance the fees related to mode of transport and the travelling time required. As public transportation system in remote villages is often limited and sometimes non-existent. Rentals of car, boat, and plane may be options. Extra allowances should also be planned for contingency in cases of transport breakdown.
3. Accommodation: planning should consider gender, cultural, and religious factors when making accommodation decisions. Safety concerns (fires, disaster risks, and security) should always be reviewed by the project teams.
4. Meals: expenses for food and meals should be included. Allowances should also be given to local helpers and recruits. Food allergy, and cultural and religious preferences should always be respected and addressed.
5. Subsidy: agreed costs and fees for local assistance (e.g. logistics, translation, and event facilitation) should be agreed in advance.
6. Contingency budget: money to cover the expenses that may be incurred due to traffic accidents or evacuation from the project site. It is approximately 5% of the budget. The contingency budget should take into consideration currency exchange costs and the ratio between cash and non-cash means of payment.

Team members who are responsible for logistic material preparation should keep expenses within budget. As credit cards or other payment methods are not common in remote villages, cash should be ready to pay expenses at the project site. The leader and at least one additional designated person should be responsible for carrying a portion of the cash to reduce the risk of loss.

Human resources

For staff management, responsibilities, tasks, and the line of authority and supervision must be defined. A job description for each of the key areas in the field work should be developed. This usually requires a title, qualifications, job summary, and a list of the duties and the relationships with other team members/stakeholders (such as the reporting authority and the communication and interaction targets). It is specifically relevant and valuable when it involves inexperienced volunteers and people in a supervisory and/or managerial role, as well as in a multicultural environment.

A lack of local expertise, capabilities, and resources, and distance from urban settings are major limitation when planning health services and programmes in rural village communities. As a result, planning for village communities should always be location-specific, realistic, and relevant, and have a clear understanding of a clear community profile and needs. Multidisciplinary teams are particularly useful in rural community-based projects, as multilevel needs are often presented. Also, the field time management will require flexibility and constant updates, as the logistics and rural living habits may affect the project/programme completion. It is important to identify the appropriate skills for the project team members during the assessments and planning of remote healthcare programmes. Furthermore, team dynamics can be affected by personalities and challenging field situations (lack of good hygienic, sleep, and food) and the team leaders should constantly reflect and regularly check on the team members to ensure good team dynamics are maintained.

"In situations where limited resources are available to invest in staff recruitment and training, staff turnover might be the main reason for a programme's failure. Moreover, a high turnover might be due to difficulties in personal circumstances, dissatisfaction over pay or poor work conditions, but essentially, the availability of the relevant staff is often a key consideration when deciding if a programme might be implemented or continued."

6.3.6 Key notes for practitioners and volunteers on rural health education programmes

Team management

Health education team members may come from diverse backgrounds. Efforts in team building is recommended through team building sessions before field departure. In the briefing sessions, the main point of the activity should be elucidated and work progress should be reported. Team members should also be given the chance to take on team building and trip preparation work.

There are different theories about personality analysis relevant to team management. The 'Team Roles' theory devised by Meredith Belbin, points out that a well-structured team should consist of nine types of people, for which each of the different personalities has its strengths and weaknesses (Belbin, 1993). The team members supplement each other to increase working efficiency. Table 6.2 describes the strengths and weaknesses of roles in a well-structured team.

Team leaders should be observant so that s/he can get to know their teammates' personalities and capacities. Tasks should be delegated in accordance with the strengths of individual personalities to reduce potential clashes among members.

Team building takes time. According to the research of American psychologist Bruce Tuckman, team development and behaviour can be broadly divided into four stages, namely forming, storming, norming, and performing (Tuckman, 1965).

Forming refers to the initiation phase of the project when members are unclear about project goals and their own roles and responsibility. Relationships among team members and team leader, and the team's system and code of conduct will be formed during this period. The team leader will need to address anxieties among members and to ensure that mutual trust can be built within the team.

Storming refers to a phase when intragroup conflicts, polarization, and power struggles arise. Members may compete with each other. They may express their discontent and frustration about the goals and expectations of the team, their roles, and their responsibilities.

Table 6.2 Roles in a well-structured team

Role	Strength	Weakness
Shaper Motivates the team to ensure it keeps moving and does not lose focus and momentum.	Willing to accept challenges, energetic, self-motivated, having the courage to overcome obstacles.	Getting angry easily, may sometimes offend others' feelings.
Resource investigator Brings the team new ideas and knowledge and ensures the thoughts of the team are expressed to the outside world.	Extrovert, enthusiastic, good at communication, sociable.	Overoptimistic, may lose interest once the initial enthusiasm has gone.
Teamworker Has the ability to glue the team together and use their versatility to identify the work required and complete it on behalf of the team.	Temperate, diplomatic, caring, willing to listen, good at averting friction.	Becoming indecisive and silent in conflicts and arguments to avoid opposing ideas.
Monitor–Evaluator Provides logical opinions to the team and can make fair judgements where required and weigh up team's options dispassionately.	Clear-headed, logical, thinks comprehensively and with insight, and having good judgement.	Lack of drive and ability to encourage others; occasionally too critical.
Specialist Brings in-depth knowledge of a main area covered by the team.	Single-minded, self-starting, and dedicated, providing the team with professional knowledge and skills.	Being able to contribute only in a particular area and may dwell on technical details.
Plant Loves thinking freely. Creative and good at using new methods to solve problems.	Creative, having a great imagination capability, smart, and good at using different strategies to solve problems.	Neglecting details and feasibility and finding it hard to cope with criticism.
Completer–Finisher Works most effectively when the task is nearly finished and can polish and scrutinize the work for errors, ensuring the quality is of the highest standard.	Perfectionist, painstaking, responsible, diligent, strong in looking for mistakes and making corrections.	Unwilling to delegate jobs to others or receive help from them; overanxious.
Coordinator Care for team's goals, arrange suitable jobs for each member.	Confident, mature, identifying talent, clarifying goals, and being able to assign jobs effectively.	Can be seen as manipulative, may offload their own share of the job.
Implementer Can plan a feasible working strategy, and implement and finish it efficiently.	Reliable, efficient, well-disciplined, pragmatic, and being able to organize work systematically and turn concepts into actions.	Inelastic, sticking to steps and principles, and responding to new opportunities slowly.

When encountering challenges and criticism from members, the team leader should resolve disputes impartially and non-judgementally. The leader should make it clear that it is normal to have differences in the team but s/he also needs to emphasize the importance of tolerance, and the fact that different opinions are important for reaching a consensus and making decisions.

Norming refers to a phase when the team reaches a consensus and performance efficiency increases. Every member accepts their own and others' roles and responsibilities, and also develops a capacity to work in harmony with others. A workflow and distinct culture gradually forms, leading to a high participation rate and a more united team. The team also starts to organize social events to strengthen bonding. Meanwhile, the leader feels able to give a greater degree of autonomy to the team, such that only big decisions are made by the team as a whole and the rest can be decentralized to individuals or subgroups.

Performing refers to a phase when the team is working together and attaining their synergic potential. They understand clearly their responsibilities and what to do. Even without supervision by the leader, members can make decisions by referring to the system. The members embrace a shared vision, work smoothly, and cooperate closely. They can resolve conflicts and consider their relationship with other members, the work culture, and the workflow when they move towards the goals. The team has a high level of autonomy. At this stage, the leader should allow the members to implement important decisions on their own.

Choosing the interventions

In addition to adopting evidence and best practices, interventions are usually chosen for their appropriateness related to the objectives, the programme's context, and the availability of resources (staff with various skills, as well as financial and logistic resources). Unfortunately, most of the available evidence might not offer a solution that will address the problem directly at the field level. For instance, published evidence might only be applicable to certain context (e.g. an urban rather than a rural setting), for specific demographic subgroups (e.g. age or gender). Frequently, there may simply be no available evidence published for the issues of concern. In addition, due to the logistical limitations in many rural settings in Asia, the delivery strategy might need to be re-tailored to fit the setting due to the geographic remoteness, lack of roads, unstable electricity, and lack of refrigerating systems, and so on. Thus, the action plan and budget will need to be tailored to provide extra provisions for time and uncertainties, as well as resource requirements. In post-natural disaster rural settings, reconstruction presents an unique opportunity to involve the community in programme development, as local resistance might be at its lowest, and political endorsements will be given when there is a true need to rebuild the community. In addition, resources are generally easier to obtain in the form of post-disaster relief assistance. Furthermore, better housing and well-being will enhance the disaster preparedness of communities facing the impact of future disasters.

With the rapid changes occurring in information technology (e.g. access to the Internet and mobile phones) in Asia, programme planners might wish to carefully consider the cost-effectiveness of direct implementation at the field level versus the option of implementing the programme online.

Other issues

Health service and programme planning in remote communities requires sensitivity to the local culture, politics, capacity constraints, and environmental limitations. 'Trust' is key to gaining access and information related to planning in these communities, and it also might be helpful to work with community partners to enhance effectiveness. It is important to foster community partners and ownership of the project. Specifically, political 'buy-ins' and community leaders (e.g. the village chief) are essential for securing the potential success of the programme. In addition, knowledgeable local workers (e.g. students, NGOs) with appropriate language skills (dialects) will be an asset when working in remote settings.

6.3.7 Preparation work

Intervention content design

When designing programme activities, the content should aim to be clear, concise, and closely related to the villagers' daily lives. Of note, rural and ethnic minority communities may have different health beliefs and understandings of health problems. It is therefore crucial to explore their knowledge level and behavioural practices when attempting to design health projects or programmes aimed at improving their health and practices. The proposed content and its format should be discussed with the villagers in order to earn their support and participation. Interactions with the villagers (such as quiz games) should be maximized to increase their sense of ownership.

Education materials

Posters, workshops, drama performances, shows, games, group discussions, and souvenirs are strategies commonly used to convey information on health promotion (see Figs. 6.3–6.7). Here are the key points for each method of disseminating information.

Posters

1. Content should be culture, gender, and age appropriate;
2. The size of the posters should be adjusted to suit the health promotion in the field context;
3. Images on the posters should be large and easily visible;
4. If posters are to be printed, check accuracy and completeness of content and allow sufficient time for reprinting should any problem be identified; choose waterproof paper that can withstand the long journey to the project site; prepare and bring along tools and materials for poster production such as scissors, colour pens, marker pens, and glue, in case the posters are damaged during the journey; and
5. Prepare a spare set of posters.

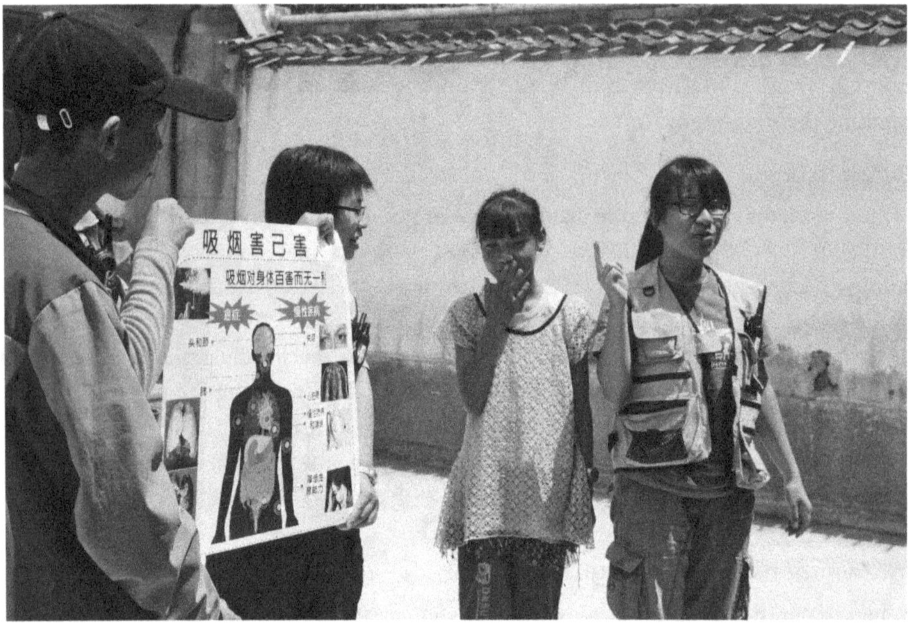

Fig. 6.3 Health promotion using a poster.
Reproduced by kind permission of Emily Ying Yang CHAN, Copyright © 2017 Emily Ying Yang CHAN.

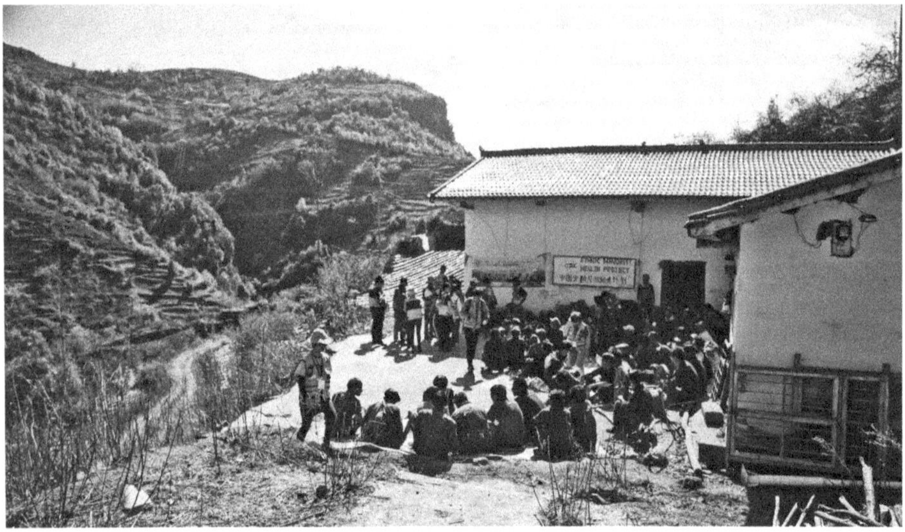

Fig. 6.4 A workshop held for some villagers.
Reproduced by kind permission of Emily Ying Yang CHAN, Copyright © 2017 Emily Ying Yang CHAN.

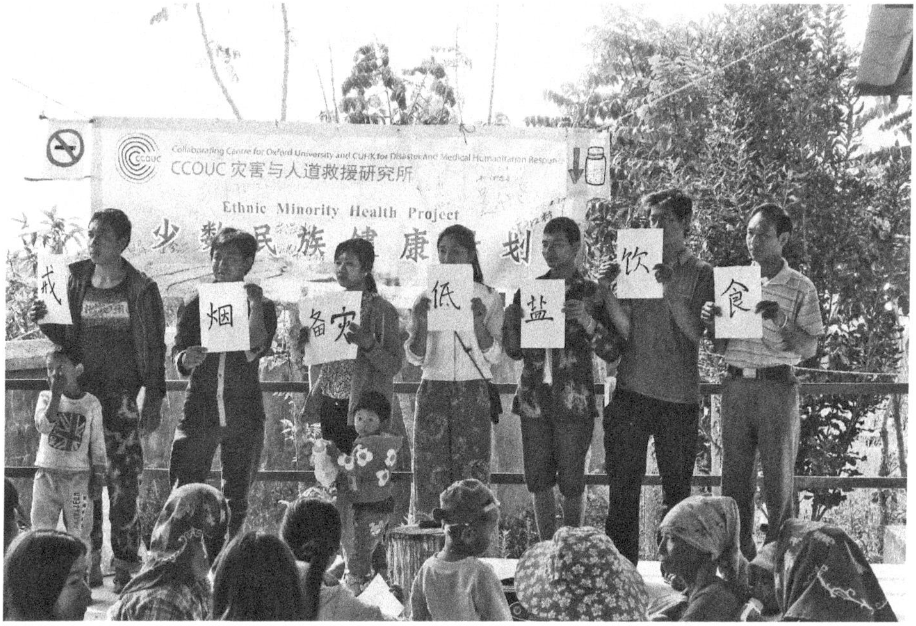

Fig. 6.5 Participation of villagers in a play.

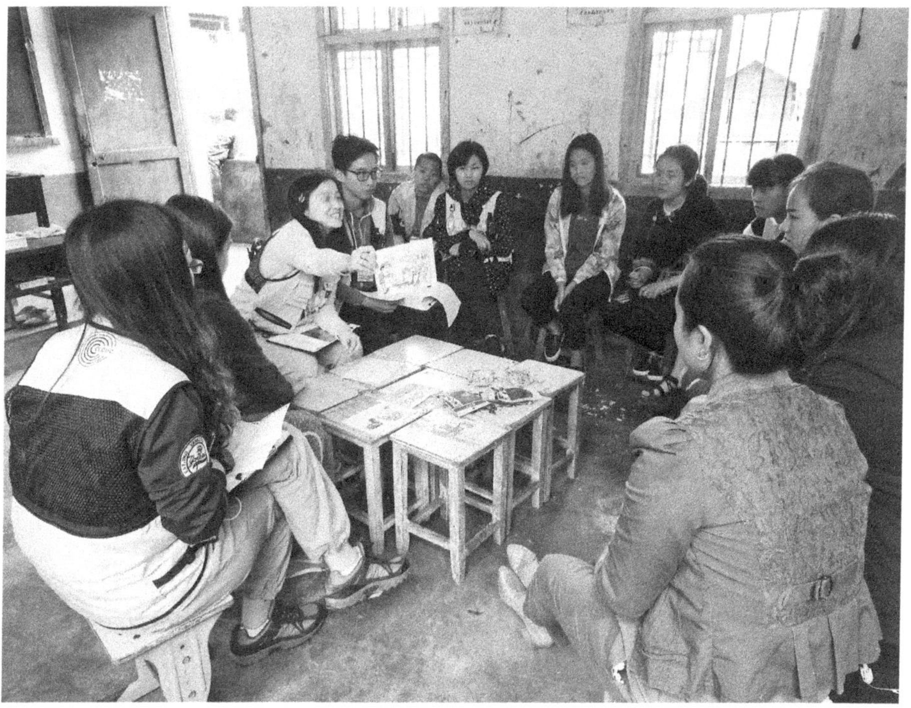

Fig. 6.6 A discussion group with villagers.

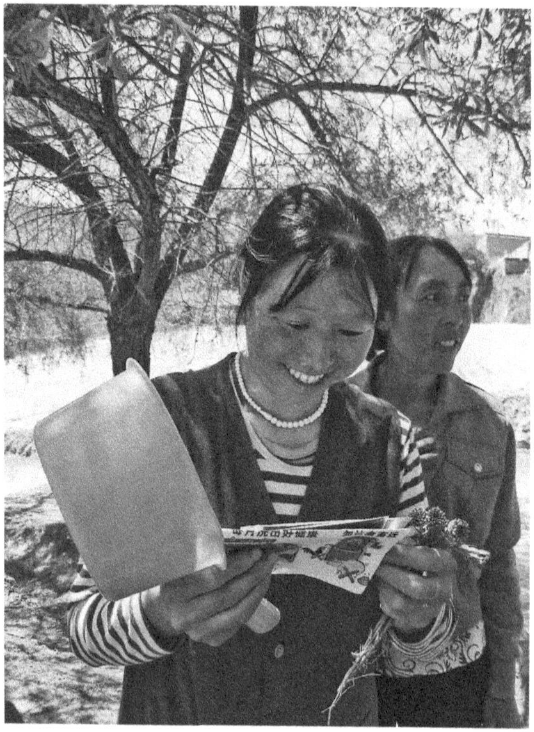

Fig. 6.7 Distribution of souvenirs to villagers.

Workshops

1. These activities have the advantage of involving more interaction with the villagers, but the preparatory work is more complex and the venue and time for the workshop and venue crowd control have to be well planned;
2. Villagers may be mobilized to offer additional workshops to their fellow community members to reinforce the health messages beyond the project period.

Dramas/shows/games

1. An overall programme plan (with an outline script at least) should be developed;
2. Team members should invite villagers to participate in the performance
3. Performance rehearse should be organized with the local interpreters and key community leaders to seek their feedbacks of the local relevance and content appropriateness of the planned events.

Group discussions

1. Group discussions facilitate better understanding of villagers' perspectives about a health issue. These events also allow villagers the opportunity to discuss and compare the health

consequences of their behaviours. If the community is very dispersed and gathering residents in one spot may be difficult, several small group discussions can be held;

2. The group size for discussion should be around six to eight people to allow sufficient time for each participant to express their view in a larger group;
3. Of note, group discussion may be dominated by talkative and opinionated villagers, hence special attention should be paid to manage the process.

Souvenirs

1. Souvenirs should have a practical use to the community.

2a. They should be durable (e.g. rechargeable or manually powered torches are preferable to battery torches in rural villages);

2b. Souvenirs such as hand fans, mugs, and calendars can carry printed health messages to sustain the effect of the education campaign afterwards;

3. If there is a large quantity of souvenirs, allow sufficient time to, for example, seek sponsorship, purchase the items, and arrange for transportation to the project site;
4. Choose locally produced or purchased souvenirs as far as possible to enhance their usefulness for local people and the possibility of getting replacements in the future.

Contingency plans should always be made when engaging in field-based activities. For example, when preparing health communication materials, duplicate copies should be made. The extra set should be kept separately during transportation (by storing it in separate luggage or in a different car) to minimize loss or damage during this process. If there are no losses or damage, the extra set can be given to the villagers for long-term display (Box 6.1).

Right timing

Health promotion activities should not interfere with the villagers' daily lives. Villagers' daily routines, festivals, communal activities, and seasonal farming schedule should be identified to maximize community participation in the health intervention activities. Contingency plans should be made in case of inclement weather conditions, or a wedding/funeral within the community. Safety of the participants should always be the priority. For instance, if the households in the village are scattered, activities should not be held at night as the villagers may need a long time to walk back home.

Suitable activity venue

The characteristics of the activity site should considered: Should the event location be indoors or outdoors? Can it support the expected number of participants? What is the availability of electricity, light, and amplifiers? If indoors, the safety and of the site should be investigated; while for outdoor sites, particular attention should be paid to environmental factors (raining and temperature extremes), the acoustics, amplifiers, illuminating devices, and canopies may need to be prepared to ensure the villagers can fully engage in the activities. It is also essential to prepare a contingency plan in the event of weather conditions.

Box 6.1 The impact of urbanization on traditional rural villages

The impact of urbanization on the villagers' daily lives should be noted. For traditional Dong minority-based villages in China, a self-sustaining ecosystem has been developed and thus no latrines are built. Villagers defecate near the family fish pond and human faeces serve as the fodder for fish, while these fish will be consumed later as food for the villagers. However, with urbanization, increased consumption of food from outside sources (including processed food and packaged food), increased population movement, and urbanized living style, risk of good safety has changed. The building of public toilets in the village could strengthen villagers' health awareness, but they may have a higher risk of consuming fish that are fed with contaminated fecal materials in the ponds.

Another more significant example of the way modernization may have changed lifestyles is in the care of children. Disposable items, such as diapers, are now commonly used. It was found in the CCOUC's rural projects that the use of diapers is causing a serious problem in waste management, and the residue of the plastic diapers may take up to 450 years to degrade if they are directly buried without treatment. If it is found in the needs assessment that diapers are making up a large portion of the disposed waste, the health promotion team may consider encouraging the villagers to use their traditional diapers during the health promotion activities. This could not only preserve their culture, but also reduce the chances of skin allergies, and it is more environmentally friendly in the sense that it reduces waste production.

Understanding the target audience

In general, the effectiveness of the health promotion depends on the characteristics of the target. For instance, simple and straightforward diagrams should be used to convey the message as education and literacy levels in rural areas are generally low and so a large amount of text should be avoided in the preparation of teaching materials. In designing the activities, the local customs, taboos, and etiquette should also be considered. For example, the materials designed for communities with Islamic beliefs should not include pigs or wine bottles.

Working in a conservative community will also require a conservative approach some examples include dressing decently and being sensitive toward community topics such as reproductive health (Box 6.2).

6.3.8 Health education activities

Activity promotion

It is important to communicate with the village chief, or the person in charge of the village, in advance and to let them help in arranging the activity and informing the target audience. The project details should be confirmed again with the village chief after the team's arrival at the site. The health promotion team may seek help from the village chief

Box 6.2 Misconceptions in disaster preparedness

Health promotion teams should remember that almost all villagers in disaster-prone communities may have some personal experience in disasters. Opinions of the villagers should be respected and programme members must be sensitive to their choice of words to avoid triggering villagers' recall of unpleasant memories.

Of note, however, experiences might not directly correlated to disaster preparedness.

Misconception of villagers in disaster-prone regions will affect how a community prepares for a disaster. According to a survey conducted in a remote Hui community in Gansu (Chan *et al.*, 2014), although previous disaster exposure was significantly associated with the perception of living in a high disaster risk area (OR = 6.16), only 10.7% of these households actually prepared for a disaster by means of possessing a disaster emergency kit. This shows that when implementing a project on disaster preparedness, the impact of the disasters and the importance of disaster preparation should be emphasized regardless of the direct experience of the communities. This could ensure that the villagers will take the necessary actions for disaster preparation.

to announce the details of the activity (such as the time, location, and target audience) during a village meeting and encourage the villagers to participate.

Before the activity, promotion team members should provide reminders about time, place, and event descriptions. Additional consideration should be planned for those in need (e.g. asking neighbours to accompany persons with disabilities to the activity venue).

If possible, public communication materials of the event should be put up in places where they can be readily seen, or at the gathering places of the villagers (e.g. ancestral halls, markets, schools, clinics, water sources, and resting places) at least a week before the activity, so that the villagers can have time to adjust their schedule to attend the activity.

Activity flow

The health promotion event may include various sessions and an activity manager should be assigned to coordinate the programme. If the event involves performance, a team member should be chosen to act as the master of ceremonies to ensure that the event runs smoothly. Contingency toward activity hindrances should also be discussed such as a poor weather, unfavourable response from the villagers, and electricity power failure.

Venue crowd control

Event crowd control is an essential aspect of organizing any public event, which also includes managing participant arrival, providing event-related information such as the rundown, and safety and emergency management.

Of note, rural women usually join an activity along with young children. If women's active participation is expected, helpers should be assigned to look after the children to enable their full participation. The youngsters can be entertained with simple educational activities, or the team members can encourage them to draw using coloured pens and paper that have been provided. In a community with many elderly individuals, it is particularly important to consider the needs of those with mobility disabilities. For example, if the activity is of a long duration, seats should be made available for older people and the disabled. It is also essential to pay attention to the weather and take this into account when scheduling outdoor activities.

Interpretation

Language barriers and cultural differences present major barriers to health promotion programmes in the diverse environments in rural Asia. Frequently, low levels of education mean that the villagers can only use local dialects and are unable to speak the country's official language or the team's spoken language. Therefore, those in charge of the project should coordinate with the village chief or a village representative beforehand, to arrange for interpretation, and to communicate with the villagers who are responsible for oral translations. All of the health promotion activities should be rehearsed at least once, to ensure that the interpreters understand the content of these activities. For promotions targeting women, a woman who can understand both the spoken language used by the promotion team and the local dialect should be sought to assist with the translation.

Communication skills

Some tips on how to communicate efficiently to villagers include:

- Be sincere and friendly;
- Use clear pronunciation and a suitable volume and tempo;
- Maintain eye contact with the audience;
- Present the message in a concise and clear manner (e.g. use straightforward words and concrete examples, and avoid jargon);
- Explain the message in a systemic way, from simple concepts to difficult ones, and emphasize the key points (e.g. by raising questions for the villagers to reinforce their memories);
- Use appropriate body language;
- Use appropriate teaching materials (e.g. use different colours or diagrams to highlight the key points), which are sensitive to cultural, religious, and gender factors;
- Keep checking whether the villagers understand the information, and listen carefully to what they say and to any questions;
- Admit if you encounter something that you do not know.

Distribution of souvenirs and materials

Health promotion team members should consider whether the materials or souvenirs that will be distributed in a health promotion activity are appropriate in the rural context. For example, asking villagers to pack extra batteries for a portable radio or torch in a disaster preparedness kit is not feasible, either economically or practically. Also, avoid distributing expensive souvenirs or materials in order to prevent the villagers from reselling them, which is not their original purpose (Box 6.3).

Box 6.3 The attitudes and principles of practitioners and volunteers

Never make casual promises

Before making any promise to the local community, field workers should examine whether they have the ability, time, and interest to fulfill and complete the expressed commitment.

Be respectful

Field workers should always respect local culture, language, religion, and customs. Before arriving at the village, the field team should attempt to understand the cultural and socioeconomic context of the village, such as the daily routines and habits of the villagers. If the target is an ethnic minority community, attention should be paid to the taboos of the ethnic group (e.g. food preference/avoidance/customs).

Be humble and thankful

Field workers should neither impose their own values on the villagers, nor behave paternalistically as though they are bestowing a favour. They should be thankful that the villagers have made time to participate in their activities which, in turn, allow them to learn about the rural culture and lives. Field workers who have the chance to stay at a villager's home will not only experience the local culture, but also have the opportunity to chat with the locals. The local wisdom acquired in this way is something that the practitioners cannot learn from textbooks.

Be a role model

If field workers want to promote health and disaster preparedness, they should act out the ideas they advocate. For example, they should not smoke or drop litter in the village, and they should also collect and classify all the waste they produce and take it away when leaving the village.

6.3.9 Health education team pre-departure preparation

For field-based health education team to function effectively, the following positions are recommended for basic field team organization:

- Team leader
- Logistic manager
- Medical support coordinator (doctor, nurse, or qualified first-aider)
- Project base support coordinator

The following are important components for pre-departure preparation.

1. Team formation:
   - Recruit and confirm with all the involved members at least six weeks before departure and collect their personal information including their full names in valid travel documents (e.g. passports), and their dates of birth to facilitate all logistic arrangements for the trip (such as purchase of travel insurance and air ticket). All information should be kept confidential to protect privacy and be compatible to rules, regulations, and guidelines of the organizing agency.
   - All travel documents should be checked for expired date/validity and confirm visa status. The copies of the travel document will only be used during crisis or emergency situations. Everything should be deleted after trip completion.
   - Invitation letter/collaboration notes from co-organizers and supporting organizations must be obtained to facilitate community endorsement and access. Such documents can also serve as proof of the collaboration in case of emergency.
   - A project invitation letter should be prepared for all the members to facilitate their application for leave from school/work and visa application.
2. Health preparation and contingency plan:
   - Identify potential health risks, infectious diseases, and hazards at the field site (e.g. altitude sickness and dengue fever).
   - Check and confirm the availability of relevant health facilities in the province/county, and check and update the locations, contacts, and update plans with collaborating partners for emergency purpose.
   - Prepare a detailed list of members' medical information (include drug and food allergy, long-term medication requirements, and blood type) to highlight the specific medical needs of each member for the medical support team.
   - For the specific trip context, the medical support team should prepare and review the appropriateness of first aid kits to ensure medical resources are up-to-date and sufficient to cater for the medical needs of the whole team.
   - Team leaders should prepare a contingency/repatriation plan for medical emergencies in the field that might require sending members to local medical facilities or transferring them to other places to receive medical treatment.
   - The group leader/medical support team should provide a health briefing to all members prior to departure, including information about:
     - o The potential health risks and the necessary precautions in the field;
     - o Immunization/vaccination, allegy (food/drugs), regular medicatioin use, and blood type; and
     - o Preparation of their own medications/medical resources to address their medical needs in the field.
   - Collect the emergency contacts of all the members, and pass the information to the supporting team. If there is an emergency case, the supporting team can assist with contacting family members.

3. Insurance:
    - All members should be required to purchase relevant travel insurance prior to departure.
    - All members should take precise note of the terms and conditions and coverage when buying insurance, including the coverage of baggage loss, flight delays/cancellations, activities at remote areas, and so on. Also, get to know the required documents for claiming procedures.
    - For projects in remote locations, it is recommended to include details of the relevant International SOS or equivalent, for emergency medical support and coverage.
    - No matter whether the insurance is purchased collectively or individually, the team leader is responsible for obtaining all the insurance information from every member and forwarding to the supporting team before departure. It should include the insurance company name, insurance policy number, and emergency call phone number.
    - If the insurance is purchased collectively, the team leader should prepare a copy of the insurance policy and distribute to all the team members, and brief all about the insurance coverage and emergency assistance hotline.
4. Team equipment:
    - Prepare a full team packing equipment list with details of the quantity, brand, and model number, and so on. The full team equipment list should be kept by the team leader and the supporting team for local custom inspection if necessary.
    - Prepare an equipment and packing list with the help of team members at least three weeks before departure (Fig. 6.8).
    - Maintain proper records of equipment, and ensure the equipment is in proper functioning and labelled for identification purpose. Replace lost or damaged items if necessary.
    - Prepare a full team final packing equipment list with details of the quantity, brand, and model number, and so on. The full team equipment list should be kept by the team leader and the supporting team for local custom inspection if necessary.
    - Prepare a banner with the organization's logo for group photos for team management, promotion, and publicity purposes.
    - Assign equipment to each team member to be cared for and carried.
5. Communication tools:
    - Compile a trip book. The content should include trip objectives, a detailed itinerary, information of the co-organizers, team members, and their respective emergency contact numbers, emergency assistance hotlines (e.g. airline company, insurance company). The trip book should be distributed to all the team members, supporting staff team, and emergency contacts before the field trip.

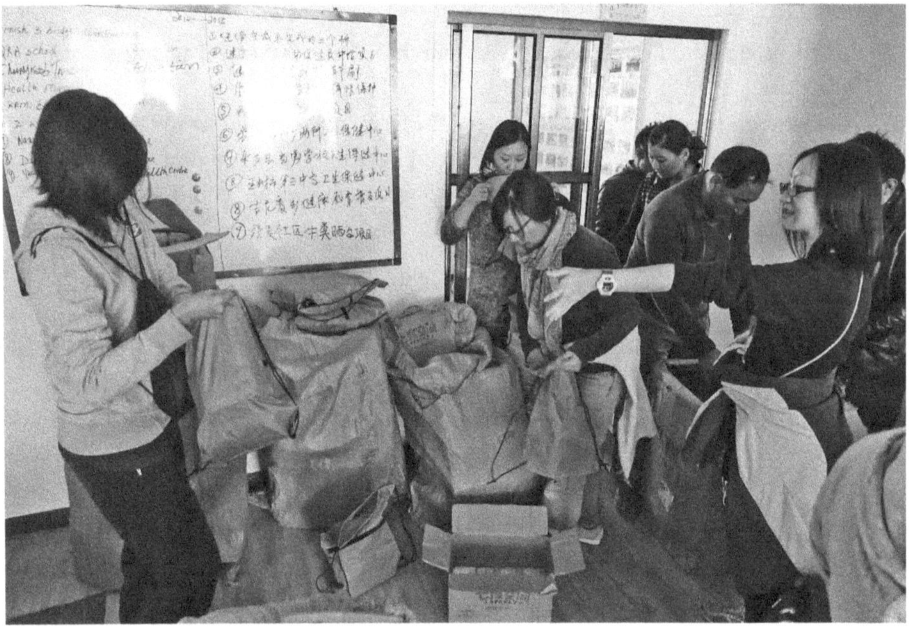

Fig. 6.8 Team equipment being checked before the team sets off.

- Equip team leaders with a mobile device with data roaming services so as to facilitate communication during an emergency or crisis.
- If walkie-talkies are chosen as field communication tools, a technical briefing should be given to all field team members before departure to ensure all devices are functioning properly and appropriate usage is discussed.

6.3.10 Safety concerns

Personal safety in field activities is crucial for the success of field-based activities. Unfortunately, incidents can still happen that threaten safety but these situations can be properly managed to minimize injuries.

6.4 Actual implementation

6.4.1 Before departure

Field-based activities in rural community have multiple risk factors that may affect personal safety. Security guidelines/protocols related to the project should be developed by the organizers to provide support in emergency situations. If there are possible safety concerns, the organizers must clarify the situation with the co-organizers and field partners. For example, if field partners avoid enquiries, the reply time is longer than usual or there is no reply, it could mean that the stability of the context needs to be reviewed. If there has been any incident which might have jeopardized the safety of team members, the trip should be cancelled.

Team members should also be responsible for finding out more about the project site before departure to enhance their safety awareness. If they notice some information which may affect the safety risk assessment, they should inform the leader or the teammate-in-charge. Group members with a non-medical background should be encouraged to obtain accredited first aid training such that they can provide timely first aid if any person gets injured or ill during the trip. Contingency and evacuation plans should be discussed with the team members before departure to the field (Box 6.4).

6.4.2 Briefing before departure

Before departure, briefing sessions should be held to allow understanding of the logistic arrangement of the trip, interaction among team members, and the opportunity for organizers to explain the project details—the division of labour, what to do, how to do it, and when. Three compulsory briefing sessions should be arranged for team members.

First briefing session

The first briefing session should be convened four to six weeks before departure. The first briefing session aims to introduce project objectives, team compositions, target audience, and outcome expectations. To manage project expectations specifically, the content of the briefing session should include:

- The project background, site background, trip objectives, any previous documents/assessment results of related trips;
- The code of conduct, role, and responsibility of all participants;
- Personal equipment, safety, and health-related preparation for the field activities;
- Project trip expenses and insurance coverage;
- Trip schedule/timetable;
- Grouping and task allocation;
- Packing list.

Box 6.4 The discipline and safety of team members

Field team should be expected to follow team safety protocol to protect the safety of the team and team members. To learn more about what should be done to keep safe at the project site, browse the 'Stay Safe–Volunteer Security Link' interactive learning platform created by International Red Cross and Red Crescent Movement: https://www.ifrc.org/learning-platform

Second briefing session

The second briefing session should be organized three to four weeks before departure. For health intervention projects, team members should have already discussed the content and programme planning. If more than one working subgroup are being formed, the organizers should try to facilitate and coordinate communication among subgroups of the project, allow exchange of information, and streamline the planning process.

In summary, the second briefing session should include the opportunity to discuss:

- Field activities content planning;
- Division of labour and details of the task assignment; and
- Specific training in trip-related tasks, e.g. household survey method, language training, and so on.

Third briefing session

The third briefing session should be organized three to four days before departure. The aim of this meeting is to:

- Confirm details of logistics related to place, time, and date of departure;
- Distribute team clothing, name badges, luggage tags, team materials and appliances, and the trip book; and
- Remind of the key updates of the project site.

6.4.3 In the field

Upon arriving at the site, the leader, or member-in-charge, should pay respect to the leadership of the local community (Fig. 6.9). Potential safety threats (such as a tense local atmosphere, and local substance abuse situation) as well as potential environmental hazards (e.g. landslides, fires, and other disaster risks) should be reviewed. In remote context when the team may be required overnight stay in the community, a daily safety review should be conducted. In addition, the project team should always ensure their visit will be environmentally friendly and waste-free to the local community. A buddy system (pairing up of team members) should also be set up to ensure safety. Team members should be advised not to bring too much cash or valuables. The leader, or the person in charge of the backup team, should ensure all the team members wear appropriate team clothing and a name badge while working at the project site. Any security concerns by team members should be taken seriously and the team should also consider whether there is a need to:

1. Activate the evacuation plan; and
2. Prepare additional security measures to guard the site where the team stays (e.g. enhanced lighting and barriers).

Team members should always have their travel documents, air tickets, drinking water, food, cash, whistles, and torches at hand. They should stay within communication reach in the field.

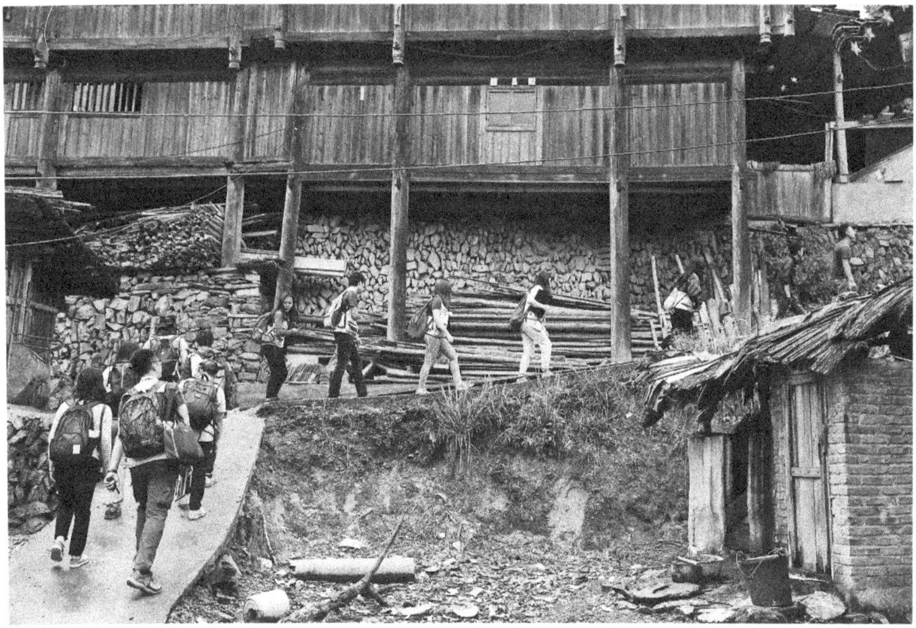

Fig. 6.9 A health promotion team arriving in a rural village.
Reproduced by kind permission of Emily Ying Yang CHAN, Copyright © 2017 Emily Ying Yang CHAN.

The team leader, or the member-in-charge, should have daily communication with the base support team. The backup team should keep track of the safety conditions at the project site and inform the team of any updates.

6.4.4 **Programme implementation**

To effectively implement field programmes (Walley and Wright, 2010), key issues to be examined include:

1. Might there be a pilot project and/or scaling up of an existing project?
2. Are there phases within the programme?
3. How will the implementation be achieved?
4. Is sustainability a concern? And if so, how?

Among the issues described above, a phase-based implementation action plan should be attempted whenever possible. It offers the participants an opportunity to chart and monitor the programme progress. In addition, adjustments might be made during a phased implementation to better reflect the field reality and also to promote local ownership and programme sustainability. In recent years, the importance of local co-shared responsibility, ownership, programme compatibility with the local norms and values, training and motivation of local staff, obtaining support for key stakeholders and opinion leaders of both genders, collaborating with local agents, and follow-up support offered by the programme implementers. Potential guidelines and support tools should also be developed to tailor the programme to the local surroundings and requirements.

6.5 Post intervention

6.5.1 Implementation and monitoring

Programme organizers should ensure the participants understand the aims and roles, responsibilities, and tasks. During the implementation, the project organizers should train team members in relevant skills and provide regular appropriate support and encouragement to motivate members to achieve the set goals (Fig. 6.10).

Processes and outcomes of a project should be monitored during implementation in accordance with the pre-designed plan. Adjustment of the implementation should also be carried out whenever necessary and feasible to ensure the goals and objectives are addressed.

6.5.2 Monitoring and evaluation consideration

Monitoring and evaluation are important tools in supporting the implementation and measuring the quality of a programme. Their main goal is to demonstrate changes resulting

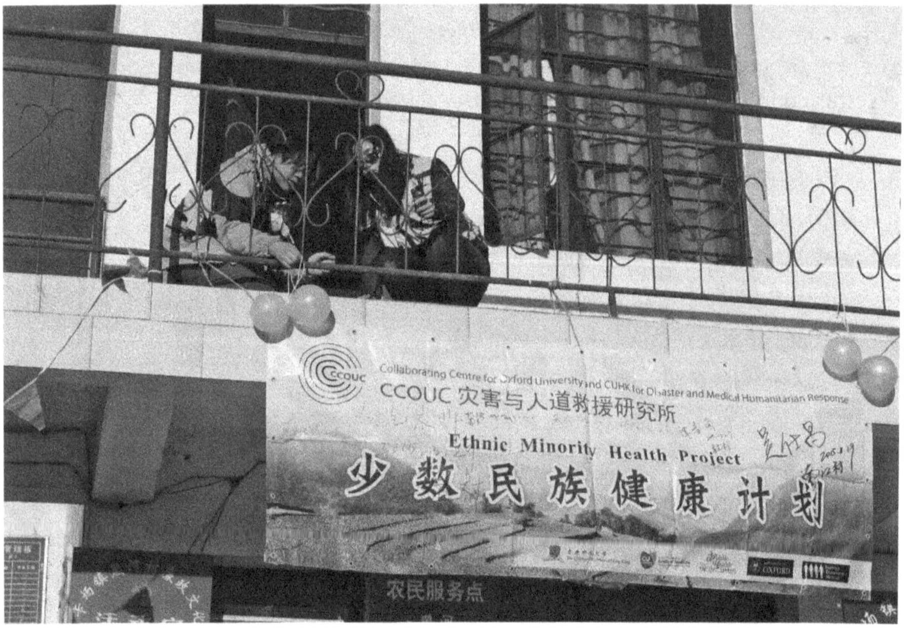

Fig. 6.10 Implementation of a health promotion programme in a Chinese rural village.

from the programme, and to determine if the programme is cost-effective. Regardless of the methods, the typical evaluation criteria include determining the effectiveness, efficiency, and processes. The objectives, methodology (i.e. design, data collection, and analysis), and staff involved should be decided at the beginning of the programme when the priorities and objectives are set.

6.5.3 Evaluation

Evaluation is an essential to programme management. The focus of an evaluation is to assess and review the project intended output and health outcome. Project results might be in terms of knowledge gains, changes in attitudes and behaviour, and community mobilization to address the health issues of interest. Evaluation also facilitates the improvement of the project design and increases the sustainability of the project. Both quantitative and qualitative methods may be used for the process. Specifically, qualitative evaluation tools, such as focus groups, help organizers find out the contributing factors to the success or failure of a project. In order to maintain transparency and accountability, project organizers should share the evaluation report with the sponsors and co-organizers of the project for reference.

6.5.4 Post-activity reports

The field team should always aim to share activity results and the related research findings with the villagers and the global academic community. Dissemination of experiences and lessons learnt will enable not only good practice, but also prevention of mistakes/pitfalls to be made by counterparts.

6.6 Alignment between global policies and field activities

Since the millennium, a number of international policy initiatives that may support the building of bottom-up health and disaster risk reduction programmes in Asia have been developed.

6.6.1 Millennium Development Goals (2000–2015) and Sustainable Development Goals (2016–2030)

The *Millennium Development Goals* (MDGs) (UN, 2016) were created as the overarching development framework for the world in 2000. During 2000 to 2015, although major strides in socioeconomic and human development have been reported, children from the poorest 20% of households, compared to those from the wealthiest 20%, were still twice as likely to have stunted growth, and four times as likely to drop out of school in the developing regions. Also, the under-five mortality rates are almost doubled for children in the poorest households when compared to children in the richest areas. In rural areas, only 56% of births are attended by skilled health personnel, compared with 87% in urban areas. Additionally, about 50% of the people living in rural areas lack improved sanitation facilities, as compared to only 18% of the people in urban areas. About 16% of the rural population do not use improved drinking water sources (compared to 4% of the urban population).

Following 15 years of progress and breakthroughs of the Millennium Development Goals mandate, the *Sustainable Development Goals* were adopted by UN Member States in September 2015 and will become one of the key global development goals to strive forwards for the next 15 years until (2030) (UNDP, 2016). When compared with its MDG predecessor (2000–2015), the SDGs embody a far more ambitious agenda and seek to bring the global civil society together to achieve their broad mandate. SDGs consist of 17 goals and 169 targets, which cover areas ranging from poverty, inequality, and health to sustainable consumption, environmental conservation, and climate change. The momentum surrounding the SDGs must not be understated: in addition to being a rallying point for mobilizing action, the actual content of the SDGs will shape the context of international development in the coming 15 years. For more information related to the SDGs, please see the related websites: https://sustainabledevelopment.un.org/?menu=1300.

6.6.2 Sendai Framework for Disaster Risk Reduction (2015–2030)

Global climate change, unplanned urbanization, increased income disparities, and environmental degradation are crucial factors that will increase the economic cost of disasters in the twenty-first century. To manage the impact of natural disasters cost-effectively, disaster risk reduction (DRR) must be made a priority for new policy making.

Disaster preparedness and DRR activities might be organized at the individual, household, community, and global levels. In recent years, the strategies and policies to address disaster preparedness have evolved from a purely 'top-down' to increasingly 'bottom-up' approach. The Hyogo Framework for Action (HFA) and the Sendai Framework are examples of top-down approach to resilience building at the global level, the promotion of community disaster health risk literacy and the implementation of early warning systems are examples of community-based, bottom-up disaster preparedness activities.

Adopted by the Member States at the Third United Nations World Conference on Disaster Risk Reduction in March 2015 in Sendai, Japan, the Sendai Framework for Disaster Risk Reduction represents a landmark framework which prioritizes DRR and resilience building within disaster management (UN, 2015). This framework creates a roadmap for countries across the world in reducing disaster risk and minimizing life loss, and enhancing livelihoods and health (Aitsi-Selmi *et al.*, 2016). Through the Sendai efforts, substantial reduction of damage to the economic, physical, social, cultural, and environmental assets of persons, businesses, communities, and countries is targeted. New risks will be prevented and existing disaster risks will be reduced through the implementation of integrated and inclusive economic, structural, legal, social, health, cultural, educational, environmental, technological, political, and institutional measures that will prevent and reduce exposure to hazards and vulnerability to disaster, as well as increasing preparedness for responses and recovery, and thus strengthening resilience.

Four priority action areas have been identified:

1. Understanding disaster risk
2. Strengthening disaster risk governance in order to manage disaster risk
3. Investing in DRR programmes for resilience purposes (Hemstock *et al.*, 2016)
4. Enhancing disaster preparedness for effective responses, and incorporating Build Back Better principles in the recovery, rehabilitation, and reconstruction processes

To support the assessment of global progress in achieving the outcomes and goals of the Sendai Framework, the following seven global targets have been agreed:

1. Substantially reduce global disaster mortality by 2030, with the aim of lowering the average global mortality figure by 100,000 between 2020–2030 compared to 2005–2015;
2. Substantially reduce the number of affected people globally by 2030, with the aim of lowering the average global figure by 100,000 between 2020–2030 compared to 2005–2015;
3. Reduce the direct economic losses from disasters in relation to the global gross domestic product by 2030;
4. Substantially reduce disaster damage to critical infrastructure and the disruption of basic services, among them health and educational facilities, including developing their resilience by 2030;
5. Substantially increase the number of countries with national and local DRR strategies by 2020;
6. Substantially enhance international cooperation in developing countries through adequate and sustainable support to complement their national actions for the implementation of the framework by 2030;
7. Substantially increase the availability of, and access to, multihazard early warning systems and disaster risk information and assessments by 2030.

The notion of disaster health risk management proposed by WHO highlights the need for the proactive management and prevention of the health impact of disasters by both the health and non-health sectors. This all-hazard approach encourages the formulation of a standard, comprehensive emergency management system that will address the health needs that are common to all types of emergencies. The introduction of the 'public health emergencies' concept in the International Health Regulations created in 2005 signifies a formal and legally binding regulation for natural and man-made hazards that is of unique significance to disaster preparedness at the global level. It attempts to minimize the unnecessary loss of health that results from service gaps and the lack of coordination of relief assistance in more fragmented and hazard-specific emergency response systems. Last but not least, the human security approach to health provides a highly relevant paradigm for conceptualizing the public health emergency and disaster preparedness in the development of global policies that have a direct influence on the allocation of relief resources, and the rights of states to claim such resources when meeting the rising challenges in medical and humanitarian responses in the decades to come.

Table 6.3 Issues to be considered for evaluation design

Principle of evaluation design	Definition	Example
Relevance	An interviewee's perception of the project relevance and relationship with him/her and the community.	Was the promotion activity relevant to your community?
Importance	An interviewee's perception of the project's importance to his/her health.	Use 'yes', 'no', 'not applicable', or 'not known'. Excessive drinking.
Knowledge/Concept	Judging an interviewee's awareness of some specific areas of health knowledge.	Which of the following is/are correct? Excessive drinking will cause fatty liver disease. Fatty liver disease can occur even after giving up smoking.
Self-efficacy	An interviewee's perceived ability to persist or control the process of behavioural change.	Do you think you can quit smoking?
Practice/Intention	Understanding an interviewee's daily routine before an intervention, whether he/she has the intention to change behaviour. Does he/she finds it difficult to practise the relevant good health behaviour after the intervention?	Have you ever attempted to quit smoking? Are you in the process of quitting smoking? Do you wish to try to quit the habit of smoking?

6.6.3 Health Emergency and Disk Risk Management (H-EDRM)

The intersection of health and disaster risk reduction (DRR) has emerged in recent years as an interdisciplinary field of paramount human consequences. Throughout several landmark UN agreements adopted in 2015-16, including the Sendai Framework for Disaster Risk Reduction 2015–2030, the 2030 Sustainable Development Goals (SDGs), the Paris climate agreement and the New Urban Agenda (Habitat III), health is recognised as an inevitable outcome and a natural goal of disaster risk reduction, the cross-over of the two fields is no doubt essential for the successful implementation of the Sendai Framework. Health Emergency and Disaster Risk Management (H-EDRM), as a joint venture of this cross-over, has emerged as an umbrella field that encompasses emergency and disaster medicine, DRR, humanitarian response, community health resilience, and health system resilience. The five focuses of H-EDRM research agenda include: 1) an all-hazards approach that incorporates the full spectrum of hazards; 2) a holistic all-needs approach, including physical, mental, and psycho-social health and wellbeing; 3) research and interventions facilitated during all phases of a disaster; 4) disaster risk identification for populations with specific health needs such as children, people with disabilities, and the elderly; and 5) research on and the building of health resilience in all communities.

Key challenges in this field include redundant research, lack of strategic research agenda, limited development of multisectoral and interdisciplinary approaches, deficiency in the science-policy-practice nexus, absence of standardized terminology and meagre coordination among stakeholders.

6.6.4 Paris Agreement

In December 2015, the twenty-first Session of the Conference of the Parties (COP21) convened in Paris, France, and the Paris Agreement was adopted on 12 December. It is the latest step in the evolution of the UN climate change framework and it builds on the work undertaken under the United Nations Framework Convention on Climate Change (UNFCCC) since its adoption in 1992.

The central aim of the Paris pact, which was agreed by 197 countries/parties, is to keep a global temperature rise for this century well below 2 degrees Celsius above pre-industrial levels, and to drive efforts to limit the temperature increase even further to 1.5 degrees Celsius. It also aims to strengthen the ability of countries to deal with climate change impacts. The mobilisation of US$100 billion a year to help developing countries cope with climate change is to extend beyond 2020 and the figure will be considered a floor until 2025. A higher financial goal is to be adopted before 2025.

Under the agreement, each country has to set its own national cap for emissions, known as "nationally determined contributions" (NDCs). The pledges made by the countries are voluntary and not legally binding, but their progress will be reviewed every five years.

The Paris agreement came into force on 4 November 2016, 30 days after the date on which at least 55 parties to the Convention deposited their instruments of ratification, acceptance, approval or accession, which accounted for at least 55% of the total global greenhouse gas emissions.

6.7 Conclusion

There are many challenges in implementing bottom-up field-based programmes in rural communities. Field programme management requires meticulous planning and implementation efforts. This chapter has discussed some of the key lessons learnt by CCOUC, and some important international initiatives which may be worthwhile to use in aligning the potential programme objectives. It should be noted that many of these international policies and efforts will also benefit from the relevant experiences and lessons learnt in the field. Communication of results through reports, scientific findings, and case studies should be attempted whenever possible to share the valuable experiences gained.

References

Aitsi-Selmi, A., Murray, V., Wannous, C. *et al.* (2016). Reflections on a science and technology agenda for 21st century disaster risk reduction. *Int J Disaster Risk Sci*, **7**, 1–29.

Belbin, R. M. (1993). *Team Roles at Work*. Oxford, UK: Butterworth-Heinemann.

Chan, E. Y. Y., Kim, J. H., Lin, C., Cheung, E. Y. L., Lee, P. P. Y. (2014). Is previous disaster experience a good predictor for disaster preparedness in extreme poverty households in remote Muslim minority-based community in China? *J Immigr Minor Health*, **16**, 466–72.

Guidry, M., Vischi, T., Han, R., & Passons, O. (2001). *Healthy People in Healthy Communities: A Community Planning Guide Using Healthy People 2010*. Office of Disease Prevention and Health Promotion, Office of Public Health and Science, U.S. Department of Health and Human Services. Available at: http://atfiles.org/files/pdf/healthycom.pdf (accessed 6 March 2017) [Online].

Hadridge, P. (2001). Strategic approaches to planning health care. In: Pencheon, D., Guest, C., Melzer, D., & Muir Gray, J. (eds), *Oxford Handbook of Public Health Practice*, pp. 342–7. Oxford, UK: Oxford University Press.

Hemstock, S. L., Buliruarua, L.-A., Chan, E. Y. Y., *et al.* (2016). Accredited qualifications for capacity development in disaster risk reduction and climate change adaptation. *Australasian Journal of Disaster and Trauma Studies*, **20**, 15–34.

Howard, G., Bogh, C., Goldstein, G., *et al.* (2002). *Healthy Villages: A guide for communities and community health workers*. Geneva, Switzerland: WHO. Available at: http://www.who.int/water_sanitation_health/hygiene/settings/hvintro.pdf (accessed 7 January 2017) [Online].

Khosh-Chashm, K. (1995). Healthy cities and healthy villages: how to tackle health and environmental problems in urban and rural areas. *Eastern Mediterranean Health Journal*, **1**, 103–1. Available at: http://applications.emro.who.int/emhj/0101/emhj_1995_1_1_103_111.pdf?ua=1 (accessed 26 January 2017) [Online].

Mahler, H. (1981). The meaning of health for all by the year 2000. *World Health Forum*, **2**, 5–22.

Tuckman, B. W. (1965). Developmental sequence in small groups. *Psychol Bull*, **63**, 384–99.

United Nations (UN) (2015). *Sendai Framework for Disaster Risk Reduction 2015–2030*. Available at: http://www.preventionweb.net/files/43291_sendaiframeworkfordrren.pdf [Online].

United Nations (UN) (2016). *The Millennium Development Goals Report 2015*. Available at: http://www.un.org/millenniumgoals/2015_MDG_Report/pdf/MDG%202015%20rev%20(July%201).pdf (accessed 27 January 2017) [Online].

United Nations Development Programme (2016). UNDP support to the implementation of the 2030 Agenda for Sustainable Development. Available at: http://www.undp.org/content/undp/en/home/librarypage/sustainable-development-goals/strategy-undp-support-to-the-implementation-of-the-2030-agenda/ [Online].

Walley, J., & Wright, J. (2010). *Public Health: An Action Guide to Improving Health*, 2nd Edition. Oxford, UK: Oxford University Press.

World Health Organization Regional Office for the Eastern Mediterranean (WHO/EMRO) (1990). *Environment health in rural and urban development and housing: a collaborative framework and strategy for WHO technical cooperation in the Eastern Mediterranean* (document EM/ES/410-E). Alexandria, Egypt: WHO/EMRO.

World Health Organization Regional Office for the Eastern Mediterranean (WHO/EMRO) (1994). *Report of the second WHO/EMRO Healthy Cities Conference, Hammamet, Tunisia* (document WHO-EM/PEH/466/E/L/07.94/115). Alexandria, Eygpt: WHO/EMRO.

Chapter 7

Issues in rural health and key messages for health and disaster risk reduction education programmes

A healthy community should have a safe and hygienic environment, with access to basic well-being-maintaining facilities and services. Key messages for education programmes related to water management, indoor environment, waste management, health-promoting behaviour, and disaster health risk reduction are presented in this chapter. Examples from the Ethnic Minority Health Project (see also Chapter 1: Introduction) will also be employed to illustrate how bottom-up resilience towards health and disaster risk in these rural communities might be established.

7.1 Water and health

Water is essential to maintain human health and well-being. Nevertheless, depending on water availability, different communities may adopt different health protection practices. In regions with scarce water resources, water storage, rainwater purification, and improving water use efficiency may be the primary strategies. In regions with sufficient water resources, water source protection and proper sanitation-related behaviours (such as handwashing) may be the main objectives of health promotion programmes. In general, safe water supply provision should satisfy the principles of quality, quantity, accessibility, cost, and reliability. According to the *Humanitarian Charter and Minimum Standards in Humanitarian Response* of the Sphere Project (2011), three major standards for water supply are advocated. These include access to water, water quality, and water facilitates.

7.1.1 Water supply standard 1: Access and water quantity

Communities should have safe and equitable access to sufficient quantity of water for drinking, cooking, and the maintenance of personal and domestic hygiene. Public water points should be at reasonable proximity to households to fulfil their minimum water requirement for sustaining well-being.

7.1.2 Water supply standard 2: Water quality

Water should be safe to use for cooking and personal and domestic hygiene without posing any significant health risks (see Fig. 7.1). Drinking water safety in turn depends on various factors such as water management, transportation, and storage.

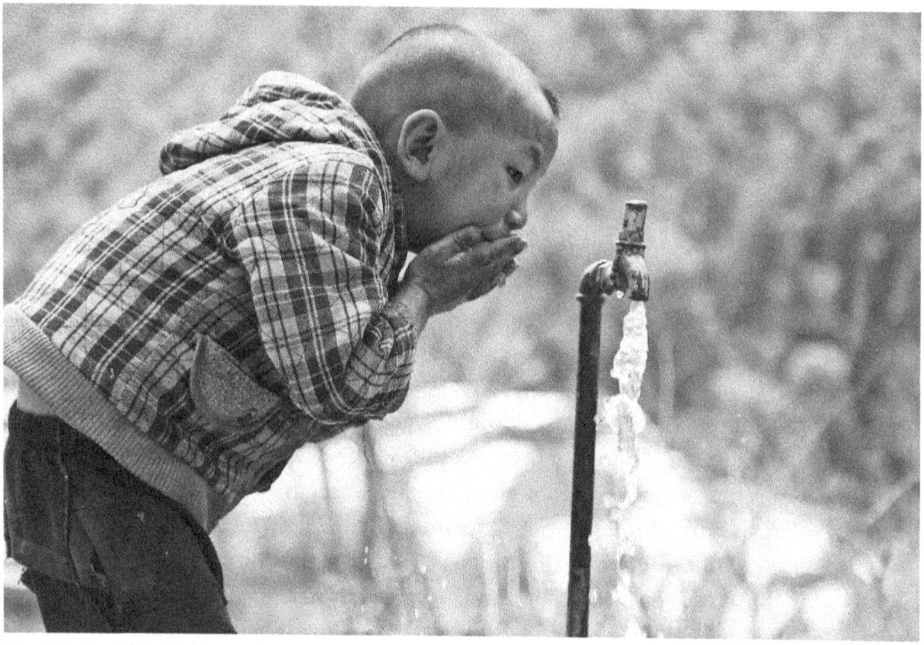

Fig. 7.1 A child drinking unboiled water directly from the tap.

7.1.3 Water supply standard 3: Water facilities

Water for regular drinking, cooking, and personal hygiene should be collected systematically and stored in appropriate facilities. Of note, drinking water should be safe at the point of consumption Box 7.1.

7.1.4 Key aspects for 'water and health' to be investigated during field needs assessments

The following pointed related to water source should be examined during the early assessment phase.

Quality

- Locations and quality of each of the sources of drinking water
- Presence of contamination or potential sources of water contamination (e.g. infrastructure, behaviours, and so on)
- Local patterns and habits of water obtainment, storage, and utilization
- The effectiveness of handwashing practice to protect health, which depends on the quality of water; and
- Prevalence and local management of diarrhoea and waterborne diseases

Box 7.1 Basic water need for survival

The amount of water used by individual depends on age, climate, society, culture, and activities. Under normal conditions, everyone should have daily access to at least 25 L of water for drinking, cooking, and personal hygiene. People with health problems will require additional water to maintain health (Howard, 2002). The minimum standard of water need among people affected by disasters and conflicts is shown in Table 7.1.

Table 7.1 Minimum standard of water usage among victims affected by disasters and conflicts

Water requirement	Reference amount of water usage
Survival	2.5–3 L daily
Hygiene	2–6 L daily
Cooking	3–6 L daily
Total	7.5–15 L daily

Source: data from The Sphere Project. *Humanitarian Charter and Minimum Standards in Humanitarian Response*, 3rd Edition, http://www.spherehandbook.org/en/the-humanitarian-charter/, accessed 11 January 2017, Geneva: The Sphere Project, Copyright © 2011 The Sphere Project.

Quantity

- The amount of water each person can have regular access to

Accessibility

- Accessibility of drinking water sources (time required to access); and
- Accessibility of each household to water sources (identify access barriers for the vulnerable community subgroups)

Reliability

- Reliability and regularity of water supply

Cost

- Daily cost for a household to obtain its water supply

The following section describes four possible health interventions related to water. These include water source protection, water quality management, proper handwashing and hygiene, and the preparation and application of *oral rehydration solution* (ORS) for diarrhoea.

7.1.5 Water source protection

Potential health risks

Most water sources in the rural Asian region are open and unprotected. Livestock, such as cows or horses, may drink from the same sources as villagers and the risk of animal faecal contamination is high. Most bacteria and parasites in the water, such as Trichuris trichiura (whipworm), Ancylostoma duodnale (hookworm), and Ascaris lumbricoides (roundworm), are invisible parasites and may cause serious infectious diseases if ingested by human beings. Furthermore, unsafe hygiene habits of infected villagers may promote disease transmission and cause grave preventable public health problems. In post-disaster settings, water source protection is crucial to avoid disease outbreaks in a densely populated suboptimal environment of displaced people.

Key aspects to be investigated during field needs assessment

A low health risk water source should have the following features:

- The water source should be completely covered or sealed.
- There should be no direct contact with surface water during water collection. If the water source is from an underground well, a hand-pump would be preferred. If it is necessary to use buckets, the water collection tool should be cleaned regularly and kept out of contact with the ground.
- Direct contact between the water source and human extremities (e.g. hands) should always be avoided.
- The water source should be distant from contamination sources (such as toilet/latrines, waste dumpsites, and animal faeces).
- There should be no accumulation of stagnant water within five metres of the water source.

Suggested health intervention messages

1. Drinking water may be contaminated during storage, collection, transport, or usage.
2. Water storage facilities should have covers to prevent potential contamination. Measures to protect open water sources are needed to avoid contamination by animals. Villagers should not defaecate, take showers, or wash anything near the water sources (see Fig. 7.2 and Fig. 7.3).
3. Measures to protect open water sources are needed to avoid contamination by animals.
4. Villagers should not defaecate, take showers, or wash anything near the water sources (see Fig. 7.2 and Fig. 7.3).
5. Wash the cups, buckets, strings, or containers which are used for water collection and storage regularly (at least once a month).

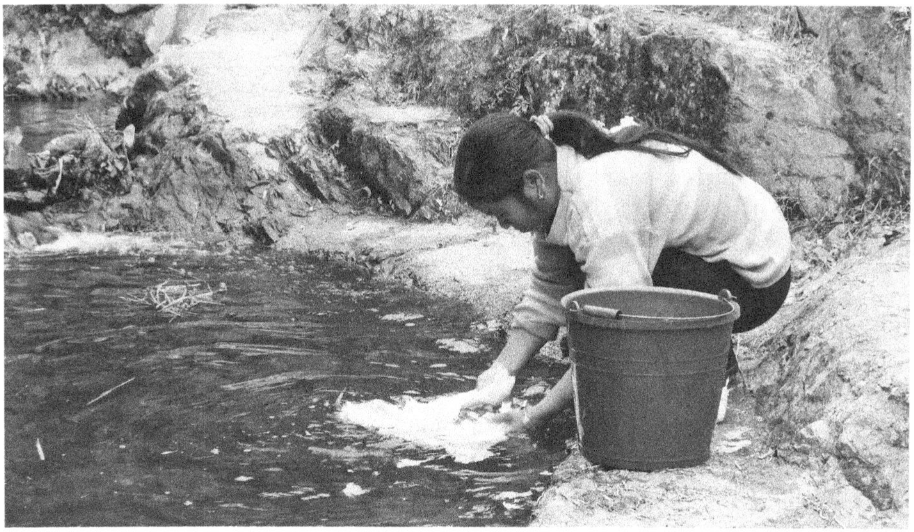

Fig. 7.2 In rural Asia, the same water source might be used simultaneously for drinking and washing.

Reproduced by kind permission of Emily Ying Yang CHAN, Copyright © 2017 Emily Ying Yang CHAN.

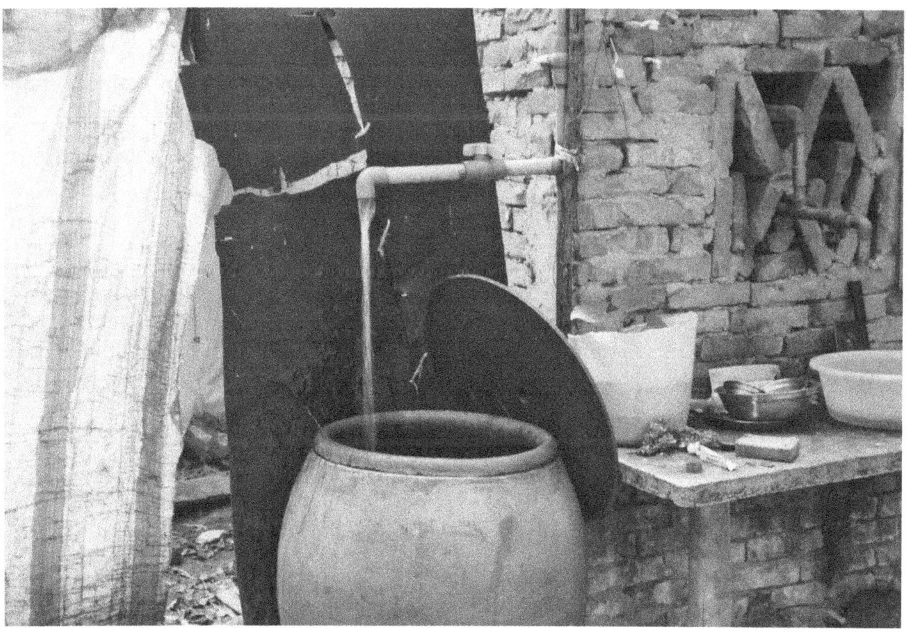

Fig. 7.3 Water storage tanks with lids help sustain water quality.

Reproduced by kind permission of Emily Ying Yang CHAN, Copyright © 2017 Emily Ying Yang CHAN.

7.1.6 Water quality management

Potential health risks

People in rural communities may believe their water sources are clean and drinkable without boiling. In summer, villagers in many communities may prefer to drink directly from the river, which is cooler than drinking boiled water. However, with modernization, lifestyle changes, and active travel, water pollution is common and harmful substances like *Escherichia coli* might exist in water that appears to be clean. In addition, in rural communities, increased use of fertilizer may lead to excess unabsorbed nitrogen and phosphorus in soil. Residual fertilizer may blend with rain and river water, which may indirectly contaminate underground water sources. The rural communities also often lack proper sewage and water treatment facilities and water sources are thus easily contaminated by detergent, faeces, and rubbish. As water boiling can destroy most waterborne pathogens (e.g. it kills most insect eggs) and lower the toxicity of chemical waste, it is a key health-promoting intervention in rural communities (Rosa *et al.*, 2010).

Suggested health intervention messages

1. Drinking unboiled water carries health risks.
2. Refrain from drinking directly from water sources, even if water appears clean. Water should also be boiled before drinking.
3. The correct way of processing drinking water is to heat the water to boiling point (100°C) and continue heating it for one more minute.

The following are some useful reference sources which provide further methods of preventing waterborne diseases and purifying water:

- *Healthy Villages: A Guide for Communities and Community Health Workers* published by the World Health Organization (WHO) (Howard *et al.*, 2002);
- 'Minimum standards in water supply, sanitation and hygiene promotion' in *Humanitarian Charter and Minimum Standards in Humanitarian Response* (The Sphere Project, 2011); and
- 'Water treatment' in *Linking Technology Choice with Operation and Maintenance in the Context of Community Water Supply and Sanitation* published by WHO and IRC Water and Sanitation Centre (Brikké and Bredero, 2003)

7.1.7 Proper handwashing

Potential health risks

'Dirty' hands is one of the major routes of disease transmission. Pathogens and parasites can stay on the skin of livestock and; direct contact with livestock can thus transmit the pathogens to humans. Contact-borne diseases and food-borne diseases may also result from lack of handwashing before eating and after toilet use. In addition, common respiratory illnesses which are droplet-borne and airborne may be transmitted if people do not wash their hands after using them to cover their mouths while coughing.

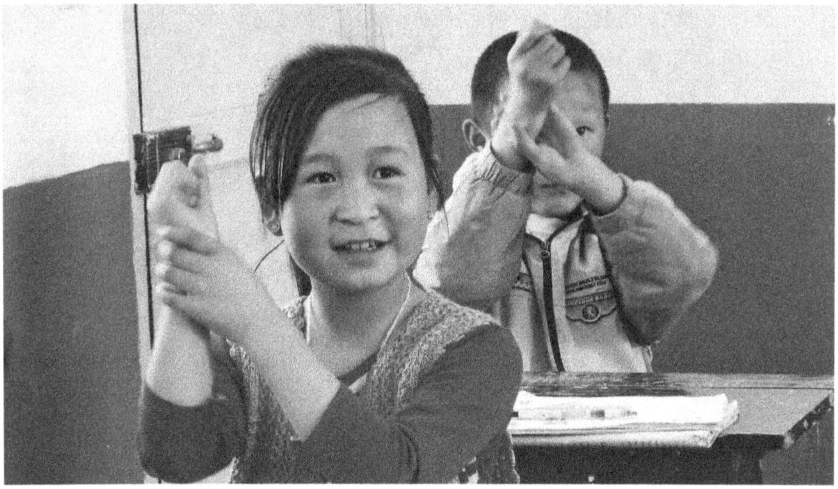

Fig. 7.4 Proper handwashing education session with primary school students.

According to the Ethnic Minority Health Project (EMHP) (see Chapter 1: Introduction) project site surveys across China, approximately a third of the villagers never wash their hands before meals. Health education practitioners however must also consider the context and limitations such as lack of resources and facilities in rural areas. In areas with water scarcity, health education activities might focus on using and regular washing of utensils (such as chopsticks/cultural appropriate utensils), rather than eating with bare hands.

Suggested health intervention messages

1. Health risks and various routes of disease transmission (contact-borne, foodborne, and droplet-borne diseases) are associated with 'dirty' hands;
2. 'Washing hands with soap and clean water' is one of the most effective methods to prevent diarrhoea and contact-borne diseases;
3. Introduction of proper handwashing: It involves the use of soap to clean and rub the palms, backs (dorsum), between the fingers, the backs of fingers, thumbs, fingertips, and wrists for 20 seconds and then rinsing the hands thoroughly (see Fig. 7.4); and
4. Important timing for handwashing should be highlighted, including before meals and after going to the toilet, coughing, sneezing, and coming into contact with animals.

The following references provide some further resources for the promotion of proper handwashing:

- 'Clean hands save lives' webpage of United Nations Children's Fund (UNICEF, 2011)
- 'Global Handwashing Day 2010' song (UNICEF, 2010); and
- 'Handwashing song' for Global Handwashing Day (Trip Creative Services, 2011)

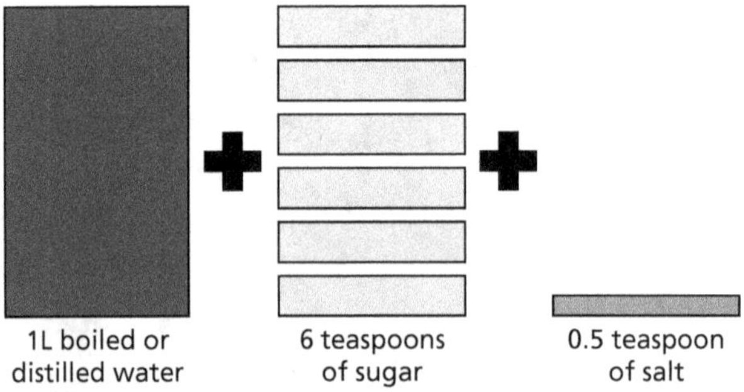

Fig. 7.5 Formula of home-made oral rehydration solution.

Source: data from the World Health Organization. *WHO position paper on oral rehydration salts to reduce mortality from cholera,* http://www.who.int/cholera/technical/en/, accessed 13 Jan. 2017, Copyright © 2017 World Health Organization.

7.1.8 **Oral rehydration solutions**

Potential health risks

Children living in rural areas were 15 times more likely to get diarrhoea compared to those living in the cities (UNICEF and WHO, 2009). In China, during the last decade, contaminated water sources and poor health infrastructure had led to pre-mature mortality of 40,000 children died of infective diarrhoea annually. According to a survey carried out by CCOUC (see Chapter 1), among disease-affected children, less than 40% received treatment from village doctors.

Oral rehydration solution (ORS) is the WHO-recommended treatment for dehydration caused by acute diarrhoea (see Fig. 7.5) in community contexts where self-care might be the only first-line treatment available (WHO, n.d.-e). It is the best non-pharmacological treatment which supports the rehydration of the affected individual with clean fluids and a mixture of electrolytes and a suitable amount of sugar. Although it cannot cure all causes of diarrhoea, ORS helps improve symptoms and support physiological function of the affected individual. It has been shown by UNICEF and WHO to be an effective way to reduce diarrhoea-related mortality by 75% and is suitable for promotion in rural and remote areas (also refer to section 7.5 on disaster preparedness for related information).

Suggested health intervention messages

1. Explain facts and symptoms of diarrhoea, e.g. typically more than three times loose or liquid defecation per day (but take note of variation of individual's bowel habit).
2. ORS is a simple and effective way to treat dehydration caused by diarrhoea.
3. ORS should be taken when vomiting or diarrhoea appears and continue until symptoms disappear.
4. Explain the ORS formula and method of preparing ORS. Highlight that the regimen of ORS may be different for various population subgroups: 1 cup (250 ml) each dose for children; 2 cups for adults. Take six times daily until the diarrhoea subsides.
5. Emphasize the importance of using clean water (distilled/boiled) and clean containers for making the ORS solution.

6. Stress the importance of the maintenance of hand and personal hygiene of both the affected individual and the carer(s).
7. Describe and highlight the importance of seeking medical help if symptoms do not improve after 48 hours or high fever persists.

7.2 Indoor environment

Indoor environmental conditions, together with behavioural habits, may pose a substantial adverse impact on health. Practices such as keeping livestock indoors may increase disease transmission. Inappropriate burning material indoors may exacerbate allergies, or even cause poisoning. Indoor smoking will increase risks of second-hand-smoke-related health issues and the improper installation of wiring in some households increases the fire hazard (see also Fig. 7.6).

7.2.1 Key aspects for the 'indoor environment' to be investigated during field needs assessments

Key focuses for the early assessment phase:

- Basic living context (such as the structure/building materials of houses)
- Location of toilets, kitchen, and cooking fuel storage
- Household ventilation system (windows)

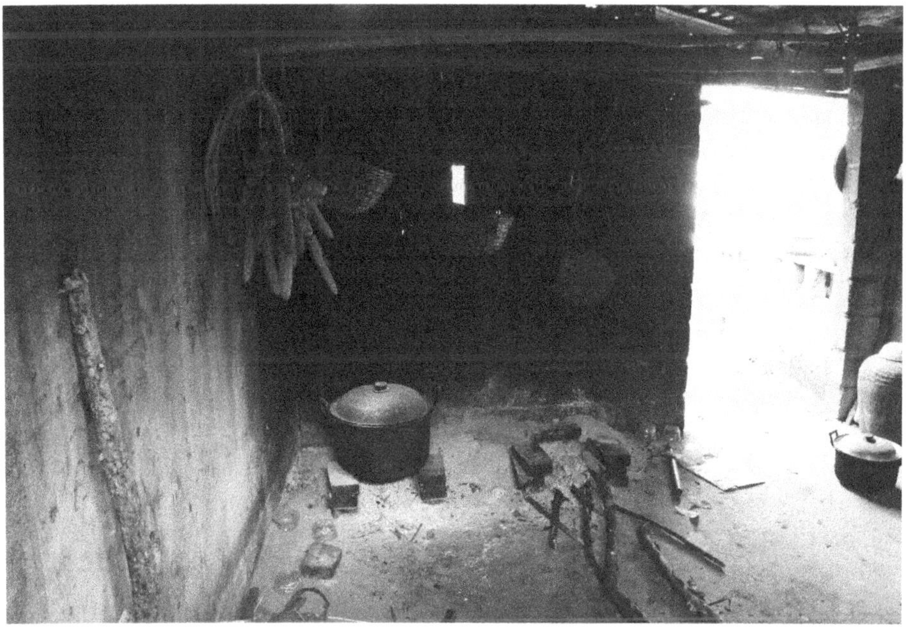

Fig. 7.6 Indoor environment in a rural house in China.

- Household fire prevention facilities
- Household heating and fuel system
- Household infrastructure with injury risks (stairs, open roof, electric wires, open fire sources, and so on)
- Whether there are smokers within the household
- If livestock and humans live within the same household compound:
  - Whether livestock is reared separately from the living quarters;
  - Whether livestock is fenced off from the rest of the living quarters.

Most of the Asian rural communities have experienced rapid changes in material access and increased urbanized living and modernized household amenities. Improved awareness of health and disaster risk reduction associated with indoor environment improvement may improve the overall well-being of a community. The following sections discuss indoor air quality, human-livestock separation, waste management, and injury prevention for rural agricultural-based households.

7.2.2 **Indoor air quality**

Potential health risks

Energy poverty in rural communities often forces village dwellers to use unrefined fuels, ranging from coal, charcoal, wood, animal faeces, and crop waste to plastics. These energy sources have low combustion efficiency (Ruiz-Mercado *et al.*, 2011) and may emit large quantities of pollutants and toxic substances which cause harm to human health (Lewis and Pattanayak, 2012). With a lack of proper ventilation, accumulation of indoor pollutants may cause a variety of human health problems. Underlying diseases such as asthma, pneumonia, and bronchitis might be aggravated and if the toxic level is high, fatal diseases like poisoning or lung cancer might be resulted. Even at its minimum impact, symptoms such as headaches, dizziness, and fatigue affect the well-being of these rural community members. According to the Department of Public Health, Environmental and Social Determinants of Health of WHO (2016), indoor air pollution caused 4.3 million deaths annually, accounting for 7.7% of death from all-cause mortality (see also WHO, n.d.-b, n.d.-c, 2014a). The problem of indoor air pollution as a public health threat is more prominent in countries where there is a lower level of development. In low- and middle-income countries, household air pollution is responsible for almost 10% of mortality, when compared with the 0.2% of deaths in high-income countries (WHO, n.d.-c). Rural women are particularly vulnerable because they are the primary caretakers of their children, cook, and spend long duration in an indoor environment. Children who are exposed to fumes are at an increased risk of developing acute respiratory illnesses, which not only affects their growth, but also increases the chance of diseases like pneumonia. The likelihood of low birth weight and poor growth and development in infants is higher if pregnant women are exposed to cooking fumes daily (Zhang and Smith, 2005). A study conducted in China found that women with prolonged exposure to cooking fumes were 4.1 times more likely to suffer from lung cancer than non-exposed counterparts (Shi *et al.*, 2005). Although there was a lack of data or reports of the impact of indoor air quality on older people and people with disabilities, the health vulnerability of these subgroups should not be neglected.

Suggested health intervention messages

1. Explain potential sources of household indoor air pollution in the target community and their effects on health;
2. Highlight the vulnerable population subgroups (such as extremes of age and people with disabilities) who tend to spend long hours within the indoor environment;
3. Advocate the benefit of improved indoor ventilation (install windows or chimneys; or simply open windows when cooking) to enhance fume discharge;
4. Discuss the possibility of renovation, e.g. separating kitchens and other rooms by walls if possible;
5. Discuss ways of improving indoor air quality:
   a. When cooking must be done in closed environments, minimize the use of 'smoke heating'-based techniques;
   b. Try to avoid overheated 'fried' food methods (e.g. deep frying, which is particularly relevant for rural Chinese and certain South-East Asian households);
   c. Stop indoor waste burning practices (see also section 7.3.1 for household waste treatment); and
   d. Avoid indoor smoking (see also section 7.4.2); and
   e. Improve stoves or fuel quality (e.g. fuel such as corn and honeycomb briquettes which produce less pollutants), thus improving combustion efficiency and reducing the discharge of hazardous substances.

Although infrastructure modification may fall out of scope of most health communication-based projects, raising awareness of the health risks associated with indoor cooking methods would be meaningful to improve well-being. For further information on indoor air pollution and related health intervention measures, refer to the WHO guidelines.

7.2.3 **Human–livestock separation**

Potential health risks

Cohabitation with livestock is common in rural areas (see also Fig. 7.7). Although most farm animals are confined in their own shelters, villagers usually allow their livestock to wander around in human dwellings. This practice not only brings hygiene issues such as bad odours, but also affects well-being of the household. For example, animal faeces can breed flies, while polluted stagnant water on the floor might promote mosquitoe breeding grounds. If hygiene practices and air ventilation within the household is suboptimal, the

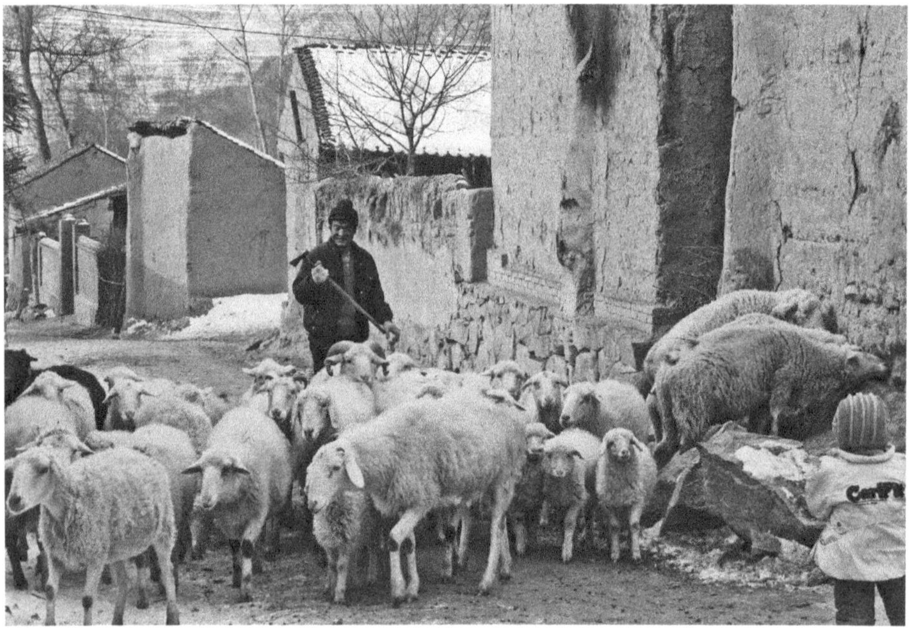

Fig. 7.7 The close contact between humans and livestock in rural Asia.

risk of the infection of villagers will increase (WHO, 2006a). Added to the poor hygiene conditions in rural areas, increased contact between humans and livestock makes humans more vulnerable to zoonotic diseases. Apart from roundworm, hookworm, and tapeworm infections, an outbreak of bird flu in recent years was also caused by frequent contact with animals. Nevertheless, most villagers do not realize the disease transmission risks and adverse health effects of living with their livestock. They include respiratory infections and allergies caused by the dust raised by the animals, and food poisoning and gastrointestinal diseases caused by contact with their faeces. In severe cases, villagers may even be infected with emerging infectious diseases.

While keeping livestock is often one of the main sources of income for rural households, there is evidence that simple measures including human and livestock separation, as well as raising local hygiene standards can effectively reduce the risk of communicable disease outbreaks thus greatly improving villagers' health status (Xiao and Fu, 2006).

Suggested health intervention messages

1. The negative impacts of living in a zoonosis-prone environment.
2. Livestock should be placed at a distance from houses, particularly kitchens and places for water storage. The ideal distance is at least 10 metres.
3. Villagers can create an isolated outdoor area for livestock by erecting simple fences to separate them from humans. Animal faeces should be disposed of carefully or used as fertilizer to prevent contamination of the indoor environment and water storage sites.

4. When promoting human–livestock separation, management of diarrhoea in the section about ORS can be introduced at the same time (see section 7.1, Water and health).

7.3 Waste management

Economic development and income increase can change consumer behaviour of villagers. For instance, there have been increasing varieties of non-biodegradable industrial products in the rural environment. In rural areas, some villages are located far from the main roads. Even if there is any centralized waste collection point, it is hard to transport waste to dumpsters nearby. New infrastructure and policy support in the middle and long term are needed to address this issue, since the construction of such things as centralized landfills or incinerators cannot be achieved in many of the Asian rural communities in the short term. In 2014, China had around 610 million permanent residents in rural villages (National Bureau of Statistics of China, 2015). Assuming everyone produces 0.5 kg of domestic waste per day, there would be 0.11 billion tons of waste produced annually. Health promotion concerning waste management should aim at minimizing the direct health impact of littering and indoor and outdoor waste burning. Health promotion may, however, target the household waste management problem at the source. Health education related to the health consequences of unfavourable waste management practices might help to raise awareness and promote habit-changing behaviours such as overall waste reduction, and reduce indoor waste burning practices.

7.3.1 Suggested health intervention strategies

1. Highlight potential health and environmental risks associated with accumulation of solid waste (see Fig. 7.8);
2. The types and amounts of typical waste produced by the villagers;
3. Examine villagers' waste disposal habits (e.g. discarding, burning, and recycling) by age, gender, and occupation;
4. Current status of waste management;
5. Principles of waste management (see Boxes 7.2 and 7.3);
6. Appropriate concepts of recycling and reuse of waste;
7. Correct methods of handling harmful waste (e.g. pesticide bottles and syringes); and
8. Explore waste disposal mechanism and opportunities in the villages.

7.3.2 Household waste treatment

Potential health risks

In a developed village, waste may be collected systematically and then transported to surrounding landfills. Littering by the roadside is common in rural villages (see Fig. 7.9) and can bring about the following harmful consequences.

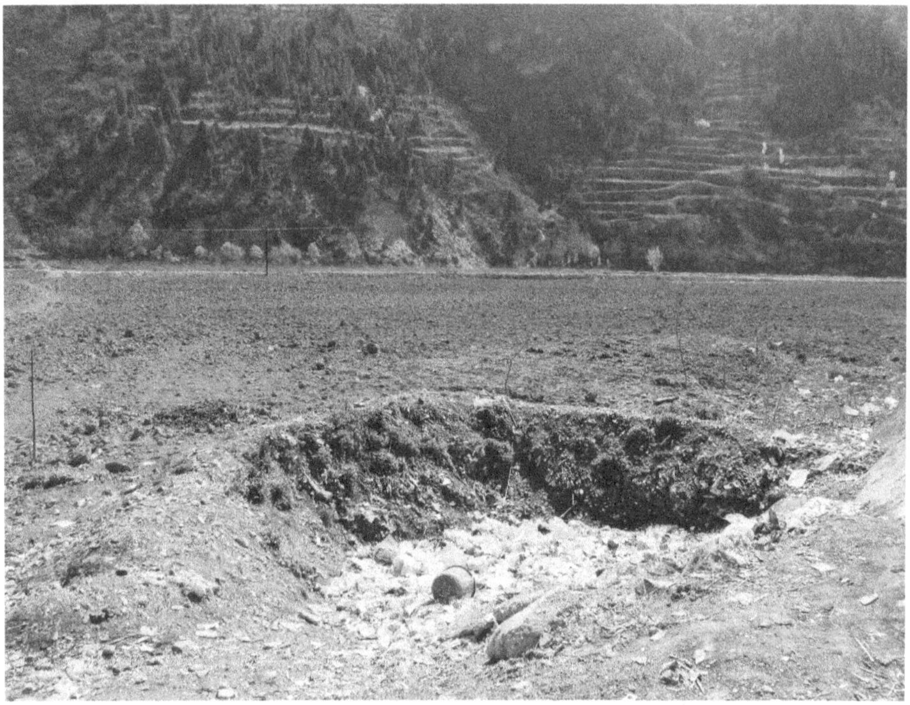

Fig. 7.8 An open area waste dump in rural China.

Box 7.2 The 4Rs principle of waste management

The 4Rs (Reduce, Reuse, Recycle, and Replace) concept is the current international principle on waste management.

'**Reduce**' refers to a reduction in waste volume at source. Currently, many countries carry out projects to minimize waste production, including regulating overpackaging, limiting private sector waste disposal and introducing waste discharge schemes. At household and individual levels, one should reduce buying or storing unnecessary items. '**Reuse**' aims to conserve resources, thus reducing the waste volume. '**Recycle**' is a process that utilizes the useful components of waste and turns them into a second resource through waste management planning. Only waste that can be separated into its separate components may be further recycled. Not only does recycling reduce waste production, but also promotes reuse of useful materials and reduces the equipment and facilities required for waste management. '**Replace**' refers to the use of more environmentally friendly alternatives to replace products that are harmful to the environment such as disposable products. It is important for the reduction of waste volume. Before disposal, efforts should be made to recycle and reuse the materials to be disposed. This is beneficial to waste reduction and facilitates recycling. It also reduces the need for waste management facilities and the burden of waste management.

Box 7.3 Effects of solid waste incineration on the human body and the environment

Potential effects of solid waste incineration include:

- Toxic substances may be released during the process:
  - Dioxin: Burning solid waste might pollute the environment and release dioxin that can accumulate in water and soil, and is readily absorbed by crops. If villagers consume these crops, they can be harmed by the toxic compound. Dioxin can enter the human body via inhalation, causing damage to various body systems such as the nervous system, the reproductive system, and the endocrine system and it can be particularly harmful to children and older people;
  - Benzopyrene: It may cause lung cancer;
  - Suspended particulate matter in smoke: It can enter the lungs by inhalation and prolonged exposure to particulate matter can increase the risk of respiratory tract infection, asthma, shortness of breath, and chest pain; and
  - Carbon monoxide: burning solid waste may generate the toxic carbon monoxide if there is insufficient oxygen or poor ventilation (e.g. indoor areas with all the windows closed or cramped outdoor areas). Inhaling carbon monoxide can reduce the oxygen-carrying capacity of red blood cells, which is particularly damaging for children with developing respiratory systems, older people, and patients with cardiorespiratory illnesses.
- Burning certain types of waste is especially dangerous, such as:
  - Plastic waste (e.g. plastic shopping bags and packaging);
  - Metal, glass, porcelain, and electric compliances.
- Burnable waste should also be collected centrally and burnt at a designated location away from village houses and livestock to reduce the potential harm.

- Environmental impact: waste decomposition can release noxious odours, pollute the air, breed rats, mosquitoes and other pests, and increase the risk of disease transmission. Moreover, many villagers unload their waste by the riverside, which may lead to water contamination. The waste may be ingested by other organisms such as fish, and disrupt the food chain and ecological balance.
- Health impacts: certain rubbish such as sharp objects, metal, and glass debris may injure villagers if they frequently walk with bare feet. Tetanus infection could be a potential serious health risk. Meanwhile, water source and agricultural field contamination by the heavy metal or toxic substances contained in the waste may indirectly and adversely affect their health.

Modern lifestyle changes and living standard improvements associated with economic development have also drastically changed the type of waste produced in rural

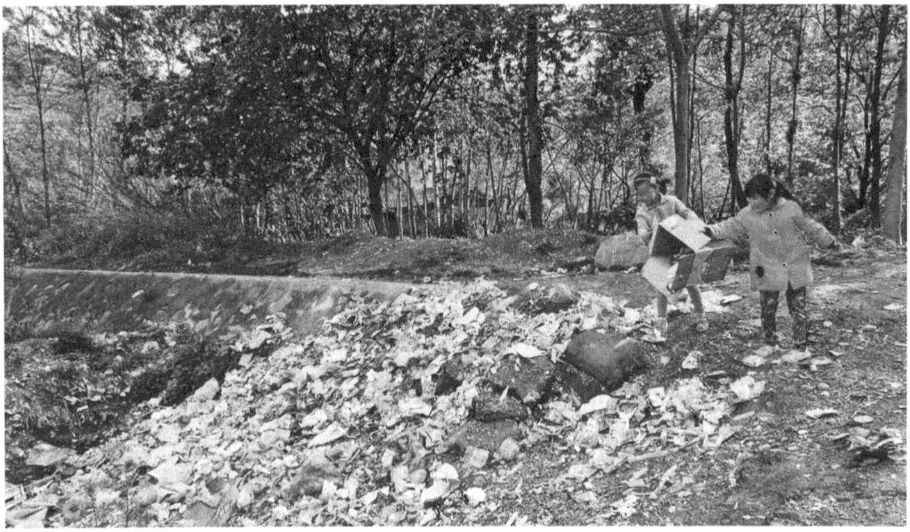

Fig. 7.9 Littering in a rural village in China.

Asia. In Asian rural communities (e.g. in India, China, Pakistan, and Indonesia), plastic food packaging becomes a significant proportion of untreated accumulated wastes. While the typical rural waste management practice is to burn refuse/ accumulated waste substances, plastic burning might may not only release irritating fumes but also produce toxic gases such as dioxins and polycyclic aromatic hydrocarbons, which are recognized carcinogens. The waste ashes may carry heavy metals, which can contaminate water sources and soil. Furthermore, waste burning indoors produces a large amount of inhalable particulate matter and with poor indoor ventilation, villagers face accumulated risks in cardiovascular, respiratory, as well as neurotoxic diseases.

CCOUC's household survey for rural China found that more than 80% of villagers burnt their waste (including plastic waste) at home, but that most of them were unaware of the health risks associated with such practices. Many villages lack the systems and resources for refuse collection and proper waste management. Burning waste thus becomes the primary choice, as this method may reduce the original waste volume by 90% and can also be a source of heat for energy poverty households (see also Chapter 1: Introduction).

Suggested health intervention messages

1. Explain the importance of waste separation. Wastes should be categorized and sorted accordingly. Improper treatment causes harm to environment and human.
2. Highlight that not all rubbish can be burnt. Burning of certain wastes (such as plastics) may case environmental damage and harms human health. Even for rubbish that is suitable for burning, it should be burnt in a designated outdoor area (where it is distant from houses, people, water sources, and animals) to reduce the impact.

Box 7.4 Waste management and vector control

'Reduce', 'reuse', 'recycle', and 'replace' are the four key principles of waste management. Proper waster management will protect against environmental pollution to water, soil, and air. In addition, to promote these practices, the co-benefits of waste management and vector control can be discussed. For example, littering may facilitate vector breeding (such as rats, mosquitoes, and insects) and might give rise to outbreak of vector-borne diseases if not controlled effectively.

3. If waste is buried in public pits, it should be covered with 10 cm of soil every day to prevent mosquitoes, insects, and mice breeding (see Box 7.4).
4. Fences should be built to isolate the waste dumping/management area to avoid children and animals getting in and to prevent accidents.
5. Of note, children's faeces management is important in communicable disease control. As the immunity of children is generally poorer, their excrement is more likely to transmit diseases via the faeco-oral route. Parents and guardians should observe safe disposal management of faeces, clothes washing, and diapers (paper diapers) and the use of bedpans (see Table 7.2).

Further information on waste burial can be found in the section 'Minimum standards in water supply, sanitation and hygiene promotion' in the *Humanitarian Charter and Minimum Standards in Humanitarian Response* (The Sphere Project, 2011).

Table 7.2 Management methods of various types of waste

Type of wastes	Example	Management method
Wastes that can be burnt	Paper, cartons	Always consider reduce/reuse/recycle before refuse. Must incinerate waste in a specific area which is far from houses, people, water sources and animals.
Kitchen waste	Fruit peels, food remains, animal faeces, or other organic waste	Use as animal feed, fertilizer or fuel. Cover the waste container for vector prevention and control.
Wastes that cannot be burnt	Plastic bags, metals, light bulbs, glass bottles, clays, electronic products, batteries	Always consider reduce/reuse/recycle before refuse. Waste should be disposed of in a specific collection point or area for burial. The collecting area should be set at locations which are far from houses, people, water sources and animals.

7.3.3 Agricultural pesticide

Potential health risks

Pesticides are widely used in agricultural systems. Thus, apart from household waste, pesticide waste is common in rural areas. Improper pesticides management can cause toxicity (acute or chronic) and damage the environment (Wang *et al.*, 2011). Four of the top ten pesticide-consuming countries are from Asia. China is the top agriculture pesticide user with a report annual use of 1,806 million kilograms (WorldAtlas, 2016).

Villagers are frequently exposed to pesticides, which account for 200,000 cases of acute self-poisonings globally each year (*The Lancet*, 2017). Of the reported 100,000 cases of pesticide poisoning in China from 1997 to 2003, non-industrial poisoning (including poisoning by accident and suicide) accounted for about 74.61% (Chen *et al.*, 2005).

Of note, pesticide poisoning is currently one of the most commonly used methods to commit suicide in Asian countries and its implication for intentional injury prevention should not be neglected (Chen *et al.*, 2012).

Industrial poisoning made up 25.39% (including the exposure to pesticides due to the absence of protective measures when applying using pesticides). In addition to direct poisoning, pesticide waste also brings environmental and health risks, and damages soil quality, water sources, and crops. Hence, labelling, storage, usage and recycling of pesticides must be handled with care. Pesticides highly toxic or labelled as such should be stored and used in strict accordance with the recommendations on the labels. Common symptoms of mild pesticide poisoning include headache, dizziness, nausea, fatigue, and stomachache whereas severe poisoning may cause muscle spasms, breathing difficulty, coma, incontinence, or even death (Chen *et al.*, 2005; Goldmann, 2004; Proceedings of Asia Regional Workshop on the Implementation, Monitoring and Observance of the International Code of Conduct on the Distribution and Use of Pesticides, 2005; Thundiyil *et al.*, 2008).

Suggested health intervention messages

1. Explain how to read illustrations and toxicity labels on pesticide packaging.
2. People should take protective measures when applying pesticides (particularly spraying). Their faces (eyes, noses, mouths) should be covered and gloves worn to avoid the toxicity of the chemicals.
3. Pesticides should be placed away from water and food sources to avoid contamination.
4. As animal feeds and pesticides might appear similar to flour, to prevent the accidental ingestion or inhalation of pesticides, these materials should not be placed near food for human consumption.
5. Pesticides should be kept out of reach of children. For example, locks are recommended for overhead cupboards with pesticides. The area where pesticides are placed should be labelled with a sign to alert family and community members.

6. Pesticides and their containers should be disposed with care. For example, they should not be discarded in fields or rivers. The packaging and containers can be buried in a landfill or recycled after use.

The following reference sources provide further information on pesticide management:

- Pesticides section under Health Topics on the World Health Organization (n.d.-d) website: http://www.who.int/topics/pesticides/en/
- WHO—Sound management of pesticides and diagnosis and treatment of pesticide poisoning:
  http://www.who.int/whopes/recommendations/IPCSPesticide_ok.pdf
- The International Code of Conduct on Pesticide Management: http://www.who.int/whopes/resources/9789251085486/en/
- 'Regulations on Pesticides Administration' by the People's Republic of China:
  http://www.gov.cn/gongbao/content/2002/content_61560.htm
- Leaflet on 'Safe Use of Agricultural Pesticides' by the Hong Kong Agriculture, Fisheries and Conservation Department: https://www.afcd.gov.hk/english/quarantine/qua_pesticide/qua_pes_safe/qua_pes_safe.html

7.4 Health behaviour

Health behaviour is closely associated with cultural, religious, environmental, and social factors. Underlying behaviour drivers should be examined before designing any intervention for a community. The following section will discuss some key health risk-related behaviours (smoking, alcohol consumption, diet issues for chronically ill patients, safe food handling, and the usage of food labelling and concepts of dental care) and some health communication approaches that may reduce the potential adverse human impact in rural settings. Of note, multiple concepts may be integrated within the same interventions to maximize the co-benefits of the health promotion efforts. For instance, the potential fire hazard should also be mentioned when introducing issues relating to smoking, while the dietary pattern and water safety concepts can be neatly incorporated into the tooth brushing promotion activity.

7.4.1 Key aspects for 'health behaviour' to be investigated during field need assessments

Focuses for early assessment

- Villagers' current smoking status and pattern;
- Villagers' knowledge about health risks associated with smoking, second-hand smoke/passive smoking;
- Villagers' drinking habits and patterns;
- Villagers' dietary and cooking habits and patterns;

- Villagers' knowledge about food labelling;
- Consult village doctors about general disease patterns, chronic disease prevalence, and medical consultation practice; and
- Community diet, snacking patterns, and tooth brushing practice.

7.4.2 Smoking

Potential health risks

Fumes produced from smoking contain more than 4,000 types of chemicals, of which over 250 were proven to be harmful to the human body and over 50 were carcinogenic. An increased risk of cardiovascular and respiratory diseases, cancers, and a low birth weight for their infants are observed among passive smokers and passive smoking causes an estimated more than 600,000 premature deaths annually (WHO Department of Public Health, Environmental and Social Determinants of Health, 2016).

Globally, the WHO Western Pacific Region (which includes the East Asia and the Pacific) has the highest smoking rate. The region accounts for one-third of all cigarettes consumed worldwide, and Asia, Australia, and the Far East are the largest consumers of tobacco (MacKay and Eriksen, 2002). Smoking prevalence among people residing in rural areas is quite significant. Taking Cambodia as an example—around 67% and 80% of men in urban and rural areas are smokers respectively. A similar pattern is also observed in Malaysia. The smoking rates are highest in rural Kelantan and lowest in urban Penang and Sarawak (WHO Regional Office for Western Pacific, 2002).

The Global Adult Tobacco Survey (GATS) conducted in 2010 as a household survey of people aged 15 and older in China, the proportion of smokers among men aged 15 or over was 52.9% (China CDC; 2010). The proportion was higher among rural males (56.1%) than urban males (49.2%). People living in different regions have adopted various smoking practices. In Yunnan Province, where tobacco growing is considered one of the economic pillars of the province, people smoke tobacco in shisha pipes. CCOUC's study also revealed that over half of the villagers did not recognize any difference in the health hazards associated with indoor and outdoor smoking (see Chapter 1). Culturally, it is common for men to greet one another with a cigarette, and most villagers have limited knowledge about the health hazards associated with active or passive smoking.

Suggested health intervention messages

1. Introduce the health risks associated with active and passive smoking for general population and high risk groups (e.g. pregnant woman, people with underlying health problems such as asthma, and so on).
2. Social and economic benefits of smoking cessation should be highlighted. Quitting cigarettes can help improve the health of smokers and the people around them. It can also save money (see Box 7.5).

Box 7.5 Health risks associated with active and passive smoking

Successful smoking cessation programmes often involve long-term smoking counselling services, clinical facilitation, as well as the support of family and friends. For long-term smokers, it is typical for them to experience multiple failures in smoking cessation attempts. However, the potential health benefits of health interventions that address the harm of smoking may be helpful to protect passive smokers in the household. For example, quitting cigarettes can reduce smoking-associated health risks and improve indoor air quality, which means a safer environment for family members. The money saved by giving up smoking can be significant financial resources for their families. Any attempts to initiate smoking should be discouraged as it is difficult to stop once the habit has started (Table 7.3).

Table 7.3 Health risks associated with active and passive smoking

Active smoking	Major carcinogen in cigarettes is tar. Smoking is a major risk factor for various life-threatening cancers: – Oral, pharyngeal and laryngeal cancer – Lung cancer – Oesophageal cancer – Kidney cancer and bladder cancer – Pancreatic cancer – Gastric cancer – Liver cancer – Cervical cancer – Leukaemia Smokers have 10 times higher risk of having lung cancer compared to non-smokers and the risk to heavy smokers is 15–25 times higher. Smoking is also related to cardiovascular diseases (e.g. coronary heart disease, aneurysm, peripheral vascular diseases, and stroke), respiratory diseases, reproductive system diseases, and an increased risk of other diseases (such as macular degeneration).
Passive smoking	Immediate health impacts: – Eye irritation, headache, coughing, sore throat, dizziness, and nausea; – Significant lung function deterioration among adult asthmatic patients; development of asthma among children and older people; and – Reduced coronary circulation after exposure to second-hand smoke for 30 minutes. Long-term health impacts: – An even higher health risk for persons exposed to second-hand smoke than cigarette smokers; – Impaired cardiovascular health and an increased risk of heart diseases and stroke; – Increased lung cancer risk among non-smokers: second-hand smoke has been classified as a Group A carcinogen by the US Environmental Protection Agency, which have been shown to cause cancer in humans; – Pregnant women exposed to second-hand smoke have an increased risk of miscarriage and giving birth to underweight and pre-term newborns;sudden infant death syndrome, as well as adverse effect on the cognitive and behavioural development; and

Box 7.5 Continued

- Infants have a higher likelihood of succumbing to sudden infant death syndrome, as well as adverse effect on the cognitive and behavioural development; and
- Children exposed to second-hand smoke may have decreased lung functions, which may lead to delayed lung development, an increased risk of respiratory diseases and irritated responses such as coughing, mucus hypersecretion and wheezing, a higher risk of otitis media, and deteriorating cystic fibrosis.

3. Introduce ways to reduce the negative impact of indoor air pollution caused by smoking. For example, no indoor smoking, or ensure ventilation before indoor smoking (see Fig. 7.10; see also Box 7.5).

For additional information on smoking and health see the section about tobacco on the World Health Organization website: http://www.who.int/topics/tobacco/en/

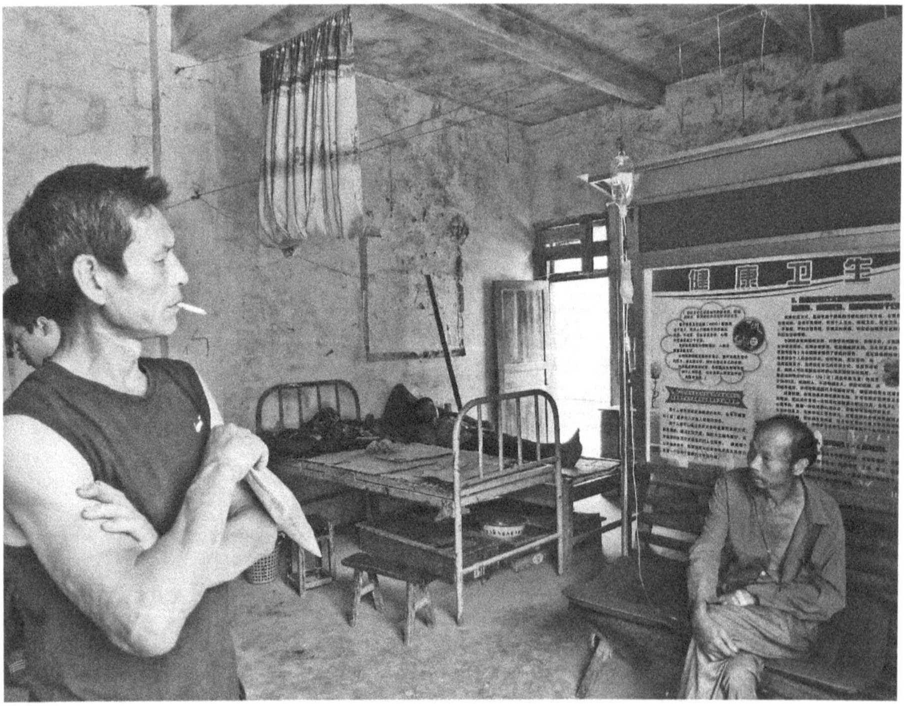

Fig. 7.10 Indoor smoking in a rural village clinic.

7.4.3 Alcohol drinking

Potential health risks

According to the World Health Organization (2015, January), 5.9% of global deaths in 2013 were associated with alcohol drinking. Excessive alcohol use is a risk factor for over 200 diseases, including cirrhosis, liver cancer, gastritis, gastric ulcers, and cardiovascular diseases, as well as mental and behavioural disorders (WHO, 2014c).

In rural villages, alcohol drinking is a common social practice and drinking habits are even more prevalent in some ethnic minority communities. In Mongolia, a national population-based survey was conducted to investigate the knowledge, attitudes, and practices (KAP) on alcohol consumption. Around 50% of males and 30% of females were found to be drinkers. In particular, morning drinking, which indicates a problematic relationship with alcohol, was found most common among males from rural areas (Demaio *et al.*, 2013). A study aiming at examining the alcohol use and consumption (with the Alcohol Use Disorder Identification Test (AUDIT)) in a rural district of Vietnam found that the prevalence of alcohol consumption-related problems was 25.5% among males and 0.7% among women. The study also found that the daily binge drinking rate was 3.6% among males, while such an issue was not identified among females (Giang *et al.*, 2008). Excessive alcohol use, in addition to being harmful to health, can also affect families and social well-being. If excessive alcohol use can be regulated through health promotion, the benefits will extend beyond the drinkers.

Among elders residing in rural India, another study found that regular alcohol intake was seen in 16.3% of the males, comparing with 0.8% of the females (Goswami *et al.*, 2005). A multisite survey on the drinking status of people in 25 provinces of China in 2007, jointly conducted by the China Health Care Association and China Medical Association, found that there was a serious lack of knowledge about drinking, the amount of alcohol that might be safely consumed, the age of drinkers, and alcohol control among Chinese citizens. The proportion of male to female drinkers was 84.1% and 29.3%, respectively, and, among all the drinkers, 65.3% of them had unhealthy drinking status. Only less than 1% understood accurately that drinking could cause physical harm, with over 30% of drinkers did not agree with the statement: 'Binge drinking harms health and it is necessary to control the amount and frequency alcohol consumption.'

A CCOUC field-based survey in its 17 sites (2017) has revealed that drinking patterns in ethnic minority areas of rural China tend to be in form of alcohol abuse than moderate drinking. Findings of alcohol drinking patterns of nine rural areas in China indicated that 58.9% of teenagers start drinking alcohol between the ages of 15 and 18 and revealed concerns about teenage drinking and the need for relevant health intervention (Wang *et al.*, 2012).

Suggested health intervention messages

As with other addictive habits, it is unrealistic to expect a drinker to completely quit alcohol after one episode of public health intervention. Yet, if villagers can understand

Table 7.4 Long-term effects of alcoholism

Physical aspect	Heart failure, high blood pressure, fatty liver (can cause cirrhosis and liver cancer), oesophagitis, gastritis, peptic ulcer, impotence, cancers, injuries, and damaged central nervous system (e.g. memory loss, loss of cognition and decision-making skills, blurred vision, poor response, loss of coordination, and hallucinations)
Psychological aspect	Emotional change, emotional instability, depression, insomnia, suicidal impulses.

Source: data from The Tung Wah Group of Hospitals: Integrated Centre on Smoking Cessation. '*Comprehensive Smoking Cessation Services*', http://icsc.tungwahcsd.org/eng21_s_smoke.html, accessed 01 Feb. 2017. Copyright © 2009 Tung Wah Group of Hospitals.

how alcohol drinking may cause physical harm, there may be augmented intention to reduce excessive drinking. Excessive use of alcohol increases disease risks and accidents and chronic excessive use may lead to irrepairable damage to health. Long-term effects of alcoholism brought about by frequent binge drinking are listed in Table 7.4. Ways to educate people on the dangers of excess alcohol drinking are listed underneith.

1. Drinking cessation may be attempted in stages, e.g. a gradual reduction in the frequency and amount of alcohol consumed. The size of the drinking glass can be changed permanently from large to small. Moreover, one can change the daily drinking habit into three times a week and then one or two times later.
2. Emphasize how excess drinking affects the people who are close to them. For example, they cannot control themselves while drinking and require assistance from others. Drinking may also affect their jobs and emotions and to reduce their ability to control abusive behaviour.

For additional resources on alcohol consumption and health:

- Fact sheet on drinking on the World Health Organization website: http://www.who.int/mediacentre/factsheets/fs349/en/

7.4.4 **Understanding and prevention of hypertension**

Potential health risks

Globally, *hypertension* is one of the most common chronic NCDss in the twenty-first century (see Table 7.5). Until recently, chronic non-communicable diseases (NCDs) such as hyptertension and diabetes mellitus have been regarded as 'diseases of urban people' and 'diseases of wealthy people' but economic prosperity and rapid urbanization have made such ailments increasingly important disease burden in rural areas (see also Chapter 1).

According to WHO guidelines, hypertension is defined as a systolic blood pressure equal to or above 140 mmHg and a diastolic blood pressure equal to or above 90 mmHg. It should be emphasized that hypertension is not diagnosed with a single over-the-limit measurement, but persistent measures of high readings alongside with clinical

Table 7.5 Some examples of hypertension prevalence in rural Asia

Country	Percentage (%)
South India	21.4 (2005–2007)
Bangladesh	13.67 (2009)
Nepal	3.3 (for female only; 2006–2008)
China	23.5 (2012)

Source: data from Kaur P *et al*. Prevalence, awareness, treatment, control and risk factors for hypertension in a rural population in South India. *International Journal of Public Health*, Volume 57, Issue 1, pp. 87–94, Copyright © 2012 Swiss School of Public Health; Khan RJ *et al*. A cross-sectional study of the prevalence and risk factors for hypertension in rural Nepali women. *BMC Public Health*, 13:55, Copyright © 2013 Khan *et al*.; licensee BioMed Central Ltd. This is an Open Access article distributed under the terms of the Creative Commons Attribution License; Khanam MA *et al*. Hypertension: adherence to treatment in rural Bangladesh–findings from a population-based study. *Global Health Action*, Volume 7, 25028, Copyright © 2014 Masuma Akter Khanam *et al*. This is an Open Access article distributed under the terms of the Creative Commons CC-BY 4.0 License; and National Bureau of Statistics of China. *China's Health Statistics Yearbook 2016*. China Statistics Publishing House, Beijing, China, Copyright © 2016.

observation. Since early-stage hypertension has no observable symptoms, villagers, many of whom have no regular health check-ups, are usually unaware of his/her conditions.

In China, hypertension, diabetes mellitus, and cerebrovascular diseases were the top 10 chronic diseases among villagers. Prevalence of hypertension among Chinese rural population was found to be about 18.6% in 2002 and had risen to 23.5% in 2012 (National Bureau of Statistics of China, 2012; 2016). The CCOUC field study found that over 40% of Chinese villagers had underlying chronic disease which required long-term medication. Only half of them could afford to buy medication with their limited resources. Some of the patients thought they could tolerate the symptoms and the disease, or were not willing to seek medical assistance. By the time their symptoms became unbearable and they needed medical support, the disease was usually advanced and complications had developed (see Chapter 1: Introduction).

Suggested health intervention messages

1. Increase awareness and knowledge of unfavourable lifestyles (diet, habits such as drinking and smoking, stressful lifestyle, and so on);
2. Describe how these habits and lifestyles might potentially cause long-term NCDs;
3. Name the common chronic NCDs in the target community;
4. Describe the characteristics of common NCDs and the potential complications (symptoms, physical functional status, care and need costs);
5. Describe hypertension (awareness of most of the cases are asymptomatic, the causes, the disease progress, complication, and the management) (Box 7.6);

Box 7.6 Hypertension

Hypertension is a chronic NCD. The blood pressure of a normal adult should be 90–130 mmHg for systolic pressure and 60–89 mmHg for diastolic pressure. The diagnosis of hypertension cannot be made by a single measurement. Only continuous measurements for a period of time (e.g. measure every morning and night for a week) showing a persistent elevation from normal can be used to diagnose hypertension. The blood pressure of children is generally lower, when compared to adults. Blood pressure depends on factors such as age, body size, sex, and health status and children's normal blood pressure increases with age to the level of normal adults.

For patients with multiple chronic diseases (such as ischaemic heart diseases and diabetes mellitus), their blood pressure may be affected by their diseases.

The symptoms and complications of hypertension include:

Major symptoms: Headache, shortness of breath, dizziness, chest pain, palpitations of the heart and nose bleeds.

Complications: Heart attack, enlargement of the heart and eventually heart failure, stroke, kidney failure, retinopathy.

(Source: WHO)

For more information about the normal value of blood pressure for different ages, refer to the National Institutes of Health (US):

Boys: http://www.cc.nih.gov/ccc/pedweb/pedsstaff/bptable1.PDF;

Girls: http://www.cc.nih.gov/ccc/pedweb/pedsstaff/bptable2.PDF.

For further information, refer to the following resources:

- Section on hypertension under health topics on the WHO website: http://www.who.int/topics/hypertension/en/

6. Understand the major behavioural related risk factors of hypertension include smoking, alcohol abuse and excessive salt intake;
7. Preventive measures for exacerbation of hypertension include regular checks on blood pressure, a low-salt diet, and stable psychological state; Use the food pyramid to explain the importance of a balanced diet (see Fig. 7.11);
8. According to WHO recommendations, every person should limit their salt intake to 5 grams per day; explain what 5 grams of salt might look like according to the local context and literacy level; and
9. If time allows, supplement the intervention with information on smoking, drinking, and healthy diet (see earlier sections 7.4.2 and 7.4.3).

7.4.5 Understanding and prevention of diabetes mellitus

Potential health risks

Diabetes mellitus is a chronic NCD. Rapid changes in diet and lifestyle, excessive consumption of alcohol, and a lack of exercise have contributed to the increase in the prevalence of

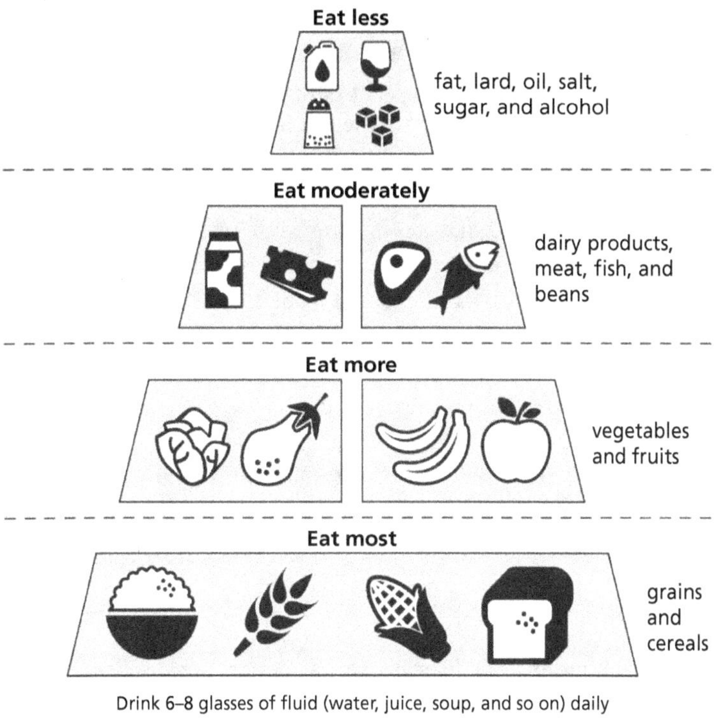

Fig. 7.11 The food pyramid.

Adapted from Central Health Education Unit of the Hong Kong Department of Health. Reproduced with permission from Department of Health, the Government of the Hong Kong Special Administrative Region (香港特別行政區政府衞生署), accessed 01 Mar. 2017, Copyright © 2014 Department of Health, the Government of the Hong Kong Special Administrative Region.

diabetes in rural Asia communities. Asia has experienced a rapidly emerging diabetes epidemic. It is estimated that India and China will remain the two countries having the highest numbers of people with diabetes by 2030. The other four Asian countries—Indonesia, Pakistan, Bangladesh, and the Philippines—are also among the top ten countries for diabetic patient numbers (Ramachandran *et al.*, 2010). Systematic review showed that the rural prevalence of diabetes in low- and middle-income countries was 5.6% in 2011. It has been increasing substantially over time, from 1.8% in 1985–89 (Hwang *et al.*, 2012). For instance, a study conducted among rural Bangladeshi population found that the prevalence of type 2 diabetes mellitus increased from 2.3% in 1999 to 7.9% in the year 2009 (Bhowmik *et al.*, 2013).

The clinical condition is caused by either insufficient production of insulin (type I diabetes) or the body cells are resistant to insulin (type II diabetes). Insulin is a hormone that regulates blood glucose levels such that the body is able to get enough glucose for energy. When the glucose cannot enter the body's cells, it accumulates in the blood and may cause harm to the body (WHO, 2016, November). Symptoms of early diabetes are not obvious. Typical complaints include dry mouth, frequent urination, a frequent sense of hunger, fatigue, weight loss, and a decline in vision. If the disease is not controlled properly, further physical complications such as retinopathy, cataracts, glaucoma, coronary artery diseases, heart failure, strokes, leg ulcers, and even gangrene may occur. Obesity, physical inactivity, smoking, and alcohol abuse are the risk factors of diabetes.

A Korea study examined the urban–rural difference in the prevalence of type 2 diabetes mellitus found that the crude-standardized prevalence was 15.4% in urban areas and 14.5% in rural areas. Type 2 diabetes mellitus was found to be significantly associated with low monthly income among urban communities and with family history among rural residents (Lee *et al.*, 2010). Studies about diabetes in China in 2010 found that diabetes prevalence among Chinese citizens aged 18 or above reached 11.6%, with the total number of diabetic patients being around 113.9 million. The prevalence in males was 12.1% and in females 11.0%. The prevalence in cities was 14.3% and in villages 10.3%. The survey also revealed that only 30.1% type II diabetic patients knew they had diabetes. The control rate was 39.7%. These statistics have resulted in the early diagnosis, early intervention, and early treatment of diabetes becoming one of the prime missions of the public health industry in China.

Suggested health intervention strategies

1. Highlight the importance of lifestyle and a diet in the development of diabetes. Villagers who suspect themselves of having diabetes should be encouraged to seek medical assistance.
2. Explain symptoms and complications of diabetes:
   Symptoms: Dry mouth, frequent urination, frequent sense of hunger, fatigue, weight loss and decline in vision.
   Complications: Retinopathy, cataracts, glaucoma, coronary artery diseases, heart failure, strokes, leg ulcers and gangrene.
3. Emphasize a healthy diet, frequent exercise, the maintenance of a normal body weight, and the avoidance of smoking as measures to prevent or delay the onset of diabetes.
4. Use the food pyramid to explain the importance of a balanced diet.
5. If time allows, supplement the intervention with information on smoking, alcohol drinking, and balanced diet.

For further information on diabetes, refer to WHO (2016, November).

7.4.6 **Food safety management**

Potential health risks

Worldwide, foodborne illnesses caused 420,000 deaths in 2010 and 40% of the food-borne disease burden was among children under five years of age (WHO, 2015b). The South-East Asia Region is one of the regions with the highest burden of foodborne diseases, having more than 150 million cases and 175 000 deaths annually; in the Western Pacific Region, contaminated food caused 125 million foodborne disease cases and more than 50,000 deaths (WHO, 2015, December 3). Food security concerns three main aspects, namely food availability, food access, and food use. Food availability refers to the abundance and sustainability of food; food access examines if people may have enough resources (such as money) to obtain food to maintain a balanced diet; and food use concerns the safety of the source, the safety measures in the food handling chain, and methods of storage, such as storage at suitable temperature.

In rural community, food safety issues often present significant health risks to its population. For example, as electronic appliances become more accessible to villagers, many have refrigerators for food storage. However, as electricity supply can be unstable in rural areas, food may become rotten in refrigerators when the freezing function shuts down. CCOUC's findings indicate that rural community members did not usually wash their hands before and after food handling. Villagers typically would use the same chopping board for both raw and cooked food, which meant cooked food might be contaminated. To protect food safety, WHO (2006b) proposes five key principles: food hygiene, raw and cooked food separation, thorough cooking, food storage at the right temperatures, safe water, and raw material use (see Table 7.6).

Table 7.6 Food safety guidelines

Food safety aspect	Key points to note
Clean	• Wash hands after toilet use • Always wash hands before and during food preparation • Wash and sterilize all used utensils after cooking • Keep the kitchen clean to prevent food contamination by pests
Separate	• Handle raw meat and seafood separately from cooked food • Use different knives and chopping boards for raw and cooked food, respectively • Store cooked food in containers to separate it from raw food
Cook	• Ensure food, especially meat, eggs, and seafood, is fully cooked and safe to eat • Packaged food like canned soup needs to be heated up to at least 70°C before eating • Cook meat juice until it becomes clear and the red colour completely fades • Reheat leftovers before eating
Storage	• Cooked food should not be kept at room temperature for more than two hours • Keep cooked and perishable food in refrigerators (below 5°C) • Even refrigerated food cannot be stored for long. Note about the expiration date. • Food should be re-heated over 60°C before use
Source	• Use safe water • Avoid eating mouldy food • Avoid eating food once the consumption date has expired • Avoid eating raw meat and livestock or birds which died for unknown reasons • Choose food that has been sterilized, such as pasteurized milk • Rinse fruits and vegetables, particularly if eaten raw • Peel fruits before eating

Suggested health intervention messages

1. Prepare before cooking (wash hands, vegetables, and cooking utensils):
   a. Wash hands thoroughly before cooking, particularly after using the toilet or feeding livestock as they may be in direct contact with food.
   b. Food maybe contaminated during the process of purchasing or transport. Even home-grown food should always be washed before being eaten.
   c. Bacteria can breed on cooking utensils, which should thus be washed before use.
2. Separate cooked and raw food:
   a. Cross-contamination between cooked and raw food increases the risk of food-borne diseases. Separation of cooked and raw food during food handling should be emphasized.
   b. Separating cooked and raw food (e.g. not using the same chopping board or knife for both raw and cooked food, washing the related cooking utensils after use for raw food before using them for cooked food).
   c. Proper food storage in appropriate facilities (e.g. refrigerators)
   d. Reheat leftovers before eating.
   e. Introduce the idea of handwashing as supplementary information.
3. Remind villagers about the use of refrigerating devices requiring stable electricity sources: intermittent electricity storage will hamper food quality and potentially risk food poisoning for dairy products.
4. Change of environmental context associated with climate change: traditional preservation practices and room temperature storage of food might need to be modified to adapt to the ambient temperature changes.

7.4.7 **Food labelling**

Potential health risks

Diet is closely associated with human health. Nutrient needs and food preferences vary according to age, gender, and special physiological need (e.g. pregnancy and extremes of age). Traditionally, villagers mainly consumed their crops and livestock and rarely ate pre-packaged food, but with modernization, pre-packaged food has become more popular in rural communities. A food label refers to information and illustrations on food packaging and is not limited to words, pictures, and symbols. It displays the product name, ingredient list, the net weight and specification, producers' and/or dealers' names, addresses and contact methods, production and expiry dates, storage instruction, and food production licence number.

Food labels enable people to understand the ingredients and nutrient value of their food so that they can decide which food they require and how much. However, in rural

Table 7.7 Example of daily intake upper limits of fat, sugar, and sodium for adults

	Daily intake upper limit	Approximately equal to	Excessive intake can increase risk of
Total fat	60 g	4 tablespoons of oil	Overweight and obesity
Sodium	2,000 mg	1 level teaspoon of salt	Hypertension and gastric cancer
Sugar	50 g	10 cubes of sugar/4 tablespoons of sugar	Overweight, obesity, and tooth decay

* With reference to a diet of 2,000 kcal

Source: data from Centre for Food Safety (Hong Kong), http://www.cfs.gov.hk/eindex.html, accessed 01 Mar. 2017, Copyright © 2017 Department of Health, the Government of the Hong Kong Special Administrative Region; World Health Organization. *Guideline: sugars intake for adults and children*, http://apps.who.int/iris/bitstream/10665/149782/1/9789241549028_eng.pdf, accessed 01 Mar. 2017, World Health Organization, Geneva, Switzerland, Copyright © 2015 World Health Organization.

communities, residents generally have a low education level and may not be able to understand the content of the food label and know how the information is related to their health. Educating villagers to understand food labels can reduce food safety risk (e.g. consuming expired food, using incorrect storage methods).

Suggested health intervention messages

1. Explain the importance and how to read the food label on pre-packaged food.
2. Explain the daily intake upper limit of fat, sugar, and sodium for adults (see Table 7.7).
3. Explain how to choose low-fat, low-sugar, and low-sodium food with reference to food labels (particularly to patients with chronic diseases like hypertension, diabetes, and obesity).
4. Explain the concept of expiry date ('use by' and 'best before').
5. Discuss some common storage methods for pre-packaged food that may be relevant to local context.

Note: The food pyramid may also be used to introduce the importance of a balanced diet.

For further information on food labelling:

- Centre for Food Safety (Hong Kong) (n.d.): https:// www.cfs.gov.hk
- *Nutrition Labels and Health Claims: The Global Regulatory Environment* (Hawkes, 2004)
- Harmonisation of food labelling regulations in Southeast Asia: benefits, challenges and implications (Kasapila & Shaarani, 2001)
- *Guide to Nutrition Labelling and Claims* (Ministry of Health Malaysia, 2010)
- *A food labeling guide: guidance for industry* (U.S. Food and Drug Administration, 2009)

7.4.8 Oral health

Potential health risks

With improvement in living standards and changes in diet, people in rural communities, similar to their urban counterparts, are consuming increasing amount of snacks. However, limited concern is placed in dental care and tooth decay is widespread. Tooth decay is damage by gradual erosion which is caused by various factors, with bacteria being one of the major culprits. Bacteria also produce toxins that damage the gingiva surrounding the teeth, causing periodontitis. Worldwide, 60–90% of school children and almost all adults have dental cavities, often leading to pain and discomfort. Oral disease is also prevalent in Asian countries (WHO, 2003, 2012).

In China, 66% of five-year-olds have tooth decay and the prevalence was 28.9% among 12-year-olds in 2005 (Hu, 2012). With population ageing in villages, periodontitis and tooth loss are common among older people and these conditions affect nutrition status, general well-being, and quality of life of the older age groups.

Suggested health intervention messages

1. Explain causes and effects of tooth decay (see Table 7.8)
2. Explain the importance of regular tooth brushing in preventing tooth decay and periodontitis.
3. Teach when and how to brush teeth properly and effectively (see Fig. 7.12)
   a. Brush teeth in the morning and at night for two to three minutes each time. Rinse mouth after meals.
   b. Using a tooth brush to remove the food debris and dental plaque on the surface and between the teeth reduces the bacteria in the mouth and other harmful substances (especially the sugar left over from sweets) and prevents a number of dental problems. The gentle massaging during brushing also stimulates the gingiva and increases blood circulation of the periodontal issues, keeping the oral cavity healthy.

For additional information on oral health see:

- Tooth Club's video showing the correct way of tooth brushing: http://www.toothclub.gov.hk/chi/home_dv_4.html#
- Oral Health Education Unit of Department of Health (n.d.): http:// www.toothclub.gov. hk/
- The global burden of oral diseases and risks to oral health (Poul, Bourgeois, Ogawa, Estupinan-Day, & Ndiaye, 2005)

7.4.9 Domestic accidents and injury prevention

Potential health risks

Injuries patterns are unevenly distributed in the world and remain an important cause of morbidity and mortality although the global injury DALY rates have been declining

Table 7.8 Causes and effects of tooth decay

Causes	Tooth decay refers to a loss of minerals from the tooth structure, which is typically caused by bacteria. The tooth surfaces are frequently covered with dental plaque. Every time food or drinks are consumed, the bacteria in the dental plaque will metabolize the sugars in the food to produce acids, which will demineralize the tooth surfaces. Although saliva can neutralize the acids and slow down the demineralizing process, it requires a long period to function effectively. If we eat and drink frequently, the acid cannot be adequately neutralized by the saliva, and the continuous demineralization will eventually result in tooth decay.
Effects	• Cavities may emit unpleasant odour and cause bad breath. This directly affects normal social life. • Tooth decay may cause persistent pain, which affects appetite, studies, work, sleep, or even general health. • When there is severe tooth decay, the bacteria may spread from the dental pulp to the surrounding periodontal tissues via the apex of the tooth, leading to inflammation or eventually the formation of dental abscesses. • If a tooth is so severely damaged that even precludes pulp treatment, an extraction is necessary. After the extraction, the neighbouring teeth may drift towards the empty space and cause a malalignment of the teeth. • If the milk teeth of children fall out due to decay, it may affect the dentition of permanent teeth such that it affects ingestion. At its worst, decay means permanent teeth cannot grow subsequently.

Source: data from Centers for Disease Control and Prevention (CDC). *Summary of Infection Prevention Practices in Dental Settings: Basic Expectations for Safe Care*, https://www.cdc.gov/oralhealth/infectioncontrol/pdf/safe-care2.pdf, accessed 01 Mar. 2017, US Department of Health and Human Services, Centers for Disease Control and Prevention, National Center for Chronic Disease Prevention and Health Promotion, Division of Oral Health, Atlanta, GA, 2016; Oral Health Education Unit of Department of Health, http://www.toothclub.gov.hk/, accessed 01 Mar. 2017; World Health Organization. *Promoting oral health in Africa: prevention and control of oral diseases and noma as part of essential noncommunicable disease interventions*, http://apps.who.int/iris/bitstream/10665/205886/1/9789290232971.pdf, accessed 01 Mar. 2017, World Health Organization, Geneva, Switzerland, Copyright © 2016 World Health Organization.

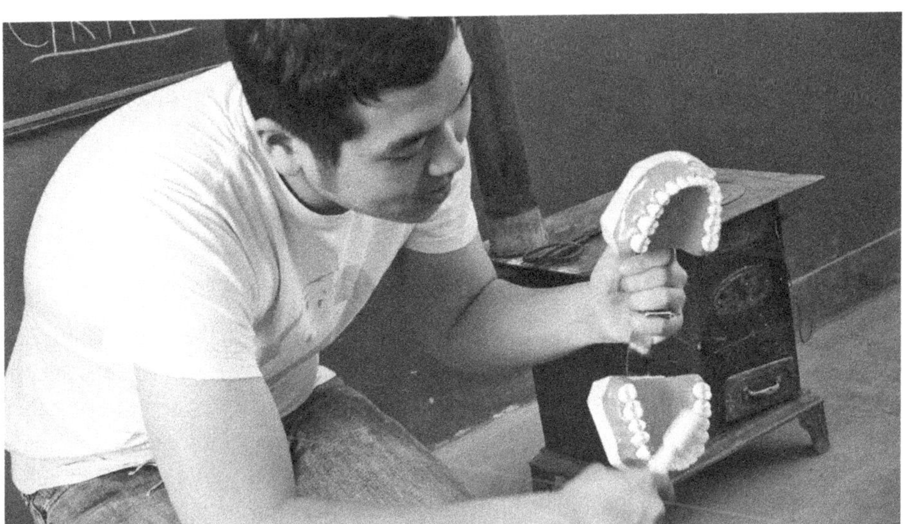

Fig. 7.12 A health promotion practitioner teaches oral health.

Reproduced by kind permission of Emily Ying Yang CHAN, Copyright © 2017 Emily Ying Yang CHAN.

(Haagsma, Graetz, Bolliger, *et al.*, 2016). In 2013, there were 973 million people across the world who sustained injuries that warranted some type of healthcare and around five million people died from injuries (Haagsma *et al.*, 2016; WHO, 2014b).

Among all types of injuries, road traffic injuries are the leading cause (24%) of injury death worldwide and are predicted to become the seventh leading cause of death by 2030 (WHO, 2014b). In South-East Asia, road traffic injuries kill approximately 316,000 people annually, which account for 25% of the global total of road traffic deaths (WHO Regional Office for South-East Asia, 2015).

Meanwhile, with the difference in their livelihoods and infrastructure rural communities have an injury pattern different from their urban counterparts. Although road traffic injuries may not be the biggest concern in rural Asia, self-harm and pesticide self-poisoning are significant concerns. In 2002, about 63% of global deaths from self-harm occurred in the Asia Pacific region and most of these deaths were in rural areas (Eddleston and Phillips, 2004). For example, in rural India, about half of injury deaths during 1997–1998 were suicides (Gajalakshmi and Peto, 2007).

In China, external causes of death such as trauma and poisoning accounted for 8.9% and were fifth among the major causes of death of villagers. Common domestic accidents included falls, drowning, poisoning by pesticides, burns, scalding, and electric shocks (National Health and Family Planning Commission of the People's Republic of China, 2013). The following section provides some prevention methods for domestic accidents (see Table 7.9).

Suggested health intervention strategies

1. Explain and discuss common rural injuries and domestic accidents.
2. Introduce injury prevention methods associated with common domestic risks in the target community.
3. Increase awareness of common injury prevention pitfalls.
4. Highlight high risk population subgroups (e.g. extremes of age and people with disabilities). Encourage villagers to help their neighbours, particularly if they are elders. If they notice that the routine and daily activities of their neighbours seem to have changed, they should check to see if any accident has taken place.

7.5 Disaster preparedness and health risk reduction

Asia has the highest number of natural disaster-prone countries in the world. Global climate change, more extreme weather events and meteorological disasters are expected in the coming decades. In remote rural communities, rural populations often rely on their own capabilities and preparations to respond to natural disasters. However, according to a survey conducted in the rural areas of China by CCOUC, only 20% to 30% of villagers perceived themselves capable of protecting themselves and their families during a disaster. In China, about half of the population lives in areas that are prone to natural

Table 7.9 Prevention methods for domestic accidents

Domestic accidents	Prevention methods	Key management principles
Injuries and bleeding	• Always clear potential injury risks at home. • Install lamps to ensure sufficient lighting. • Repair uneven floors to prevent falls. • Keep the floor dry. • Place sharp objects (scissors and agricultural tools) in an appropriate location. • Keep children out of reach of tools and poisons that may potentially cause injury. • Do not leave babies unattended on raised surfaces. Rails should be installed round cots and stairs. • If older people can barely walk, disability-friendly passages should be created. • Make sure sleeves and trousers for extremes of age are not too long.	1. Check to see if the person is conscious. 2. Check to see if the skin is intent. Check for the presence of bleeding, fractures/dislocations and injuries such as head and neck, torso, and limbs. 3. If the skin is intact in the affected area, apply cooling and rest/stabilization to soft tissue injuries to reduce swelling and pain. 4. In case of bleeding, apply firm direct pressure to stop the bleeding. If bleeding is controlled, check there is no foreign body in the wound. If none, use a clean wound dressing to cover the wound and add pressure with hand. Elevate the injured limb to reduce bleeding. In case of uncontrollable bleeding, seek urgent medical help. 5. If there is any deformity on the injury site, stablize the injury and seek help. 6. In the case of unconsciousness after a head injury, or there is headache, vomiting and confusion, please seek urgent medical assistance.
Drowning	• Explain the danger of playing near water sources. • Water wells and large water storage facilities should be covered and kept out of reach of children. • Avoid or prohibit children to play or swim in ponds, creeks or rivers alone. • Teach swimming skills.	1. Remove the victim from water. Assess if the affected individual is conscious. Assess whether rescue breaths and cardiopulmonary resuscitation (CPR) are necessary. 2. If CPR is not necessary, lay the victim on their side with no pressure on the chest. Provide a head-down position to allow free drainage of fluid. Then seek medical help.
Poisoning	• Medications and chemicals should be kept within their original containers. Avoid using containers for food to store them. • Label the container such that the children understand the danger of the chemical.	1. Assess consciousness of the affected individual. Call for immediate help if in doubt. 2. Assess safety. Avoid direct contact with the gases, fluids, or other material containing poisons. 3. Ensure ventilation of the site.

(continued)

Table 7.9 continued

Domestic accidents	Prevention methods	Key management principles
	• Keep children out of reach of medication, chemicals (such as pesticides) and other dangerous substances (such as alcohol and petrol). The ideal location would be locked cupboards.	4. Ask details of the poison/medications taken and share the information with the health professionals who manage the case.
	• Never describe medication to children as 'candy' or 'sugar solution' to avoid misconception. • Always check the name, dose, dosage, and expiration date of the medication regularly. • Avoid using medications prescribed for others. • Avoid storing more than one medication in the same container to avoid confusion.	
Burns/scalds	• Handling boiling oil, water and soup with care. • Pay particular attention to the stove. The handles of cooking pots should point inwards. • Check the food temperature before feeding for extremes of age. • Check the water temperature before giving children a bath. • All hot food and tools should be placed in the middle of the table. Prevent children from climbing onto the table. Avoid using a table cloth to prevent pulling and spillage. • Take measures to manage open fire sources indoors. • Tell the children not to go to the kitchen and to stay away from fire. • Keep children out of reach of tools that can produce fire. • Warn children not to play with fire.	1. Assess consciousness of the affected individual. 2. Assess burns to the face/ airway, if the patient breathes abnormally, loses consciousness, or becomes confused, seek medical care immediately. 3. Hold burnt skin under running water for 10 minutes. If the patient feels cold or shakes, stop. 4. Use clean dressing to dry the wound. Use dressing to cover the wound and hold it with bandage. 5. Never burst the blister or remove any material or clothing on the wound. 6. Never apply soy sauce, toothpaste, or other pastes to the wound.
Electric shock	• Pay attention to children and teach them to avoid electricity sources such as sockets. • Roll up wires that are too long to avoid children playing with them. • Make sure electrical appliances are inaccessible to children. • Use plug socket covers for sockets not in use.	1. Assess consciousness of the affected individual. 2. Turn off the electricity supply immediately. Avoid touching the victims. Use electrical insulators such as wooden sticks, brooms, or plastic sticks to separate the victims from the electricity source. Seek medical care immediately.

Table 7.9 continued

Domestic accidents	Prevention methods	Key management principles
	• If there is any suspicion that wires, sockets, or plugs are damaged, stop using them. • Check the integrity of electric appliance and supply regularly.	3. When it is safe to do so, assess if the victim is breathing or if they have a pulse. If not, state CPR immediately. 4. If the patient is breathing with difficultly and is unconscious, position them face upwards to ensure the airway is clear. 5. Electric shocks may burn a deep layer of the skin and other injuries.
Choking/Suffocation	• To serve food for older people and children, food should be prepared in smaller pieces and deboned. • Tell children not to eat while playing. • Do not allow children or infants to use milk bottles without adult supervision. • Choose toys that are appropriate to the age of children. Ensure there is no tiny part that will fall off easily. • Keep tiny objects, string, and plastic bags out of reach of children. • Beware of dental issues affecting older people. • Beware of the risks of post-stroke and head injury patients.	1. Assess consciousness of the affected individual. Call for help immediately. 2. Encourage the victims to cough the object out. 3. If the victim (older than one year) has complete obstruction of the airway and is conscious, apply up to five back blows. 4. If five back blows fail to relieve the airway obstruction, give up to five abdominal thrusts by standing behind them with arms around their abdomen. Clench one fist. Grasp the clenched fist with the other hand and place it on the victim's upper abdomen. Press the fist against the victim's abdomen with a quick upward thrust five times. Then forcefully slap the middle of the back. 5. For infants with signs of complete airway obstruction and is conscious, lie the infant prone on the forearm. Support the head with one's thigh and grip the lower jaw with a hand to make its head drop. Slap the infant between the shoulder blades five times with the heel of the other hand. 6. If strangled, unknot the rope or string. Check for breathing and obstruction in the mouth. Seek medical help immediately.
Animal bites/insect stings (such as dogs, snakes, scorpions, bees, and red fire ants)	• Vaccinate all pets and livestock (e.g. rabies vaccines for dogs).	1. Assess consciousness of the affected individual. 2. Use a large amount of clean water to wash bite wounds.

(continued)

Table 7.9 continued

Domestic accidents	Prevention methods	Key management principles
	• When walking through forest undergrowth or jungles, wear protective clothing (waterproof boots, gloves, and long trousers) to prevent snake bites. • Use bed nets and insect repellents.	3. If there is suspected poisoning or anaphylaxis, send the person to hospital immediately. 4. If there is bleeding, compress the wound to stop bleeding. 5. Healthcare professionals may vaccinate the victims with rabies or tetanus vaccine if necessary. They will offer medication and wound care. 6. Never cut open, suck, or squeeze the wound. Never tie the injured limbs.

Source: data from Hong Kong Centre for Health Protection, http://www.chp.gov.hk/en/index.html, accessed 01 Mar. 2017; Hong Kong Fire Services Department, http://www.hkfsd.gov.hk/eng/ accessed 01 Mar. 2017; Collaborating Centre for Oxford University and CUHK for Disaster and Medical Humanitarian Response (CCOUC), http://ccouc.org/home, accessed 01 Mar. 2017. For further information on the key management principles, please refer to *International first aid and resuscitation guidelines* 2016 by International Federation of Red Cross and Red Crescent Societies: http://www.ifrc.org/Global/Publications/Health/First-Aid-2016-Guidelines_EN.pdf

disasters and a significant proportion are ethnic groups living in rural village areas. Economic development, education and the quality of life are relatively low in these villages. Combined with a scarcity of resources, these communities experienced increased risk of casualties and property loss in disasters.

7.5.1 Key aspects for 'disaster preparedness and health risk reduction' to be investigated during field need assessments

The following issues should be explored for the target community to understand the context of specific disaster experiences, risks, and potential programmes that might address the local needs.

- Typical disaster type(s) which affect the target community;
- Disaster frequency;
- Recent disasters;
- Disaster impact (most recent disaster, most serious disaster in history for the area); previous experience in disasters and extreme events; any casualties, damages, and economic losses;
- Explore the high disaster risk areas (e.g. near river banks for floods) within the community/village;
- Identify the vulnerable subgroups (extremes of age, living alone, orphan children/older people, physically/mentally handicapped individuals, pregnant woman, and so on) within the community.

- Existing disaster contingency plan and warning system in the village;
- Villagers' or citizens' awareness of issues related to existing contingency plan and alarming system; and
- Climate change and its specific impact on the target community;

This section focuses on disaster preparedness and useful information about disaster preparation in the event of earthquakes, flooding, mudslides, fire, and related health risks. It also includes disaster preparedness kits. Practitioners are also encouraged to consider activities involving making ORS (see the section 'Oral rehydration solutions') and disaster preparation education.

7.5.2 **Earthquake**

Potential health and disaster risks

Asia is one of the most earthquake-prone continents in the world. Although it is not possible to prevent or change the likelihood of earthquakes, the chance of survival and safety can be greatly increased by actively promoting disaster preparedness awareness.

Suggested health intervention strategies

1. Explain typical injury and disease risks associated with earthquakes;
2. Identify areas with high earthquake risk within the target community.
3. Identify vulnerable groups within the target community and encourage the community to set up emergency contingency plan (evaluation plans and surge capacity to support rescue). Arrange extra support to ensure the vulnerable subgroups (children, pregnant women, elderly living alone or physically challenged individuals) are evacuated and post disaster help might reach them.
4. If people happen to be indoors during an earthquake, there are three principles that might help to decrease casualties:
    - Drop: both knees and hands down on the floor;
    - Cover: both hands and arms should protect the head and neck from being hit by the surrounding solid objects. If there is a reliable cover nearby (e.g. desk), then hold on to it firmly and stay under it; and
    - Hold on: protect the head and neck until the end of the earthquake. If the cover is moving because of the earthquake, then hold it firmly and keep covered by moving with it.

If the building is not earthquake-resilient, then the three principles are not applicable, and victims should escape to an outdoor open area immediately.

5. If one happens to be outdoors during an earthquake:
    - Remember to wear shoes and bring along the disaster kit while escaping;
    - Do not try to take a large amount of belongings or equipment;

- Stay away from destroyed buildings, fallen windows, and proceed to an open area if possible;
- Stay away from voltage transformers, overhead power lines, high-voltage poles, and light poles;
- Stay away from slopes, trees, rivers, and beware of rockfalls and landslides;
- Be cautious about the aftershocks; and
- Do not go back to the destroyed or even partially collapsed houses/tunnels.

6. What to do when trapped after an earthquake:
   - Stay calm;
   - Protect one's airway: cover nose and mouth for protection against foul odours or suspended dust in the air;
   - Preserve body energy;
   - Remove the surrounding debris carefully if the collapsed building is instable;
   - Remove the debris and clutter but avoid causing further collapse or there are any dangerous structures nearby;
   - Use any materials nearby or hit stones together to make some noise to draw attention and call for rescue; avoid shouting to preserve energy; if possible, look for a water and food supply; and
   - Never give up hope.
7. Consider also teaching how to use disaster preparedness kits (see the section 'Disaster preparedness kits') and ORS (see the section 'Oral rehydration solutions').

7.5.3 **Flood**

Potential health and disaster risks

Flood is the most common natural disaster globally. With global climate change, extreme weather events will occur more frequently in Asia, such as the flooding in the Philippines ensuing Super Typhoon Haiyan (Yolanda) in 2013 and the flooding and landslide in Taiwan following more than 3,000 mm of rainfall brought about by Typhoon Morakot in 2009. Both are the deadliest in the two countries' history. Villagers living in the disaster-prone regions know more about preparation work for rainstorms and flooding and emergency responses in flooding (WHO, n.d.-a).

Suggested health intervention strategies

1. Explain typical injury and disease risks associated with flooding.
2. Identify areas with high flood risks within the target community.
3. Identify vulnerable groups within the target community and encourage the community to set up emergency contingency plan (evaluation plans and surge capacity to

support rescue). Arrange extra support to ensure the vulnerable subgroups (children, pregnant women, elders living alone, or physically challenged individuals) are evacuated and post-disaster help might reach them.

4. Preparation for flooding:
   - Stay away from low-lying areas. If houses are located in low-lying areas, evacuate to higher ground or other safe areas when there is a flooding warning;
   - Avoid building houses on flood plains whenever possible. Try to elevate buildings and reinforce them when resources are available;
   - Pay attention to weather forecasts;
   - If houses are located near slopes or areas with loose soil and rocks, evacuate quickly when there is a flooding warning;
   - People working near rivers, ponds, or coasts should evacuate quickly;
   - Move livestock to a safer area;
   - Place boards or a heap of sand to maintain conduit whenever possible to ensure water drainage;
   - Design a suitable venue for evacuation such that people can evacuate quickly during flooding; and
   - Prepare disaster preparedness kits and an adequate supply of energy food;
   - Explain typical diseases post flooding, and methods of their prevention.
5. Coping response in flooding
   - Prepare to:
     i. Evacuate to higher ground; do not attempt to climb up electric cable posts;
     ii. Secure oneself to any fixed or floating objects (such as boats, wooden boards, doors, wooden beds) if trapped in a flood; look for opportunities to ensure survival; and
     iii. If evacuation is impossible, climb up to rooftops, high-rise buildings, tall trees or walls, to ensure survival. Wait for rescue. Never try to swim in the flood.
   - Stay away from the following places:
     i. Electric cable posts or power lines and surrounding areas;
     ii. Slopes, fish ponds, reservoirs and river confluences; and
     iii. Do not attempt to swim unless the water level rises above the roof.
   - Post-flooding reminders:
     i. Maintain personal hygiene as far as possible;
     ii. Avoid drinking contaminated water;
     iii. Always attempt to boil;
     iv. Do not consume contaminated food;
     v. For people with allergies and underlying respiratory problems, beware of exacerbation in the post-disaster phase;

vi. Environmental health risk management: beware of power lines and unstable infrastructure; and

vii. Reduce stagnant water to prevent insects and mosquitoes breeding; these efforts might reduce the risk of infectious diseases.

6. Consider also teaching how to use disaster preparedness kits (see the section 'Disaster preparedness kits') and ORS (see the section 'Oral rehydration solutions').

7.5.4 Mudslides and landslides

Potential health and disaster risks

Mudslides and landslides involve the mass movement of mud, sand, and rocks on a slope after other disasters such as heavy rain or heavy snow in mountainous or hilly areas. With climate change, rainstorms are likely to be more frequent even in drought-prone regions as loose and dry soil will be flushed down slopes by the rainwater causing a slide. Asian countries like China, India, Indonesia, Nepal, Pakistan, and the Philippines are among the most mudslide-prone countries in the world. In China, provinces such as Yunnan, Sichuan, Gansu, Shaanxi and Tibet are the most severely affected. The most severe mudslide disaster in the country occurred in Zhugqu County, Gansu in 2010. More than 1,000 people died or were reported missing, with huge economic loss and damage to infrastructure.

Suggested health intervention strategies

1. Explain typical injury and disease risks associated with mudslides/landslides.
2. Identify areas with high flood risks within the target community.
3. Identify vulnerable groups within the target community and encourage people to set up an emergency contingency plan (evaluation plans and surge capacity to support rescue). Arrange extra support to ensure the vulnerable subgroups (children, pregnant women, elders living alone, or physically challenged individuals) are evacuated and post-disaster help might reach them.
4. Uncommon sounds (such as strong wind or trees cracking) and sights (such as rock or sand flow) may be early signs of a mudslide. If mudslide risks are recognized, the higher the chance of survival. If someone is stuck in the mud, they should call for rescue by blowing the whistle in the disaster preparedness kit. Shouting is not recommended as it requires a bigger effort.
5. Mudslide and landslide warning signs include:
   - Tilting, cracking, or distortion in the buildings on the slope. Escape immediately if they are seen.
   - Visible changes in the river level such as a sudden increase or decrease in water flow, loud noises, and sense of vibration originating from gullies. These are the signs of mudslides.

- Debris flowing from the hill slopes, cracking sounds from slopes and trees. Pay attention to these sounds.

6. Response to mudslides in mudslide areas:
   - Look for any nearby safe zone as soon as possible;
   - Escape sideways out of the path of the mudslide rather than running away downhill in the same direction as the slide;
   - Hold on to any fixed objects (e.g. trees) when it is not possible to evacuate; and
   - Use hands to protect one's head.
7. Consider also teaching how to use disaster preparedness kits (see section 7.5.6 'Disaster preparedness kits') and ORS (see section 7.1.8 'Oral rehydration solutions').

7.5.5 **Fire**

Potential health and disaster risks

Fire creates one of the most important injury risks in rural areas. Although the housing density in rural areas is usually low, building materials are of low resistance to fire. Kitchens are often built indoors and indoor smoking also increases the risk of indoor fires. In addition to this, ageing and damaged residential electric wires can trigger fires easily.

Suggested health intervention strategies

1. Explain typical injury and disease risks associated with fire.
2. a. Identify areas with high fire risks within the target community.

   b. Explore the common fire hazards in the target community.
3. Identify vulnerable groups within the target community and encourage the community to set up an emergency contingency plan (evaluation plans and surge capacity to support rescue). Arrange extra support to ensure the vulnerable subgroups (children, pregnant women, elders living alone, or physically challenged individuals) are evacuated and post-disaster help might reach them.
4. Different types of fires require different management (see Table 7.10). In the case of a small fire, put it out yourself as soon as possible. However, escape immediately when a major fire occurs.
5. Fire management:
   - When fire breaks out in an enclosed environment, do not rush to open the windows as this might exacerbate the fire.
   - When the fire gets out of control, leave immediately. Once out of the house, stay out. Do not attempt to go back to retrieve any possessions that have been left behind.

Table 7.10 Methods of putting out fires arising from different materials

Material that catches fire	**How to put out the fire**
Wooden materials and buildings	Use abundant amounts of water.
Electrical appliances	First cut off the electrical supply then put out the fire with fire extinguishers. If there is no fire extinguisher, use a wet blanket instead. If a TV catches fire, put it out from the side to avoid injury from a bursting cathode ray tube.
Wok with burning oils	Cover the wok with a lid.
Inflammable materials such as petrol, diesel, or alcohol	Use fire extinguishers, sand, or wet blankets.

Note: Beware of the health hazards of smoke, fume, and gas emitted from the fire.

- Suffocation is the major cause of death in fires. The fumes in the area will pervade the entire space. As hot air rises, a lot of smoke would stay in the top layer. Hence, do not walk upright but crawl and use a wet towel that is folded several times to cover the nose and mouth to prevent smoke inhalation.
- During an escape, if people encounter a fire blocking their way, they should wet their clothes, hat, and shoes and envelop themselves with wet towels or clothes (and then rush out through the fire).

6. Management if one's clothes catch fire
    - Four major steps: stop, lie down, roll, cool down.
    - Stop running. Lie down and roll continuously with your face covered by your hands. Use water to cool the burnt area.
7. Burns management:
    - Four steps: rinse, remove, cover, and transfer.
    - Rinse: rinse the wound with running water.
    - Remove: remove the clothing that covers the wound. If that is not possible, cut the clothes to expose the area.
    - Transfer: transfer to the hospital after emergency wound management. If the burn involves a large surface area, try to cover the affected area with 'sterile' dressing.

For additional information on handling burns, see:

- 'International first aid and resuscitation guidelines 2011' by the International Federation of Red Cross and Red Crescent Societies: http://www.ifrc.org/PageFiles/53459/IFRC%20-International%20first%20aid%20and%20resuscitation%20guideline%202011.pdf
- 'First aid management of people with burns' on the website of the Chinese Ministry of Public Security: http://www.mps.gov.cn/n2256228/n2256229/n2256230/n2256237/c4148827/content.html

7.5.6 Disaster preparedness kits

Potential health and disaster risks

Although the occurrence of natural disasters cannot be completely eliminated or prevented, adequate disaster preparedness and effective emergency response may minimize the human impact of disasters. In remote and inaccessible communities. Disaster preparedness kits are essential to support bottom-up resilience. Nevertheless, less than 5% of these villagers' homes possessed disaster preparedness kits. This poor preparedness puts them in greater danger when facing a natural disaster. In this section, the use of disaster preparedness kits and the importance of preparing these kits are discussed.

Suggested health intervention strategies

1. Explore the common disasters in the target community.
2. Identify high disaster risk areas within the target community.
3. Identify vulnerable groups within the target community. Extra support in evacuation and post-disaster help might likely be needed.
4. Disaster preparedness kits should include items that may support and maintain the basic requirements of health. Recommended items include water, whistle, flashlight, flint, money, identity documents, family portraits, and daily or essential medication for patients with chronic diseases (see also Fig. 7.13 and Table 7.11).

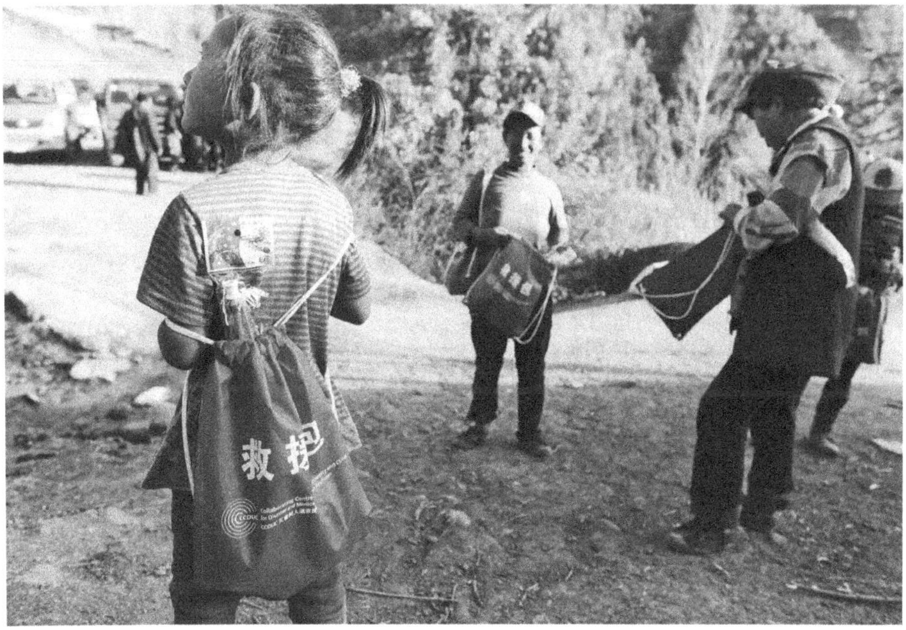

Fig. 7.13 Rural villagers with CCOUC disaster preparedness kits.
Reproduced by kind permission of Emily Ying Yang CHAN, Copyright © 2017 Emily Ying Yang CHAN.

Table 7.11 Basic content of a CCOUC disaster preparedness kit

Basic needs for survival and health	Item
1. Water and sanitation	**Soap** It helps maintain personal hygiene and prevent diseases. **Towels** It can be used as bandage to control bleeding. If soaked in cold water, it can be used as a cold pack for an injured area. **1.5 L Water bottle** Water is essential for life. In addition to drinking, it is also used for cooking and personal hygiene. An intake of 2.5–3 litres of water per day from drinking and food meets the survival needs of an individual, while the total basic water needs including cooking and hygiene should be 7.5–15 litres per day. The bottle can be used to contain clean drinking water and make an oral rehydration solution.
2. Food	**Non-perishable food** Can be used for allaying hunger in the short term. Pay attention to the nutrition of the food. 1. Infants: breastfeeding is always preferred if possible. 2. Pregnant women: avoid eating uncooked food. They should have sufficient intake of calcium-rich and whole-grain food, vegetables, fruits, and meat. They should also have an adequate water intake. 3. Elderly: avoid eating high-sodium food. They should have sufficient intake of calcium-rich food, vegetables, fruits, fish, and meat. They should also have an adequate water intake. **Dietary guidelines for people with chronic conditions** 1. Hypertension: avoid eating high-sodium food. They should have sufficient intake of fibre-rich, potassium- and magnesium-rich food (e.g. vegetables and fruits). 2. Diabetes: avoid eating high-sugar and high-fat food. They should have sufficient intake of whole-grain food, vegetables, and fruits. Eat smaller but frequent meals.
3. Shelter and clothing	**Emergency blanket** 1. It is made of heat-reflective plastic sheeting. It can be used at low temperatures to maintain body temperature. 2. Use the blanket to cover the body to reduce heat loss and prevent a sudden drop in body temperature. 3. The metallic surface of the blanket flashes in the sun. This can be used as an improvised locator beacon for search and rescue. 4. The blanket can also be used as a raincoat if there is rain or storm. **Manual dynamo torch** 1. The torch can be used for lighting as well as signalling. 2. Manual dynamo torches are better than torches which require batteries. **Multipurpose penknife** This should be multifunctional, small in size, and easy to carry. The penknives should have the following functions: 1. Can opener: usable for opening packaged can food; 2. Bottle opener: suitable for removing the bottle caps;

Table 7.11 continued

Basic needs for survival and health	Item
	3. Screwdriver: as equipment and for construction; 4. Sharp knife blade: as equipment and for construction; 5. Other uses: as a ruler, spanner/monkey spanner or direction indicator **Flints** To light the fire, even in an extremely cold or humid environment. Sparks from a flint are also effective for sending signals in darkness, even in extreme conditions.
4. Health services	**First aid equipment and common drugs** To support immediate medical care for bleeding or other common diseases (such as flu). **Picture of current medications** The medication names should be included for reference. If possible, pictures of traditional medicines, herbs, and other health-maintaining medications should also be included. **Guide on first aid and ORS preparation** Detailed procedures and relevant graphic illustration for reference.
5. Information and communication	**Whistle** To help responders to locate the person; more effective and energy-saving than shouting. **Family portrait** To help responders to look for any missing family member. **Copy of identity document** For identification and registration purposes. **Emergency contact information** Information including name, contact number and so on, for contact tracing. **Others** Petty cash should be prepared for emergency.

* Other items required depend on local culture, religious beliefs and resources availability.

5. Introduce the principle of the key functions of the disaster kits (water/sanitation, food/nutrition, shelter/non-food items, healthcare essentials, and information) and how to use each of the included items in the kits.
6. Disaster preparedness kits should be kept in readily accessible locations, for example, near the door or on the table that is most frequently used. In case of disaster, the kit can then be reached as quickly as possible.
7. Pay attention to the expiry date for the items in the kits and replace expired items regularly.
8. Due to culture and resource limitations, each community might have its own version of the disaster preparedness kit. Local knowledge and culture should always be consulted.

For more information on disaster preparedness and disaster preparedness kits, see:

- *Public Health Humanitarian Responses to Natural Disasters:* https://www.routledge.com/Public-Health-Humanitarian-Responses-to-Natural-Disasters/Chan/p/book/9781138953703
- *Handbook for disaster preparedness in residents living in the capital:* http://96181.bjhd.gov.cn/yjgl_59627/fzcs/201209/W020120905642740006387.pdf

7.6 Conclusion

This chapter discusses some common topics in health communication and education topics that support bottom-up resilience building efforts in health and disaster health risk reduction in rural communities. In the next three chapters, the challenges for rural health and disaster preparedness and response will be discussed.

References

Bhowmik, B., Afsana, F., My Diep, L., *et al.* (2013). Increasing prevalence of type 2 diabetes in a rural Bangladeshi population: a population-based study for 10 years. *Diabetes Metab J*, **37**, 46–53.

Brikké, F. & Bredero, M. (2003). *Linking Technology Choice with Operation and Maintenance in the Context of Community Water Supply and Sanitation: a reference document for planners and project staff.* Geneva, Switzerland: WHO and IRC Water and Sanitation Centre. Available at: http://www.who.int/water_sanitation_health/hygiene/om/wsh9241562153.pdf (accessed 13 January 2017) [Online].

Centers for Disease Control and Prevention (2016). *Summary of Infection Prevention Practices in Dental Settings: Basic Expectations for Safe Care.* Atlanta, GA: U.S. Department of Health and Human Services, Centers for Disease Control and Prevention, National Center for Chronic Disease Prevention and Health Promotion, Division of Oral Health.

Centre for Food Safety (Hong Kong) (n.d.). Available at: https://www.cfs.gov.hk [Online].

Chen, S. Y., Wang, H. F., & Yin, Y. (2005). [The reporting system of acute pesticides poisoning and general situation of pesticides poisoning in China]. *Chinese Journal of Industrial Hygiene and Occupational Diseases*, **23**(5), 336–9 (Chinese).

Chen, Y. Y., Wu, K. C. C., Yousuf, S., & Yip, P. S. (2012). Suicide in Asia: opportunities and challenges. *Epidemiol Rev*, **34**, 129–44.

Chinese Center for Disease Control and Prevention (China CDC) (2010). *Global Adult Tobacco Survey (GATS): fact sheet (China: 2010).* World Health Organization, Geneva, Switzerland. Available at: http://www.who.int/tobacco/surveillance/en_tfi_china_gats_factsheet_2010.pdf (accessed 12 January 2017) [Online].

Demaio, A. R., Dugee, O., De Courten, M., Bygbjerg, I. C., Enkhtuya, P., & Meyrowitsch, D. W. (2013). Exploring knowledge, attitudes, and practices related to alcohol in Mongolia: a national population-based survey. *BMC Public Health*, **13**, 178.

Eddleston, M. & Phillips, M. R. (2004). Self-poisoning with pesticides. *BMJ*, **328**(7430), 42–4.

Gajalakshmi, V. & Peto, R. (2007). Suicide rates in rural Tamil Nadu, South India: verbal autopsy of 39,000 deaths in 1997–98. *Int J Epidemiol*, **36**, 203–7.

Giang, K. B., Allebeck, P., Spak, F., Van Minh, H., & Dzung, T. V. (2008). Alcohol use and alcohol consumption-related problems in rural Vietnam: an epidemiological survey using AUDIT. *Subst UseMisuse*, **43**, 481–95.

Goldmann, L. (2004). *Childhood Pesticide Poisoning: Information for Advocacy and Action.* Chatelaine, Switzerland: UNEP Chemicals.

Goswami, A., Reddaiah, V. P., Kapoor, S. K., Singh, B., Dwivedi, S. N., & Kumar, G (2005). Tobacco and alcohol use in rural elderly Indian population. *Indian J Psychiatry*, **47**, 192.

Haagsma, J. A., Graetz, N., Bolliger, I., *et al.* (2016). The global burden of injury: incidence, mortality, disability-adjusted life years and time trends from the Global Burden of Disease study 2013. *Inj Prev*, **22**(1), 3–18.

Hawkes, C. (2004). *Nutrition Labels and Health Claims: The Global Regulatory Environment*. Geneva, Switzerland: WHO.

Howard, G., Bogh, C., Goldstein, G., *et al.* (2002). *Healthy Villages: A Guide for Communities and Community Health Workers*. Geneva, Switzerland: WHO. Available at: http://www.who.int/water_sanitation_health/hygiene/settings/hvintro.pdf (accessed 7 January 2017) [Online].

Hu, D. Y. (2012). [*Report on the Development of Oral Health in China*]. Beijing, China: Social Science Literature Publishing House (Chinese).

Hwang, C. K., Han, P. V., Zabetian, A., Ali, M. K., & Narayan, K. V. (2012). Rural diabetes prevalence quintuples over twenty-five years in low-and middle-income countries: a systematic review and meta-analysis. *Diabetes Res Clin Pract*, **96**, 271–85.

Kasapila, W. & Shaarani, S. M. D. (2011). Harmonisation of food labelling regulations in Southeast Asia: benefits, challenges and implications. *Asia Pac J Clin Nutr*, **20**, 1–8.

Kaur, P., Rao, S. R., Radhakrishnan, E.., Rajasekar, D., & Gupte, M. D. (2012). Prevalence, awareness, treatment, control and risk factors for hypertension in a rural population in South India. *Int J Public Health*, **57**, 87–94.

Khan, R. J., Stewart, C. P., Christian, P., *et al.* (2013). A cross-sectional study of the prevalence and risk factors for hypertension in rural Nepali women. *BMC Public Health*, **13**, 55.

Khanam, M. A., Lindeboom, W., Koehlmoose, T. L. P., Alam, D. S., Niessen, L., & Milton, A. H. (2014). Hypertension: adherence to treatment in rural Bangladesh–findings from a population-based study. *Glob Health Action*, **7**, 25028.

The Lancet (2017). Phasing out harmful use of pesticides. *The Lancet*, **380**, 1076.

Lee, H. Y., Won, J. C., Kang, Y. J., *et al.* (2010). Type 2 diabetes in urban and rural districts in Korea: factors associated with prevalence difference. *J Korean Med Sci*, **25**, 1777–83.

Lewis, J. J. & Pattanayak, S. K. (2012). Who adopts improved fuels and cookstoves? A systematic review. *Environ Health Perspect*, **120**, 637–45.

MacKay, J. & Eriksen, M. (2002). *The Tobacco Atlas*. Geneva, Switzerland: WHO. Available at: http://www.who.int/tobacco/publications/surveillance/tobacco_atlas/en/ [Online].

Ministry of Health Malaysia (2010). *Guide to Nutrition Labelling and Claims*. Ministry of Health Malaysia, Putrajaya, Malaysia: Food Safety and Quality Division.

Ministry of Health of the People's Republic of China, Standardization Administration of the People's Republic of China (2007). [*Standards for Drinking Water Quality*]. Standards Press of China, Beijing, China (Chinese). Available at: http://www.moh.gov.cn/open/db_query/new/20070628143525.pdf (accessed 13 January) [Online].

National Bureau of Statistics of China (2012). [*China's Health Statistics Yearbook 2012*]. Beijing, China: China Statistics Publishing House (Chinese).

National Bureau of Statistics of China (2015). Statistical Communiqué of the People's Republic of China on the 2014 National Economic and Social Development. Available at: http://www.stats.gov.cn/enGliSH/PressRelease/201502/t20150228_687439.html (accessed 11 January 2017) [Online].

National Bureau of Statistics of China (2016). [*China's Health Statistics Yearbook 2016*]. Beijing, China: China Statistics Publishing House (Chinese).

National Health and Family Planning Commission of the People's Republic of China (2013). [*China Health and Family Planning Statistical Yearbook 2013*]. China: Pecking Union Medical College Press.

Oral Health Education Unit of Department of Health (n.d.). Available at: http://www.toothclub.gov.hk/ [Online].

Poul, E. P., Bourgeois, D., Ogawa, H., Estupinan-Day, S., & Ndiaye, C. (2005). The global burden of oral diseases and risks to oral health. *Bull World Health Organ*, **83**, 661–9.

Proceedings of Asia Regional Workshop on the Implementation, Monitoring and Observance of the International Code of Conduct on the Distribution and Use of Pesticides (RAP Publication 2005/29) (2005). Bangkok, Thailand: FAO.

Ramachandran, A., Ma, R. C. W., & Snehalatha, C. (2010). Diabetes in Asia. *Lancet*, **375**(9712), 408–18.

Rosa, G., Miller, L., & Clasen, T. (2010). Microbiological effectiveness of disinfecting water by boiling in rural Guatemala. *Am J Trop Med Hyg*, **82**, 473–7.

Ruiz-Mercado, I., Masera, O., Zamora, H., Smith, K. R. (2011). Adoption and sustained use of improved cookstoves. *Energy Policy*, **39**, 7557–66.

Shi, H. L., He, Q. C., Dai, X. C., & Zhou, B. S. (2005). [Study on risk factors of lung cancer in non-smoking women]. *Chinese Journal of Lung Cancer*, **8**, 280–3. (Chinese).

The Sphere Project (2011). *Humanitarian Charter and Minimum Standards in Humanitarian Response*, 3rd Edition. Geneva, Switzerland: The Sphere Project.

Thundiyil, J. G., Stober, J., Besbelli, N., & Pronczuk, J. (2008). Acute pesticide poisoning: a proposed classification tool. *Bull World Health Organ*, **86**, 205–9.

Trip Creative Services (2011). Handwashing song [Video at youtube]. Available at: https://www.youtube.com/watch?v=hHY7P0TXlaU [Online].

United Nations Children's Fund (UNICEF) (2010). Global Handwashing Day 2010; Chen Kun teaches how to sing handwashing song [Video on Internet]. Available at: http://www.unicef.cn/cn/index.php?m=content&c=index&a=show&catid=49&id=71 [Online].

United Nations Children's Fund (UNICEF) (2011). 'Clean hands save lives'—Global Handwashing Day 2011 is celebrated by millions of people worldwide [Internet]. Available at: http://www.unicef.org.hk/en/clean-hands-save-lives-global-handwashing-day-2011-is-celebrated-by-millions-of-people-worldwide/ [Online].

United Nations Children's Fund (UNICEF), World Health Organization (WHO) (2009). *Diarrhoea: Why children are still dying and what can be done*. UNICEF, New York, NY, WHO, Geneva, Switzerland. Available at: http://apps.who.int/iris/bitstream/10665/44174/1/9789241598415_eng.pdf (accessed 11 January 2017) [Online].

U.S. Food and Drug Administration (2009). *A food labeling guide: guidance for industry*. Department of Health and Human Services. Available at: http://www.fda.gov/Food/GuidanceRegulation/GuidanceDocumentsRegulatoryInformation/LabelingNutrition/ucm2006828.htm (accessed 14 July 2015) [Online].

Wang, C., Zhang, W., Guo, Y. H., & Zhao, S. H. (2011). [Hazardous classification and label on the package and transport of pesticides]. *Agrochemicals*, **50**, 534–8 (Chinese).

Wang, H. L., Sun, H., Pan, X. Y., Jiang, Z. G., Cao, J. Z., & He, Z. (2012). Alcohol use among rural residents in Guizhou province. *Guizhou Medical Journal* (Chinese).

WorldAtlas (2016). Top Pesticide Using Countries. Available at: http://www.worldatlas.com/articles/top-pesticide-consuming-countries-of-the-world.html [Online].

World Health Organization (WHO) (n.d.-a). Flooding and communicable diseases fact sheet: risk assessment and preventive measures. Available at: http://www.who.int/hac/techguidance/ems/flood_cds/en/ (accessed 12 January 2017) [Online].

World Health Organization (WHO) (n.d.-b). Household (Indoor) Air Pollution. Available at: http://www.who.int/indoorair/en/ (accessed 13 January 2017) [Online].

World Health Organization (WHO) (n.d.-c). Mortality from household air pollution. Available at: http://www.who.int/gho/phe/indoor_air_pollution/burden/en/ (accessed 11 January 2017) [Online].

World Health Organization (WHO) (n.d.-d). Pesticides. Available at: http://www.who.int/topics/pesticides/en/ (accessed 13 January 2017) [Online].

World Health Organization (WHO) (n.d.-e). WHO position paper on oral rehydration salts to reduce mortality from cholera. Available at: http://www.who.int/cholera/technical/en/ (accessed 13 January 2017) [Online].

World Health Organization (WHO) (2003). *The World Oral Health Report 2003*. Available at: http://www.who.int/oral_health/media/en/orh_report03_en.pdf

World Health Organization (WHO) (2006a). *The Control of Neglected Zoonotic Diseases: A route to poverty alleviation: report of a joint WHO/DFID-AHP meeting, 20 and 21 September 2005, WHO Headquarters, Geneva, with the participation of FAO and OIE*. Geneva, Switzerland: WHO. Available at: http://apps.who.int/iris/bitstream/10665/43485/1/9789241594301_eng.pdf (accessed 11 January 2017) [Online].

World Health Organization (WHO). Department of Food Safety, Zoonoses and Foodborne Diseases (2006b). *Five keys to safer food manual*. World Health Organization, Geneva, Switzerland. Available at: http://www.who.int/foodsafety/publications/consumer/manual_keys.pdf (accessed 12 January 2017) [Online].

World Health Organization (WHO) (2012). *Oral health*. Available at: http://www.who.int/mediacentre/factsheets/fs318/en/ [Online].

World Health Organization (WHO) (2014a). *Indoor Air Quality Guidelines: Household Fuel Combustion*. Available at: http://apps.who.int/iris/bitstream/10665/141496/1/9789241548885_eng.pdf?ua=1 [Online].

World Health Organization (WHO) (2014b). *Injuries and Violence: The Facts 2014*. Available at: http://apps.who.int/iris/bitstream/10665/149798/1/9789241508018_eng.pdf?ua=1&ua=1&ua=1 [Online].

World Health Organization (WHO) (2014c). Global status report on alcohol and health 2014. World Health Organization, Geneva, Switzerland. Available at: http://www.who.int/substance_abuse/publications/global_alcohol_report/en/ (accessed 12 January 2017) [Online].

World Health Organization (WHO) (2015a). *Guideline: Sugars Intake for Adults and Children*. Geneva, Switzerland: WHO.

World Health Organization (WHO) (2015b). *WHO Estimates of the Global Burden of Foodborne Diseases: Foodborne Disease Burden Epidemiology Reference Group 2007–2015*. Available at: http://apps.who.int/iris/bitstream/10665/199350/1/9789241565165_eng.pdf [Online].

World Health Organization (WHO) (2015, January). Alcohol: Fact sheet. Available at: http://www.who.int/mediacentre/factsheets/fs349/en/ (accessed 12 January 2017) [Online].

World Health Organization (WHO) (2015, December 3). WHO's first ever global estimates of foodborne diseases find children under 5 account for almost one third of deaths. Available at: http://www.who.int/mediacentre/news/releases/2015/foodborne-disease-estimates/en/ [Online].

World Health Organization (WHO) (2016). *Promoting Oral Health in Africa: Prevention and control of oral diseases and noma as part of essential noncommunicable disease interventions*. Geneva, Switzerland: WHO. Available at: http://apps.who.int/iris/bitstream/10665/205886/1/9789290232971.pdf [Online].

World Health Organization (WHO) (2016, November). Diabetes: Fact sheet. Available at: http://www.who.int/mediacentre/factsheets/fs312/en/ (accessed 12 January 2017) [Online].

World Health Organization (WHO), Department of Public Health, Environmental and Social Determinants of Health (PHE) (2016). *Burning Opportunity: Clean Household Energy for Health,*

Sustainable Development, and Wellbeing of Women and Children. WHO, Geneva, Switzerland. Available at: http://apps.who.int/iris/bitstream/10665/204717/1/9789241565233_eng.pdf?ua=1 (accessed 11 January 2017) [Online].

World Health Organization (WHO) Regional Office for South-East Asia (2015). *Road Safety in the South-East Asia Region 2015. 2015*. Available at: http://www.who.int/violence_injury_prevention/road_safety_status/2015/Road_Safety_SEAR_3_for_web.pdf [Online].

World Health Organization (WHO) Regional Office for Western Pacific Region (2002). Smoking Statistics. Available at: http://www.wpro.who.int/mediacentre/factsheets/fs_20020528/en/ [Online].

Xiao, Q. Y. & Fu, Z. F. (2006). [Newly discovered viral zoonoses and related risk factors, prevention and control]. *Chinese Journal of Epidemiology*, 27, 1089–92 (Chinese).

Zhang, J. & Smith, K. R. (2005). *Indoor Air Pollution from Household Fuel Combustion in China: A Review*. Paper presented at: The 10th International Conference on Indoor Air Quality and Climate, 2005 Sep 4–9, Beijing, China.

Chapter 8

Special topics in rural health I

Natural disasters and climate change

The following three chapters will examine some contemporary topics in rural health. This chapter will look into two related topics: natural disasters and climate change.

8.1 Natural disasters

Key points

Asia, which is characterized by high-population density living and wide socioeconomic disparities among its countries, has the highest number of natural disasters in the past three decades. Most of the countries had limited disaster response capacities and for the first decade following the millennium; four out of five of the world's most populous countries (China, India, Indonesia, and Pakistan) are in Asia, which can be considered as the most disaster-prone continent globally. Traditional emergency health responses after disasters include the emergency treatment and service for injuries, communicable diseases, management and care for acute life-threatening diseases, surveillance and emergency preparedness for disease outbreaks, nutritional support, water supplies, and sanitation (Landesman, 2012; The Sphere Project, 2004, 2011). In recent years, despite the epidemiological and demographic transitions, the management of non-communicable chronic diseases and the health needs of older people and people with disabilities are usually forgotten, or left out of these action plans (Chan and Sondorp, 2007).

8.1.1 Global burden of natural disasters and mortality pattern in developing countries

Globally, natural disaster occurrence has significantly increased in the past two decades (Centre for Research on the Epidemiology of Disasters [CRED], 2016c). Asia, which is characterized by high population density living and wide socioeconomic disparities among its countries, had the highest number of natural disasters in the past three decades. Most of the countries had limited disaster response capacities and for the first decade following the millennium, four out of five of the world's most populous countries (China,

Table 8.1 Mortalities related to major disasters around the world (1900–2016)

Country	Start date	Killed	Disaster type
Bangladesh	12/11/1970	300,000	Storm
People's Republic of China	27/7/1976	242,000	Earthquake
Haiti	12/1/2010	222,570	Earthquake
People's Republic of China	22/5/1927	200,000	Earthquake
People's Republic of China	16/12/1920	180,000	Earthquake
Indonesia	26/12/2004	165,708	Earthquake
Japan	1/9/1923	143,000	Earthquake
Bangladesh	29/4/1991	138,866	Storm
Myanmar	2/5/2008	138,366	Storm
Soviet Union	5/10/1948	110,000	Earthquake

Source: data from Centre for Research on the Epidemiology of Disasters (CRED). '*Disasters list*', http://www.emdat.be/disaster_list/index.html, accessed 06 Feb. 2017,

India, Indonesia, and Pakistan) are in Asia can be considered as the most disaster-prone continent globally. In 2015, 152 out of 346 global natural disasters occurred in Asia, which represented 44% of the total number of disasters (CRED, 2015, 2016a). The large landmass with its many river basins, flood plains, mountains, active seismic and volcanic zones, combined with its densely populated cities, presents both topological and human factors which will affect the climate in Asia, and the continent reported 2,778 disasters during the 1994–2013 period, with 3.8 billion people affected, and approximately 841,000 deaths. Between 1994 and 2013, China, the Philippines, India, Indonesia, and Bangladesh have remained near the top of the list of the 10 most disaster-affected countries in the world. Among all natural disasters, earthquakes have been the least predictable and most lethal (Guha-Sapir *et al.*, 2004), while meterological disasters have constituted 86% of global disasters since 1995-2004 (CRED, 2016c). Table 8.1 describes the mortality pattern associated with the major disasters during the last century.

8.1.2 **Impact of the epidemiological transition in medical disaster relief**

Most developing countries have entered into their demographic and epidemiologic transition. Healthcare needs and healthcare systems in these countries often encounter the pressure to cater for population ageing as well as have to face the double-burden of both infectious diseases and chronic illnesses. Table 8.2 shows the burden of chronic diseases and natural disasters in selected middle-income countries (1900–2016).

The epidemiological transition has affected disease patterns in multiple levels and will impact on disaster response effectiveness. Disruptions in routine medical care during the disaster may exacerbate pre-existing diseases through environmental pollution (dust resulting

Table 8.2 Burden of chronic diseases and natural disasters in selected middle-income countries (1900–2016)

Country	Total number of natural disasters 1900–2016	% Deaths caused by NCDs					% NCDs deaths among the total deaths
		Cardiovascular diseases	Cancer	Chronic respiratory diseases	Diabetes	Other NCDs	
China	858	45	23	11	2	6	87
India	679	26	7	13	2	12	60
Indonesia	476	37	13	5	6	10	71
Pakistan	199	19	8	6	3	15	51

Source: data from Centre for Research on the Epidemiology of Disasters (CRED). *'Country profile'*, http://www.emdat.be/country_profile/index.html, accessed 07 Feb. 2017, Copyright © 2016 CRED; World Health Organization. *Noncommunicable diseases country profiles 2014*, http://www.who.int/nmh/publications/ncd-profiles-2014/en/, accessed 07 Feb. 2017. Geneva: World Health Organization, Copyright © 2014 World Health Organization.

from the disaster), stress, and the inability of the health service providers to adapt to resource constraints and to deal with chronic disease management in a disaster field setting.

The absence or disruption of treatment for chronic diseases such as hypertension, diabetes mellitus, mental illness, and HIV/AIDS following a natural disaster is not only life-threatening for disease-affected vulnerable groups, but may also give rise to disability-related complications (e.g. diabetes retinopathy or strokes) that result in a reduction in the quality of life, impaired livelihood, and the costs of complicated treatments and avoidable deaths. Table 8.3 provides some of the key mechanisms through which populations with chronic conditions might be affected during natural disasters (Case Study 8.1).

In general, although most frontline practitioners agree that life-saving treatments should be given, it is unclear whether regular treatments should also be offered in those locations where the pre-disaster medical treatment of chronic disease is limited or non-existent. For NCD, although medical services provision may be attempted (see Table 8.4), major gaps in the field level response include the lack of an operational mandate, resources, awareness, and technical know-how among the relief agencies and health workers on the management of chronic diseases during an emergency relief operation.

8.1.3 Impact of the demographic transition in medical disaster relief

Population ageing is a major global healthcare challenge in coming decades (WHO, 2015, September; Beaglehole *et al.*, 2007, 2008). Researchers have suggested 80% of older adults in developed countries have at least one underlying chronic medical condition, and many also have some level of disability (Aldrich and Benson, 2008). With potential underlying vulnerability in socioeconomic status, health, and activities of daily living, the post-emergency needs of older people in disasters and crises can be overwhelming (Chan *et al.*, 2017; Wells, 2005). (Case Study 8.2).

Table 8.3 Some key mechanisms and possible outcomes of disasters that may affect populations with chronic diseases

Mechanisms	Possible outcomes
Communicable conditions	
Suboptimal hygiene and living environment.	Increase risks of infection for population with underlying vulnerability (e.g. people with subimmune status).
Discontinuation of a drug intake (e.g. TB).	Failure of the treatment compliance. Increased risk of multidrug-resistant TB strains in the community.
AIDS (a population may have existed before the occurrence of the natural disaster, but their needs have not been met (Spiegel, 2004)).	Increased incidence and vulnerability of transmissions.
Pre-existing structure/availability of resources and capacity.	Prioritization of other medical conditions for treatment.
Non-communicable conditions	
Direct impacts through disaster-induced stress (e.g. cardiovascular disease) (Kario et al., 2003).	Increased incidence and prevalence of stress-induced manifestations and complications of chronic conditions.
Interruption of health services.	Higher risk of disease complications due to the lack of follow-up/resources.
Inappropriate post-disaster diet and lifestyle– particularly since the health of patients who have underlying chronic conditions is often sensitive to changes in the lifestyle and diet (Kirizuka et al., 1997).	Increased risk of the manifestations and complications of chronic medical conditions.
Complications from diabetes and other chronic conditions due to an inability to conduct operations.	Affected disease prognosis and survival.
Lack of information on a patient's medical history, and losses of medical record.	Care providers are unaware of potential complications and problems. Issues with resource allocations (drug and treatment planning).
Unstable NCD status increases the risk of medical treatments for injuries.	Affected disease prognosis and survival.
Local willingness to accept a technical transfer (of knowledge and know-how).	Lack of competency and a platform for the knowledge transfer.

Source: data from Spiegel PB. HIV/AIDS among conflict-affected and displaced populations: dispelling myths and taking action. *Disasters*, Volume 28, Issue 3, pp. 322–39, Copyright © 2004 Overseas Development Institute; Kario K, McEwen BS, and Pickering TG, Disasters and the heart: a review of the effects of earthquake-induced stress on cardiovascular disease. *Hypertension Research*, Volume 26, Issue 5, pp. 355–67, Copyright © 2003 The Japanese Society of Hypertension; Kirizuka K, Nishizaki H, Kohriyama K, *et al.* Influences of The Great Hanshin-Awaji Earthquake on glycemic control in diabetic patients. *Diabetes Research and Clinical Practice*, Volume 36, Issue 3, pp. 193–6, Copyright © 1997 Elsevier Science Ireland Ltd. Published by Elsevier Inc.

Case Study 8.1 The forgotten healthcare needs during natural disasters in post-millennium middle-income countries

Immediate trauma and infectious diseases are often the only health needs identified and managed post natural disaster. On 12 May 2008, an 8.0 Richter scale earthquake hit the Chinese province of Sichuan. More than 70% of the earthquake survivors had management needs for their underlying chronic conditions during the emergency period. Reports from the frontline medical teams found that up to 38% of the survivors needed clinical management for their pre-existing chronic medical conditions before any further surgical interventions could be performed for their physical trauma. General lack of awareness of NCDs, absences of clinical guidelines, relevant drugs and equipment, limited technical know-how, concern over lack of reimbursement of treatment costs, and logistic arrangements (confusion over the healthcare entitlement of migrant workers within the disaster area) and as the appropriate platform for case follow up.

Table 8.4 Issues to consider when providing non-communicable disease services

To act	Not to act
Affected population	
Population need	Local population resistance due to a different cultural understanding of the problem
Demand from the recipient population	Competition (the local service providers' and physicians' financial incentives are being threatened)
Pre-existing structure/availability of resources and capacity	Prioritization of other acute medical conditions for treatment
Capacity of the relief agencies versus local capacity	
Resources (medication, human resources, equipment)	Competing medical priorities
Operational mandate	Lack of an operational mandate for long-term health-related issues
Humanitarian imperatives (emergency/life-saving measures for patients)	Lack of required drugs and technical capacity/competency
Technical challenges	
Technical capacity Treatment standards/best practices guidelines	Lack of training and accreditation of qualifications Lack of field relevant guidelines/standards/protocols
Sustainability/continuity because of an available local partnership	Unwillingness or lack of cooperation from the stakeholders
Willingness to accept technical transfers (of knowledge and know-how)	Concern for the management continuity and sustainability

Case Study 8.2 Differences in older people health needs between urban and rural clinics post disaster

Significant differences were found between the health needs and utilization patterns of rural and urban clinics four months after the Pakistan Kashmir earthquake. Regardless of clinical locations, older people with chronic medical needs were the predominant rural clinic users.

Measuring 7.6 on the Richter scale, the earthquake occurred on 8 October 2005 and struck Pakistan's autonomous state of Kashmir, as well as part of the Indian-administrated Kashmir. The official death toll in Pakistan was 79,000 and reached nearly 1,400 in Indian-administered Kashmir. When comparing health services usage in rural and urban clinics, there were fewer older people and notable gender differences in remote mountainous clinic attendance (Site 1) when compared with the number who attended the urban internally displaced person (IDP) clinic. Given that older people belong to the predominant age group in the rural communities, this suggests that barriers including geographic access were significant in these remote areas (Chan and Gainey, 2006). In particular, men were the predominant service users (70%) at the mountainous clinic; while the service utilization by older women was found to be inversely related to the travel distance to the clinic (i.e. the use of the services was greater the shorter the distance to the clinic from home). Table 8.5 demonstrates the utilization of healthcare services by older people in different settings.

Table 8.5 Utilization pattern of services by older people in the two healthcare settings according to clinical records#

Location	Rural mountainous clinic*	Urban IDP camp**
Total attendees	2942	392
Services received by older people+	14%	26%
Male/Female	7:3	3:4

#Clinical records review for January-February 2006
*Merlin's P3, Sarli Saccha Clinic
** Muslim Hand IDP camp in Chella Bandi
+ According to UNHCR, the population aged 45 or above constituted about 19% of the population in that area.
Reproduced with permission from Chan EYY and Griffiths S. Comparison of health needs of older people between affected rural and urban areas after the 2005 Kashmir, Pakistan earthquake. *Prehospital and Disaster Medicine*, Volume 24, Issue 5, pp. 365–71, Copyright © 2009 World Association for Disaster and Emergency Medicine.

Access issues

As the service provision was free in both of the study settings, treatment cost was not a barrier to the access of health/medical services for any part of the studied population. However, unintended service access barriers, such as the gender of the service providers, were found. The clinic attendance records in the mountainous clinic showed that during the days when clinical services were provided solely by male doctors, the overall utilization of the medical services decreased by 30%. Meanwhile, men were also found to have reverse access barriers to psychosocial support that mostly targeted exclusively at women and children. A recurrent theme found among the men during the discussions that took place in both clinics (rural and urban) was 'a feeling of limited access to international relief services because they were only available for the "vulnerable groups: women and infants"'. See also Case Studies 8.3 and 8.4.

Source: data from Chan EYY and Griffiths S. Comparison of health needs of older people between affected rural and urban areas after the 2005 Kashmir, Pakistan earthquake. *Prehospital and Disaster Medicine*, Volume 24, Issue 5, pp. 365–71, Copyright © 2009 World Association for Disaster and Emergency Medicine.

8.1.4 Rural and urban differences in medical needs in post-relief settings

Major sociodemographic differences exist between urban and rural clinic service utilization post disaster. Service planners should consider service utilization patterns and the underling access barriers for rural communities. Case Studies 8.3 and 8.4 describe examples of healthcare needs after an earthquake.

Case Study 8.3 Comparison of the demographic and disease profiles of the health service users in rural stationery and remote mobile clinics after the 2005 Kashmir, Pakistan earthquake

The destruction in the earthquake-affected region closest to the earthquake's epicentre was almost 100%. The characteristics of the patients/attendees of various relief clinics around the Neelum Valley, Pakistan Kashmir six months after the 2005 earthquake were examined.

Overall, significant differences were found between a stationary clinic versus a mobile clinic, after the acute relief phase of the 2005 Kashmir earthquake in the remote areas. Patients of an older age, female gender, and those living far from a clinic, as well as patients with earthquake-related trauma, wound infections, and gastrointestinal conditions were found to be more significantly associated with use of the mobile clinic even four months after the disaster. Conversely, the users of the stationary clinic tended to be younger, lived closer to the clinic site, and had disease profiles which were predominantly chronic in nature.

The mobile clinic had twice as many patients who were older than 65 years old (stationary: 3%; vs. mobile: 6%, $P = 0.03$). Furthermore, 56% of the mobile clinic users were female compared to 30% at the stationary clinic ($P < 0.0001$). Respiratory disease constituted 20–22% of the case load in both the clinics and was found to be the commonest single diagnostic group during the study period. Despite being four months after the earthquake, those who attended the remote mobile clinic still presented with medical needs associated with unmanaged earthquake related trauma (mobile: 18%; vs. stationary 10%, $P < 0.01$), wound infections (mobile: 15%; vs. stationary: 5%, $P < 0.01$), and gastrointestinal diseases (mobile: 15%; vs. stationary: 5%, $P < 0.01$). Nevertheless, the stationary rural clinic had almost triple the number of patients who presented chronic conditions when compared with the mobile clinic. In addition, more non-specific medical conditions were presented at the stationary clinic in comparison with the mobile clinic (stationary: 8%; vs. mobile: 3%, $P = 0.02$).

Case Study 8.4 Comparison of the health needs between a rural mountainous clinic and the urban IDP medical services following the 2005 Kashmir, Pakistan earthquake

During the study period four months after the earthquake, 2,942 and 392 consultations from the rural mountainous clinic (Site 1) and the urban IDP medical services (Site 2) were reviewed, respectively. More males were reported as rural clinic users; while for the urban clinic, female users were found to be predominant patients.

Significant differences in self-perceived well-being were found between the older people in the remote mountainous area when compared with the urban IDP counterparts. While none of the respondents sustained any major injuries due to the earthquake, twice as many older people (68%) in the remote mountain area reported worse health outcomes post disaster than those in the IDP camps. Table 8.6 shows the results of the selected self-reported health problems and well-being of the older people between urban and rural settings (Fig. 8.1).

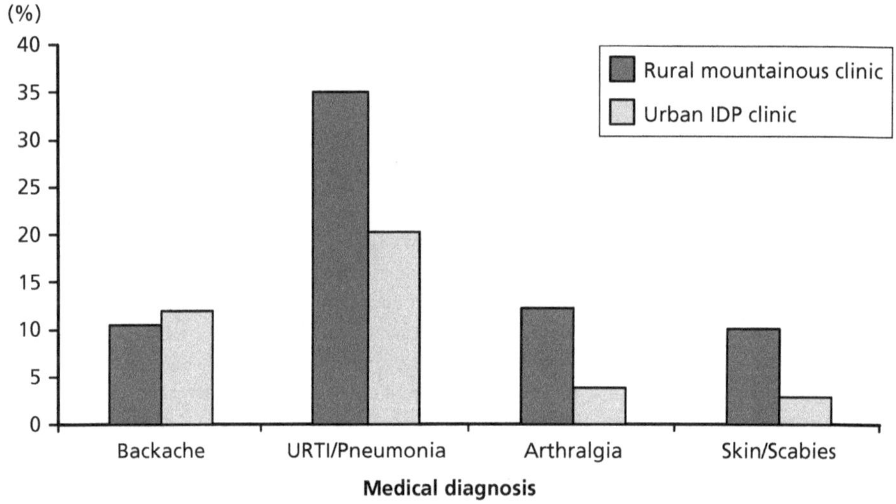

Fig. 8.1 Comparison of the commonest medical diagnoses* between the rural and urban clinics as recorded in the medical consultation records from January to February 2006.

* Rural: Among 2,942 medical records at the Sarli Saccha mountain clinic; Urban: Among 392 medical records at the urban MH Chella Bandi IDP clinic.

Disparities were found in the access to care for chronic medical conditions among the post-earthquake population groups. Before the disaster, only 35% (30) of the older people living in the mountains had received medical management for their underlying chronic medical problems, compared to 70% (28) of the older people living near the city in the IPD camps. Post earthquake, among those who had received chronic medical treatment prior to the disaster, 80% (68) of those living in the remote mountain regions reported losing access to their chronic medical treatment in comparison to 40% (16) of those who were living near the city in the IDP camp. Of note, the clinical records showed discrepancies between the diagnoses and the drugs prescribed, including an overprescription of antibiotics across all age groups.

Table 8.6 Comparison of selected self-reported health problems of older people in two different settings

	Rural site mountainous clinic* % (N = 85)	Urban site IDP camp**% (N = 40)	Chi-square P value
Selected physical health-related problems			
Dental problems	100% (85)	25% (10)	<0.0001
Visual problems	75% (64)	38% (15)	<0.0001
Weight loss	75% (64)	50% (20)	0.001
Eating problems (indigestion, lack of appetite)	87% (74)	50% (20)	0.002
Hearing problems	54% (50)	40% (16)	0.043
Other physical complaints Headache Dizziness Joint/muscle pain	40% (34) 34% (29) 54% (50)	23% (9) 20% (8) 50% (20)	0.043 0.07 0.10
With known underlying medical problems Discontinued treatment post disaster	25% (21) 80% (68)	38% (15) 40% (16)	0.02 <0.001
Selected psychosocial health-related problems			
Experienced the death of at least one family member/close relative	90% (77)	40% (16)	<0.001
Loss of possessions Some All Refused to answer	30% (26) 50% (43) 20% (17)	30% (12) 40% (16) 30% (12)	0.1 0.07 0.06
Feeling depressed and helpless	72% (61)	44% (18)	<0.001
Sleeplessness	65% (55)	44% (18)	<0.001
Feeling a lack of resources: Medical Food Clothes/not enough clothes Shelter Financial support Social support **Most cited other needs:** Cooking utensils	60% (51) 25% (21) 20% (17) 70% (60) 90% (77) 60% (51) 40% (34)	20% (8) 5% (2) 5% (2) 50% (20) 55% (22) 20% (8) 5% (2)	<0.001 <0.001 <0.001 <0.001 <0.001 <0.001 <0.001
Overall worsening of health after the earthquake (4 months later)	68% (58)	35% (14)	<0.001
Social related issues			
Currently living alone Living with family Living with friends/neighbours	10% (9) 50% (43) 40% (34)	2% (1) 70% (28) 28% (11)	<0.001 0.04 <0.01

(continued)

Table 8.6 continued

	Rural site mountainous clinic* % (N = 85)	Urban site IDP camp**% (N = 40)	Chi-square P value
Living in: Houses Tents	30% (26) 60% (51)	10% (4) 90% (46)	0.03 0.02
Had received any assistance after the earthquake (aside from medical services)	50% (43)	100% (40)	<0.01

*Results abstracted from the mountainous clinic; **Results abstracted from the IDP camp clinic

8.1.5 Addressing needs post disaster: Bottom-up resilience to address health and disaster risks

To address the vulnerability of older people and the health needs of the population with chronic diseases, stakeholders must prepare, plan, and respond according to the underlying demographic patterns and needs of their communities. In general, emergency health and medical responders should always attempt to review the demographic and epidemiological profiles of the disaster-affected populations. Approaches to address increase bottom-up health resilience and disaster risk reduction are discussed next.

Health delivery considerations for chronic diseases after a natural disaster in developing countries

Management and provision of healthcare for chronic conditions after disasters is a complex topic. Population beliefs and receptivity, pre-disaster service availability, local technical capacities, availability of resources in terms of finances and materials, and the commitment and duration of the involvement of the intervening agency and possible partnerships should all be taken into consideration. The timing of the intervention (in terms of the stage of the disaster), its goals, where the operations should be set up, the availability of a referral system, and the technical capacity of the relief agencies are all important factors to be considered (Fig. 8.2).

When studying why the older people and chronic medical needs were forgotten by the medical providers, key issues identified include the lack of sensitivity among relief and health workers about post-disaster health needs of older people; the lack of provision and accreditation of field-relevant technical training; the absence of field-based clinical guidelines for chronic diseases and post-disaster geriatric disease management in developing countries; and advocacy for including geriatric as well as chronic-disease-specific components in the natural disaster medical relief programmes.

8.1.6 Pathway of care

Using the concept of 'Pathway of Care', there are a range of possible health-related interventions that may be carried out in disaster-affected settings to support bottom-up resilience-building and response attempts (see Fig. 8.3).

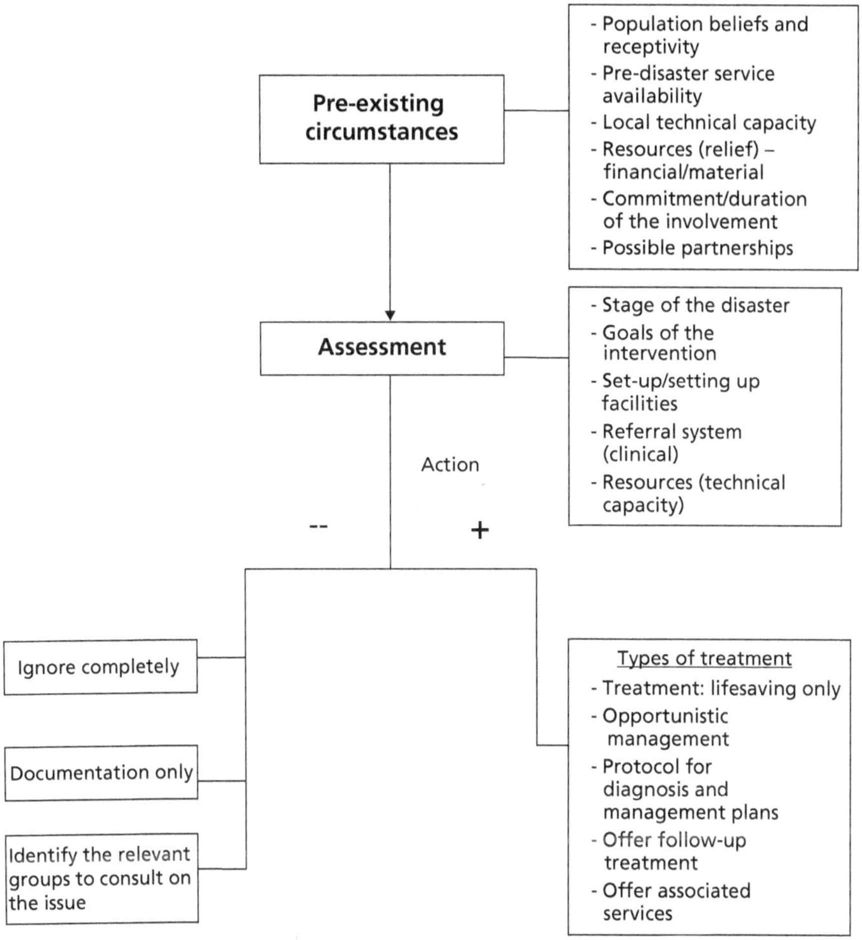

Fig. 8.2 A conceptual model to guide the decision-making on whether or not to provide chronic medical services during post-disaster emergency responses in developing countries.

The hierarchy of prevention

Using the hierarchy of prevention, health relief programmes and activities can be built in low cost and have a profound effect on reducing the impact on the long-term health of the affected population. Even for populations with no pre-existing or regular access to services for chronic non-communicable diseases (NCDs), low cost, primary prevention programmes that target behaviour modifications such as dietary advice and exercise would create benefits for the health of the general population in the long run. Table 8.7 shows some potential low-cost activities and programmes that might prevent, as well as support, the populations with chronic medical needs in developing countries.

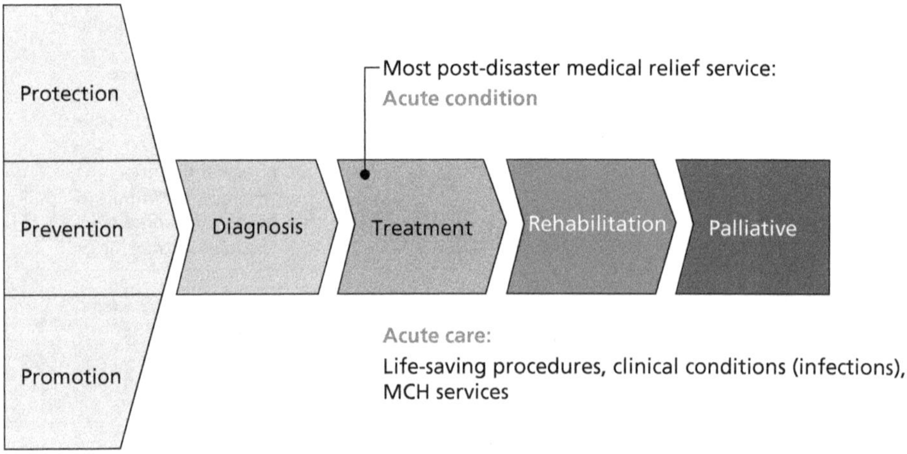

Fig. 8.3 Application of the 'Pathway of Care' concept for disaster preparedness planning and disaster responses.

Health protection: Food aid provision with balanced nutritional values, food items suitable for patients on a specific diet needs (e.g. diets for diabetic patients and low-salt diets), medical supplies (provided pre-disaster) for patients with chronic illness, issuing medical cards with a simple NCD information for patients in emergency;

Health prevention: Vaccinations (for the groups of extreme ages), communicable disease prevention (e.g. bed nets in malaria- and dengue-prone areas), water, and sanitation maintenance;

Health promotion: Health education programmes to increase awareness of NCDs and prevention education on the transmission of chronic communicable diseases (e.g. TB and HIV);

Diagnosis: Simple screening for hypertension and high cholesterol levels, as well as blood glucose levels, in clinic settings;

Treatment: Supply of life-supporting medications for chronic diseases and stabilization of a patient's condition;

Rehabilitation: Immediate health needs are usually focused on providing emergency care and operations. There is a major need for rehabilitation centres to follow-up medical and surgical cases treated during disasters;

Palliative care: Comfort and dignity of patients should always be viewed as an integral part of disaster response and medical care. Palliative care is thus crucial, but it is often not addressed as part of the healthcare needs in disasters.

8.1.7 **Implications for bottom-up health resilience and disaster risk reduction**

Despite the changes in the underlying health and medical needs of disaster-prone communities globally, the current international post-disaster medical humanitarian aid practices and policies remain based upon the assumptions from a couple of decades ago (Chan and Sondorp, 2007; Spiegel *et al.*, 2010b; Spiegel, 2017). With the ageing global population and the increasing burden of non-communicable, chronic diseases, a rethink is necessary of how medical and healthcare needs can be provided following a natural disaster in the twenty-first century (Chan, 2008; Chan and Griffiths, 2009; Chan and Kim, 2011; Ford *et al.*, 2006; see Chapter 6 for policy implications).

8.1.8 **Conclusion**

For the decades ahead, non-communicable chronic medical conditions and population ageing will become too significant a burden to ignore during emergency preparedness

Table 8.7 Some potential low-cost activities and programmes that might prevent and support the populations with chronic medical needs in developing countries

Primary prevention
Educate the affected population about chronic disease prevention and awareness (e.g. dietary /habits, exercise, smoking cessation, alcohol use, injury prevention)
Secondary prevention
Identify and assess the health risk (cardiovascular risk) during opportunistic consultations
Opportunistic screening of chronic medical conditions (hypertension, DM)
Establish patient management plans for chronic medical problems based on the availability of local resources
Support the establishment of chronic medical services through training and coordination
Tertiary prevention
Educate healthcare workers on the prevention and detection of chronic disease complications through training and coordination efforts
Act as a liaison to support the development of a multidisciplinary service among different sectors in order to promote communication and partnerships
Establish disease target monitoring systems, according to the local service availability
Support the development of disease surveillance programmes in the local setting

Adapted with permission from Chan EYY and Sondorp E. Medical interventions following natural disasters: missing out on chronic medical needs. *Asia Pacific Journal of Public Health*, Volume 19, pp. 45–51, Copyright © 2007 Asia-Pacific Academic Consortium for Public Health.

and field response operations. Experience, documentation, and research evidence are urgently needed to stipulate up-to-date and the most feasible preparedness and response plans to support bottom-up health resilience and disaster risk reduction efforts.

8.2 Climate change

Key points

- Climate change has caused significant impacts on living environment and human health for the twenty-first century.
- Major health-related concerns include changes of disease patterns, frequency increases in disasters, sustainability of water supply, food security, and agricultural-based livelihood, as well as loss of biodiversity.
- Rural areas and remote communities are vulnerable to the adverse impact of climate change.

Climate change is a global environmental challenge and has caused a huge impact on ecosystems, economies, and human well-being. As defined by the Intergovernmental Panel on Climate Change (IPCC), climate change refers to a change in the state of the climate that can be identified (e.g. by the use of statistical tests) by changes in the mean and/or the variability of its properties, and that persists for an extended period of time, typically decades, or longer. It refers to any change in the climate over time, whether it is due to natural variability or as a result of human activity (IPCC, 2007; UN, 1992). Changes in ambient temperature, rainfall patterns, melting of glaciers and sea ice, rising sea levels, and more frequent and severe extreme weather events such as floods, droughts, storms, heatwaves, and cold spells are reported across the world for the past few decades.

Increased human activities are regarded as a major contributor to the rise in the amount of greenhouse gas (GHG) emissions, which intensifies the Earth's natural greenhouse effect and results in a rise in the global average surface temperatures—the result of global warming. Records show that the global average for the combined land and ocean surface temperature has increased by 0.85°C (0.65–1.06°C) over the period from 1880 to 2012. It is projected that by 2100, the global surface temperature change will likely exceed 1.5°C in comparison with the pre-industrial period (IPCC, 2014).

In rural communities, climate change impact on water supply, food security, and agricultural income, as well as economic loss resulting from infrastructure destruction by extreme events (such as destruction of the roads, buildings, dams, and irrigation systems). Secondary and tertiary industries (such as manufacturing and tourism) that depend heavily on natural resources will also be substantially affected. With a strong dependence on agriculture and natural resources, rural populations are particularly vulnerable and are highly sensitive to climate variability and extreme weather conditions (IPCC, 2014).

8.2.1 Impact on health

Research evidence has already demonstrated a significant impact of climate change on human health. The altered climate patterns, extreme weather events, and climate-related disasters affect patterns of food production, water access, as well as foodborne, waterborne, and vector-borne diseases transmission, which will bring adverse impact on human health. Cholera, influenza, meningococcal meningitis, malaria, and dengue fever are examples of climate-sensitive diseases. Research findings also found associations between climate variables and the patterns of NCDs (cardiovascular, respiratory, injuries, mental health outcomes). Table 8.8 highlights some selected health impacts of climate change.

8.2.2 Impact on water availability

In rural areas, availability of irrigation water is crucial for sustaining agricultural activities and people's livelihoods. In Africa, studies indicate that not only would climate change lead to a widespread catastrophic failure of rural groundwater supplies, but also 90 million people who live in rural areas where the annual rainfall is between 200–500 mm are sensitive to changes in its intensity, or other seasonal variations of annual rainfall may cause problems for the groundwater supply (MacDonald *et al.*, 2009). Climate change

Table 8.8 Possible health impacts of climate change with confidence ratings

Effect	Exposure affected by climate change	Changes in the environment and ecosystem	Potential health outcomes	Confidence rating*
Direct	↑ Frequency and intensity of temperature and precipitation extremes	- Excessive heat - Increased ozone and other pollutants	↑Mortality and morbidity Cardiovascular/respiratory diseases Mental health issues	Very high
	↓ Number of cold days and nights	- Warmer winters	↓ Cold-related mortality and morbidity	Low
Indirect through the ecosystem	↑ Temperature and humidity Altered precipitation patterns ↑ Sea levels and temperature of sea/fresh water	- Changes in the biology and transmission of pathogens - Lack of safe water and food - Contamination of fresh water with flood water or sea water	↑Mortality and morbidity from food- and waterborne diseases	Very high
	↑ Temperature and humidity Altered precipitation patterns	↑ Parasite replication Prolonged transmission seasons Changing distribution of the disease vectors	↑Mortality and morbidity from vector-borne disease	Medium
	↑ Temperature and humidity Altered precipitation patterns	Change in pollen production	↑Mortality and morbidity from respiratory diseases	Likely
Indirect through human systems	↑ Temperature Altered precipitation patterns	↓ Food production in tropical regions ↑ Food insecurity due to the reduced supply and higher prices	↑Mortality and morbidity from undernutrition, particularly in poor regions	High

* The confidence rating corresponds to the confidence level in the evidence for the potential health impact from IPCC AR5.

Source: data from De Blois J, Kjellstrom T, Agewall S, *et al.* The effects of climate change on cardiac health. *Cardiology*, Volume 131, Issue 4, pp. 209–17, Copyright © 2015 S. Karger AG, Basel; Intergovernmental Panel on Climate Change. *Climate change 2014: impacts, adaptation, and vulnerability*. Cambridge: Cambridge University Press, Copyright © 2014 Cambridge University Press; World Health Organization. *Strengthening health resilience to climate change: Technical briefing for the World Health Organization*, http://www.who.int/phe/climate/conference_briefing_1_healthresilience_27aug.pdf, accessed 10 Jan. 2017, Copyright © 2014 World Health Organization.

is expected to have a similar impact on water resources and human access in the Asian region for the decades to come. The following case study shows the impact of climate change in Himalayas and Bhutan (see Case Study 8.5; see also Case Study 8.6).

Case Study 8.5 The Himalayas region (Bhutan and China's Tibetan areas)

The Hindu Kush-Himalayan (HKH) is the origin source of 10 large Asian river systems. HKH provides water and ecosystem services, as well as being the basis for the livelihoods of a population of 210 million people in the region. Around 1.3 billion people, or one-fifth of the world's population, rely on these water sources for their survival (International Centre for Integrated Mountain Development, n.d.).

In the Himalayas, the temperature rise in the last three decades has been between 0.15°C and 0.60°C per decade (Shrestha *et al.*, 2010). A study that examined about 15,000 glaciers and 9,000 glacial lakes across the five countries (Bhutan, Nepal, Pakistan, and selected basins of China and India) in the region (Asia-Pacific Network for Global Change Research, 2005) between 1999 and 2003 found that with global warming, the glaciers have been retreating at an increased rate since the 1970s, and the glacial lakes are increasing in both number and size (Bajracharya *et al.*, 2006). For instance, there has been a 5.5% shrinkage in the volume of China's 46,928 glaciers, which is equivalent to a loss of more than 3,000 sq. km of ice (Bajracharya *et al.*, 2007). Similar shrinkages have also been observed in Nepal, India, and Bhutan. Valley glaciers and small glaciers are retreating at an even faster rate (Bajracharya *et al.*, 2006). Globally, up to half could be lost by 2100 (Kuhn, 1993; Oerlemans, 1994). It has been predicted that if the climate continues to change at the present rate, two-thirds of China's glaciers will disappear by 2050, and almost none will remain by 2100 (Yao, 2004).

As the glaciers retreat, the rapid accumulation of water in the lakes formed behind moraine or ice dams can lead to a sudden breach of these weak and loose moraine dams. The resulting rapid discharge of a huge amount of water and debris is known as a *glacial lake outburst flood* (GLOF). GLOFs can be catastrophic to the areas and populations located downstream, as they may cause the loss of human lives and the serious destruction of infrastructures and properties. Over the years, a number of GLOF events have been documented in the HKH region, some of which have a transboundary impact. Typically, GLOF events are recorded in the Asian Himalayas region at least once in 3–10 years (Bajracharya *et al.*, 2006).

Bhutan is a small, landlocked country that is located in the eastern Himalayas. In the Kingdom of Bhutan, 24 glacial lakes have been identified as being potentially dangerous. Eight of these are located in the Pho Chu basin, making this basin a 'hotspot' for potential GLOF activities (Bajracharya *et al.*, 2006). In China, satellite images acquired in 2000–2001 showed that 24 of the glacial lakes in the Pumqu river basin in Tibet (Xizang) can be identified as being potentially dangerous for GLOF events (Che *et al.*, 2004). In addition to the increased risk of outburst floods from the glacial lakes, climate change can have implications for a region's hydrological regime. Firstly, the increase in GLOFs and other flash floods in the headwater regions will adversely affect the development of hydropower in some Himalayan countries, such as Nepal and Bhutan (Chalise *et al.*, 2006). This is particularly important as hydropower is the backbone of the Bhutanese economy. About 80% of the power generated by the hydro resources in Bhutan is exported to neighbouring India after domestic consumption needs have been met. These power exports account for more than 40% of the country's national revenue and 25% of the gross domestic product (GDP). Another 25% of the GDP comes from the development of the hydropower infrastructure. The country's revenue from exporting hydropower is also the primary source of its socioeconomic developments in health, education and agriculture (Organisation for Economic Co-operation and Development, 2011). Secondly, the base of the water resource—the ice reserve—is likely to shrink and may have a serious impact on the water supply in the dry season. The livelihood of the population, as well as the agricultural and industrial developments will be profoundly affected (Chalise *et al.*, 2006).

To minimize the adverse impact of flash floods and GLOFs on the rural populations of Bhutan and the other Himalayan countries, regular glacier and glacier lake monitoring and an early warning system to predict GLOFs have been established. With an early warning system and a GLOF simulation model, the authorities may be able to predict the arrival time of the floods and the locations of flooded areas downstream, so as to activate relevant precautionary measures to reduce the damage (Bajracharya *et al.*, 2006; Kumar and Murugesh Prabhu, 2012).

Ambient temperatures change pose increased risks in vector-borne diseases contol in Bhutan. Over 50% of the country's population resides in malarial areas (the more severe *Plasmodium falciparum* (30–60% of cases) and *Plasmodium vivax* are prevalent in Bhutan), and dengue fever becomes an emerging vector-borne infectious disease in Bhutan. Specifically, dengue fever was first documented in the country in 2004, and is now endemic during the monsoon period, sometimes appearing in the form of explosive outbreaks (Kumaresan and Sathiakumar, 2010). Diarrhoeal diseases, which contribute to about 10–15% of the burden of diseases, represent another climate-related health risk in Bhutan. With climate impact on water resources (drying up of water sources, contamination caused by flooding), risk of diarrhoeal diseases are also likely to increase (WHO, n.d.a).

Case Study 8.6 Drought risk reduction engaged by women in Sri Lanka

In Sri Lanka, women were trained to engage in better land use, water management, and livelihood diversification to lessen impact brought by climate-change-related drought and landslides in their rural communities (Dueñas i Cid and Ochoa i Cañigueral, 2016; UN Educational, Scientific and Cultural Organization, 2012). Not only have these programmes reduced community vulnerability to the economic risks associated with disasters, but also improved female participation to engage in economic development and climate change hazard reduction.

8.2.3 Impact on food security

Climate change affects all dimensions of food security. Food availability (production and trade), food access (lower agricultural output and higher food prices), food utilization (nutritional problems and hunger), food stability (fluctuations of the food supply), and food safety are all sensitive to climate variation (World Food Programme, n.d.; Schmidhuber and Tubiello, 2007). Global ambient temperature changes from 1980 to 2008 were associated with reduction of global yields of maize and wheat by 3.8 and 5.5%, respectively. Although this impact had been offset by some gains resulting from improved agricultural technologies in developing countries (Lobell *et al.*, 2011), reductions in yields or crop failures have directly affected the incomes of the farmers and deteriorate rural livelihoods (Morton, 2007).

8.2.4 Impact on disaster occurrence

Epidemiological analysis of the global disasters that have occurred during the past three decades shows a substantial rise in the number of climate-related disasters, such as storms and floods, which has contributed to an increase in the disaster frequency. In total, an average of 335 weather-related disasters were recorded each year between 2005 and 2014, which was an increase of 14% from 1995 to 2004, and almost twice the level recorded during 1985–1994 (United Nation International Strategy for Disaster Reduction & CRED, 2015). Flooding alone accounted for 47% of all weather-related disasters (1995–2015) and affected 2.3 billion people, the majority of whom (95%) live in Asia.

Case Study 8.7 Health and disaster resilience building in rural DPRK

Ryongchon is the most north-west county in the Democratic People's Republic of Korea (DPRK), which borders with China by the Yalu River (also known as Amnok River). Susong Farm is a collective farm located in the delta area of the Yalu River. The farm consists of 470 households and 1,800 villagers (Collaborating Centre for Oxford University and CUHK for Disaster and Medical Humanitarian Response, 2016).

Disaster-related health risk and potential strategies

Natural disasters, particularly flooding, are one of the major challenges for Susong Farm. A tributary of Yalu River passes through the cropping field the farm. The higher riverbed makes the field very valuable to flooding during the monsoon. Alike other areas in the northern DPRK, single cropping is usually practised due to the lower temperature. Rice, maize, and soybean are typical crops of this farm, which are expected to be harvested in autumn. However, a major disaster during the summer could severely affect their livelihood in the upcoming year. Some acute health impact, such as injury and gastrointestinal infections (e.g. caused by unclean drinking water) are often reported after flooding. With the effect of climate change, the frequency and intensity of extreme weather events such as typhoons, flooding, and drought are likely to be exacerbated in the future. In light of these threats, DRR is the core concept of adapting to climate change and related health impacts.

Healthcare needs in rural communities

In this farm, villagers have access to free healthcare services through its clinic. Although there is a shortage of equipment and medicine, basic clinical, dental care, midwifery, and public health services are being provided. Each doctor responsible for about 100 households. Patients with more severe conditions are referred to the county-level hospital (10 km away) for further care. Clinic records showed an average daily outpatient visit of 15 patients, who are mostly young children, women, and elders. Due to the heavy manual workload, musculoskeletal conditions are the most commonly reported complaints. Summer is considered the peak season for skin problems, gastrointestinal tract diseases, and injuries. The local doctor estimated that 30% of patients have hypertension. Patients with tuberculosis are not treated locally but transferred to higher level hospital for at least six months. Due to lack of medical supply, needles and some other medical disposables are reused by the clinic. The lack of diagnostic equipment (e.g. microscope) and power supply make it difficult to diagnose some certain diseases or pathogen (e.g. virus, bacteria, parasite, or fungus).

To reduce the impact of health emergency and, the Sendai framework on disaster risk reduction 2015–2030 may be used to plan for programmes that might enhance community health resilience and reduce disaster risks.

Priority 1: Understanding disaster risk

A good understanding of local disaster risk is the basis of successful DRR. The farm lacks systematic assessment and regular information should be collected to support relevant planning and disaster warning (floods) and risk communication. Focus group discussions were conducted and community risk awareness programmes were proposed in DPRK.

Priority 2: Strengthening disaster risk governance to manage disaster risk

A farm-based disaster management committee (DMC), which is responsible for contingency plans and coordination mechanism for disasters might be established. All stakeholders (youths and elders, men and women, farmers and leaders) who are engaged in farm-related activities should be involved in the process. Regular training and education on disaster and health should be organized by the DMC to update latest lessons learnt in DRR in the community.

Priority 3: Investing in disaster risk reduction for resilience

Financial and material investments are recognized internationally as key elements in disaster risk reduction. Given the limited resources, the local school and clinic should share the higher priority when considering an investment. Two potential 'safe facilities' in Susong Farm, namely the health clinic and the local school, were identified. Both were located in the elevated area, and had rarely been flooded even in the major flood episodes in the area. Suggested investments include the reinforcement of the physical structure and the lifeline infrastructure support to these structures (e.g. water, electricity and heating facilities) to enhance the capacity of healthcare professionals (disaster-related knowledge/skills and proper equipment). When there is a major disaster, the school may act as an emergency shelter for people affected. Before external assistance arrives, local emerging medical needs mainly rely on the farm doctors and nurse. Therefore, it is vitally important to improve their resilience and ensure they are functional to response during and after the disaster.

Priority 4: Enhancing disaster preparedness for effective response and to 'build back better' in recovery, rehabilitation, and reconstruction

Enhancing disaster preparedness ensures capacities are in place for effective response and recovery when a disaster occurs. In the Susong Farm, except for a basic school manual-operated metal bell at the school to inform the community, there is currently no other early warning system or communication mechanism. Although this traditional manual approach has proven effective, especially with consideration to electricity shortage, there are several limitations which might be of local concern. These include the coverage, protocol of alert triggering, and regular drill exercises.

Potential disaster and health risk reduction programme has been initiated in 2016 (CCOUC, 2016). Results of this programmes will be checked in the coming years.

8.2.5 Impact on population movement

Climate change may exacerbate the pace of rural–urban migration (IPCC, 2014). According to the Asian Development Bank (2012), 42 million people were displaced by extreme weather events in Asia and the Pacific during 2010–2011. Socioeconomic problems associated with climate and environmental migrants are important issues to be addressed for the coming decades to climate-affected regions globally.

8.2.6 Implications for bottom-up health resilience and disaster risk reduction

Although various global initiatives (see Chapter 6) have been launched to address the impact of climate change, developing countries and particularly their rural communities, which are affected by poverty and socioeconomic vulnerability, have less resilience to these climate challenges (IPCC, 2014; see Case Study 8.7; see also Chapter 7 for policy implications and Chapter 9 for plantation and health).

8.3 Conclusion

Climate change presents major challenges to maintain human well-being and secure habitats in the twenty-first century. People living in rural and remote areas, with a high dependence on agriculture and natural resources, coupled with their existing vulnerabilities (such as poverty, and lower skill levels and education), face multiple vulnerabilities in health and disaster risks associated with this global environmental phenomenon. Both mitigation and adaptation approaches must be considered simultaneously to mitigate and to minimize adverse human impact in rural areas.

References

Asian Development Bank (2012). *Addressing Climate Change and Migration in Asia and the Pacific: final report*. Manila, Philippines: Asian Development Bank.

Asia-Pacific Network for Global Change Research (2005). *Inventory of Glaciers, Glacial Lakes and the Identification of Potential Glacial Lake Outburst Floods (GLOFs) Affected by Global Warming in the Mountains of India, Pakistan and China/Tibet Autonomous Region*. Available at: https://www.apn-gcr.org/resources/files/original/d71dea72bc764245642e7d047c095463.pdf (accessed 10 January 2017) [Online].

Bajracharya, S. R., Mool, P. K., & Shrestha, B. R. (2006). The impact of global warming on the glaciers of the Himalaya. *Proceedings of International symposium on Geo-disasters, infrastructure management and protection of world heritage sites, 25–26 November 2006, Nepal Engineering College, Ehime College and National Society for Earthquake Technology Nepal*, pp. 231–42.

Bajracharya, S. R., Mool, P. K., & Shrestha, B. R. (2007). *Impact of climate change on Himalayan glaciers and glacial lakes: case studies on GLOF and associated hazards in Nepal and Bhutan*. Available at: http://condesan.org/mtnforum/sites/default/files/publication/files/1369.pdf (accessed 9 January 2017)[Online].

Beaglehole, R., Ebrahim, S., Reddy, S., Voute, J., & Leeder, S. (2007). Prevention of chronic diseases: a call to action. *Lancet*, **370**(9605), 2152–7.

Beaglehole, R., Epping-Jordan, J., Patel, V., *et al.* (2008). Improving the prevention and management of chronic disease in low-income and middle-income countries: A priority for primary health care. *Lancet*, **372**(9642), 940–9.

Centre for Research on the Epidemiology of Disasters (2015). *The Human Cost of Natural Disasters 2015: A Global Perspective*. Available at: http://reliefweb.int/sites/reliefweb.int/files/resources/PAND_report.pdf (accessed 9 January 2017) [Online].

Centre for Research on the Epidemiology of Disasters (2016a). *2015 Disasters in numbers*. Available at: http://www.unisdr.org/files/47804_2015disastertrendsinfographic.pdf (accessed 9 January 2017) [Online].

Centre for Research on the Epidemiology of Disasters (2016b). Country profile. Available at: http://www.cred.be (accessed 7 February 2017) [Online].

Centre for Research on the Epidemiology of Disasters (2016c). Disasters list. Available at: http://www.cred.be/ (accessed 6 February 2017) [Online].

Chalise, S. R., Shrestha, M. L., Bajracharya, O. R., *et al.* (2006). Climate change impacts on glacial lakes and glacierised basins in Nepal and implications for water resources. *Climate Variability and Change—Hydrological Impacts* (Proceedings of the Fifth FRIEND World Conference held at Havana, Cuba, November 2006), IAHS Publ.308.

Chan, E. Y. Y. & Gainey, V. (2006). *Health Needs Assessment post Pakistan Kashmir Earthquake 2005*. London, UK: HelpAge International.

Chan, E. Y. Y. & Griffiths, S. (2009). Comparison of health needs of older people between affected rural and urban areas after the 2005 Kashmir, Pakistan earthquake. *Prehosp Disaster Med*, **24**, 365–71.

Chan, E. Y. Y. & Kim, J. (2011). Chronic health needs immediately after natural disasters in middle-income countries: the case of the 2008 Sichuan, China earthquake. *Eur J Emerg Med*, **18**, 111–4.

Chan, E. Y. Y. & Sondorp, E. (2007). Natural disaster medical intervention: missed opportunity to deal with chronic medical Needs? an analytical framework. *Asia Pacific Journal of Public Health*, **19**(Special Issue), 45–51.

Chan, E. Y. Y. (2008). The untold stories of Sichuan earthquake. *Lancet*, **372**(9636), 359–62.

Chan, E. Y. Y., Hung, H., & Chan, G. K. W. (2017). *Policy Implications for Managing Older People in Disaster* (Policy Brief). Hong Kong: CCOUC.

Chan, E. Y. Y. & Sondorp, E. (2008). Including chronic disease care in emergency responses. *Humanitarian Exchange Magazine*, **41**, 43–5. Available at: http://odihpn.org/wp-content/uploads/2008/12/humanitarianexchange041.pdf (accessed 7 February 2017) [Online].

Che, T., Jin, R., Li, X., *et al.* (2004). Glacial lakes variation and the potentially dangerous glacial lakes in the Pumqu basin of Tibet during the last two decades. *Journal of Glaciology and Geocryology*, **26**, 397–402.

Collaborating Centre for Oxford University and CUHK for Disaster and Medical Humanitarian Response (CCOUC) (2016). *Potential Strategies on Health Related Community Disaster Risk Reduction: Needs Assessment Report of Susong Farm in DPRK by CCOUC.* Hong Kong, China: CCOUC.

De Blois, J., Kjellstrom, T., Agewall, S., *et al.* (2015). The effects of climate change on cardiac health. *Cardiology*, **131**, 209–17.

Iueñas i Cid, D. & Ochoa i Cañigueral, L. (2016). Climate change and health related challenges as trigger for education opportunities to foster social knowledge and action. In: Filho, W. L., Azeiteiro, U. M., & Alves, F. (eds), *Climate Change and Health: Improving Resilience and Reducing Risks* (Climate Change Management Series), pp. 297–313. Cham, Switzerland: Springer International Publishing.

Ford, E. S., Mokdad, A. H., Link, M. W., *et al.* (2006). Chronic disease in health emergencies: in the eye of the hurricane [Internet]. *Preventive Chronic Disease*, **3**(2). Available at: http://www.cdc.gov/pcd/issues/2006/apr/pdf/05_0235.pdf (accessed 7 February 2017) [Online].

Guha-Sapir, D., Hargitt, D., & Hoyois, P. (2004). *Thirty Years of Natural Disasters 1974–2003: The Numbers.* Louvain, Belgium: Presses universitaires de Louvain.

Intergovernmental Panel on Climate Change (2007). *Climate change 2007: synthesis report.* Available at: https://www.ipcc.ch/publications_and_data/ar4/syr/en/mains1.html (accessed 10 January 2017) [Online].

Intergovernmental Panel on Climate Change (2014). *Climate Change 2014: Impacts, Adaptation, and Vulnerability.* Cambridge and New York: Cambridge University Press.

International Centre for Integrated Mountain Development (n.d.). River basins. Available at: https://www.icimod.org/?q=rps_riverbasins (accessed 10 January 2017) [Online].

Kuhn, M. (1993). Possible future contribution to sea level change from small glaciers. In: Warrick, R. A., Barrow, E. M., & Wigley, T. M. L. (eds), *Climate and Sea Level Change: Observations, Projections and Implications*, pp. 134–43. Cambridge, UK: Cambridge University Press.

Kumar, B. & Murugesh Prabhu, T. S. (2012). *Impacts of climate change: glacial lake outburst floods (GLOFs).* Available at: http://www.sikkimforest.gov.in/climate-change-in-sikkim/6-Chapter-Impact%20of%20Climate%20Change%20%20Glacier%20Lake%20Outburst%20Floods%20(GLOFs).pdf (accessed 9 January 2017) [Online].

Kumaresan, J. & Sathiakumar, N. (2010). Climate change and its potential impact on health: a call for integrated action. *Bulletin of the World Health Organization*, **88**, 163.

Landesman, L. Y. (2012). *Public Health Management of Disasters: The Practice Guide* 3rd Edition. Washington, DC: American Public Health Association.

Lobell, D. B., Schlenker, W., & Costa-Roberts, J. (2011). Climate trends and global cropproduction since 1980. *Science*, **333**, 616–20.

MacDonald, A. M., Calow, R. C., MacDonald, D, *et al.* (2009). What impact will climate change have on rural groundwater supplies in Africa? *Hydrolog Sci J*, **54**, 690–703.

Morton, J. F. (2007). The impact of climate change on smallholder and subsistence agriculture. *P Natl Acad Sci USA*, **105**, 19680–5.

Oerlemans, J. (1994). Quantifying global warming from the retreat of glaciers. *Science*, **264**, 243–5.

Organisation for Economic Co-operation and Development (2011). Case story on cross-border power export from Dagachhu Hydropower Development. Available at: https://www.oecd.org/countries/bhutan/48651659.pdf (accessed 9 January 2017) [Online].

Schmidhuber, J. & Tubiello, F. N. (2007). Global food security under climate change. *P Natl Acad Sci USA*, **105**, 19703–8.

Shrestha, B. B., Nakagawa, H., Kawaike, K., Baba, Y., & Zhang, H. (2010). Glacial lake outburst due to moraine dam failure by seepage and overtopping with impact of climate change. *Annuals of Disaster Prevention Research Institute, Kyoto University*, **53B**, 569–82.

The Sphere Project (2004). *Humanitarian charter and minimum standards in disaster response*, 2nd Edition. Geneva, Switzerland: The Sphere Project. Available at: http://www.refworld.org/docid/3d64ad7b1.html (accessed 6 February 2017) [Online].

The Sphere Project (2011). *Humanitarian Charter and Minimum Standards in humanitarian response*, 3rd Edition. Geneva, Switzerland: The Sphere Project. Available at: http://www.spherehandbook.org/en/the-humanitarian-charter/ (accessed 6 February 2017) [Online].

Spiegel, P. B. (2004). HIV/AIDS among conflict-affected and displaced populations: dispelling myths and taking action. *Disasters*, **28**, 322–39.

Spiegel, P. B. (2017). The humanitarian system is not just broke, but broken: recommendations for future humanitarian action. *Lancet*. Published online 8 June 2017: http://dx.doi.org/10.1016/S0140-6736(17)31278-3

Spiegel, P. B., Checchi, F., Colombo, S., & Paik, E. (2010). Health-care needs of people affected by conflict: future trends and changing frameworks. *Lancet*, **375**, 341–45.

United Nations (UN) (1992). *United Nations Framework Convention on Climate Change*. Available at: https://unfccc.int/resource/docs/convkp/conveng.pdf (accessed 6 February 2017) [Online].

United Nations (UN) Educational Scientific and Cultural Organization (2012). *Education Sector Response to Climate Change: Background Paper with International Examples*. Bangkok, Thailand: UNESCO Bangkok.

United Nation (UN) International Strategy for Disaster Reduction; Centre for Research on the Epidemiology of Disasters (2015). *The Human Cost of Weather Related Disasters: 1995–2015*. Available at: http://www.unisdr.org/files/46796_cop21weatherdisastersreport2015.pdf (accessed on 9 January 2017) [Online].

Wells, J. (2005). Protecting and assisting older people in emergencies (Network Paper No. 53). Available at: http://odihpn.org/wp-content/uploads/2005/12/networkpaper053.pdf (accessed on 14 July 2017) [Online].

World Food Programme (n.d.). Climate impacts on food security. Available at: https://www.wfp.org/climate-change/climate-impacts (accessed on 9 January 2017) [Online].

World Health Organization (WHO) (n.d.a). Climate Change Adaptation to Protect Human Health: Bhutan project profile. Available at: http://www.who.int/globalchange/projects/adaptation/en/index2.html (accessed 11 January 2017) [Online].

World Health Organization (WHO) (2014a). *Noncommunicable diseases country profiles 2014*. Geneva, Switzerland: WHO.

World Health Organization (WHO) (2014b). *Strengthening Health Resilience to Climate Change: Technical Briefing for the World Health Organization.* Available at: http://www.who.int/phe/climate/conference_briefing_1_healthresilience_27aug.pdf (accessed 10 January 2017) [Online].

World Health Organization (WHO) (2015, September). *Ageing and Health.* Available at: http://www.who.int/mediacentre/factsheets/fs404/en/ (accessed 22 December 2016) [Online].

Yao, T. (2004, September 23). Research and environment news from China 2004. *China Daily*, **3**, 1–40.

Chapter 9

Special topics in rural health II

Border towns, plantations, and nomadic pastoralists

This chapter examines health issues associated with population living in border town, plantation, and nomadic environment.

9.1 Border towns

Key points

- Border towns, due to their geographical location, culture, and frequent population movement, present complex public health issues to be tackled by policymakers and public health practitioners.

A border town typically refers to a town or city that lies close to the geographic boundary between two countries. Some countries have multiple border neighbours (e.g. China has 14), and health issues and challenges associated with each of these communities might be different. Due to the proximity of the populations and the sharing of environmental resources, border towns often depend on their neighbourhood community for mutual coexistence. For example, two border towns may share the same water supply but as their use of the water and drainage systems are different, disputes of access and water pollution may result. While border towns offer work opportunities and socioeconomic prospects, workers may be affected by the working environments, policies, and conditions of another country. In many Asian borders, the population that has settled in the border area are ethnic minorities and tends to be marginalized and neglected by the larger society (Freeman, 2011). The general health status of the country might not reflect the health needs/status of people living in these border town areas. Border town population may have health needs/status that resemble more to their counterparts across the border.

9.1.1 Marginalization, security, and safety issues

Border controls can vary greatly in different countries and different political contexts and maintaining security may be a major challenge in these areas. When a disturbance or crisis occurs in the neighbouring countries, incidents may have an effect across the border

(Freeman, 2011), which can all cause public health and disease control concerns. For border areas that are sparsely populated and with poor infrastructure support, there might be a lack of border control or a limited capacity for law enforcement. Cross-border criminal activities (such as illegal immigration, smuggling, drug trafficking, organized crime, and even terrorism) can be rampant (Freeman and Thompson, 2011). In more developed border areas, people may commute daily for work, trade, education, travel, and other activities. Porous borders may pose heavy burden in tracking movement and in controlling health risks.

9.1.2 Health in border towns

Population movements may increase public health and medical risks. The diverse disease profiles of migrants or transient visitors may pose pressures on the healthcare and health systems of border areas. Differences in health standards and socioeconomic disparities in the border countries may reduce the effectiveness of health protection measures and pose a burden on border health services. For example, at the China–Myanmar–Thailand border, Burmese, tend to seek medical services and treatment in China (Kunming, the provincial capital of Yunnan Province) and Thailand. Meanwhile, at the China border, despite its efforts to control local communicable diseases, suboptimal governance and a lack of public health services in Myanmar have continued to render population vulnerable and susceptible to untreated diseases (Freeman and Thompson, 2011), and thus reduce the human health security of the border towns in China (Griffiths *et al.*, 2005; Xiao *et al.*, 2007) (see Case Study 9.1).

9.1.3 Health protection

Population movement may import infections and lead to local transmissions (Edwards *et al.*, 2015). Cross-border movements of populations have contributed to the high rates of disease transmissions along international borders (Cotter *et al.*, 2013; Edwards *et al.*, 2015). With population movement, drug resistance and the dispersal of drug-resistant parasites may be spread by mobile populations, for whom there are often delays in diagnoses and treatment, as well as improper health-seeking or self-medicating behaviours (Edwards *et al.*, 2015). With lower levels of capacity following up and tracing diseases, borders become crucial entry points for communicable diseases such as influenza, SARS, HIV/AIDS, and vector-borne diseases (e.g. malaria, dengue, and zika) if they are not properly managed (Kamel, 2009). Case Study 9.2 describes the effort to manage cross-border health in India. Disease surveillance and control in border towns will need to meet both the health needs of the local residents and the health issues associated with a transient and high health risk subpopulation.

Cross-border collaborations are important for health protection efforts (e.g. managing vector-borne diseases such as malaria and dengue fever). In the Greater Mekong Subregion of Thailand,[1] malaria management is a public health priority, especially in the areas adjacent to the borders of Myanmar and Cambodia (Thailand Bureau of Epidemiology, 2011). Population mobility has been identified as a key determinant for malaria multidrug resistance development and suboptimal control in these areas (WHO, 2016).

Case Study 9.1 Golden Triangle: China and Thailand–Laos–Myanmar border

China's border is shared by 14 countries, which include Afghanistan, the Kingdom of Bhutan, India, Kazakhstan, the Democratic People's Republic of Korea, Kyrgyzstan, Laos, Mongolia, Myanmar, Nepal, Pakistan, Russia, Tajikistan, and Vietnam. With the increase of global trade and international travel, China's border towns are crucial locations for interactions and exchanges with these neighbouring countries.

Situated in Southeast Asia, Myanmar is bordered on the north and north-east by China, on the east and south-east by Laos and Thailand, and on the west by Bangladesh and India. As part of the Golden Triangle region, Myanmar is the world's second largest opium producer after Afghanistan. In some areas of the country's rugged north, there are lawless conflicts and vast amounts of opium, heroin, and methamphetamine are produced and smuggled through the border towns into China, Thailand, and India. Drug abuse was reported to have reached a crisis level among some of Myanmar's ethnic communities in the states of Kachin and Shan, as well as in the country's transport nodes and border towns such as Lashio, Muse (bordering Ruili, in China's Yunnan Province), Kalay, and Tamu (bordering Moreh, in India's Manipur State) (Thompson, 2009).

When there are security incidents at one country's border, consequences will be felt across the neighbouring border town (Griffiths *et al.*, 2005). For example, in 2009 a series of skirmishes broke out, followed by a small military operation, in the northern Shan State of Myanmar. More than 35,000 civilians and armed soldiers escaped to the bordering area of Yunnan Province in China. The Yunnan provincial government responded by providing medical assistance such as food, water, and medical services in the refugee camps (Centers for Disease Control and Prevention, 2014).

In China, border areas are mostly populated by ethnic minorities, who may have similarities or even kinships with the culture of its neighbouring countries (Freeman, 2011). Ruili, Yunnan Province, is a Chinese Burma border area which faces major public security problems in terms of border policing. One-third of the robbery offences in Ruili City were reported to be committed by outsiders (Freeman and Thompson, 2011).

Marginalized people who may engage in the commercial sex trade, cross-border drug trafficking, and drug use, have limited access to public health services, education and social services (Freeman and Thompson, 2011). The control of sexually transmitted diseases and HIV/AIDS remains suboptimal (Xiao *et al.*, 2007). Yunnan Province, where the first official case of HIV/AIDS was identified and reported in China in 1989, still has the highest incidence rate of HIV/AIDs among all the provinces in China.

Measures of the Chinese government and their impact on border health

To effectively prevent the spread of HIV/AIDS, coordinated efforts must be made with the bordering countries such as Vietnam and Myanmar (Des Jarlais *et al.*, 2005). For example, since long-distance container truck drivers are at a high risk for HIV/AIDS, the Chinese province provides voluntary HIV testing at its border crossings, and regular cross-border training and technical exchanges are also organized in the border areas (Freeman and Thompson, 2011; Hu and Guo, 2014; Yang, 2015). However, while the public awareness of HIV/AIDS has increased, the transient migrants continue to engage in high-risk behaviour at an alarming rate (Xiao *et al.*, 2007), resulting in more than 10,000 new cases being diagnosed (Hu and Guo, 2014).

Targeted projects in its border areas were developed to manage border health and security risks. The 1998 Border Action Campaign, the Western Development Program in 1999, and the Revitalization of the Old Industrial Base in Northeast China in 2003 are examples of projects which aim to promote economic development and infrastructure constructions, as well as finance social construction projects along the border (Baidu Baike, n.d.-a, n.d.-b; Freeman and Thompson, 2011). The initiative of developing the border town Ruili of Yunnan Province adjacent to Myanmar also funded health education programmes and health checks to reduce the cross-border transmission of HIV/AIDS; while the same initiative in Erlian town, bordered with Mongolia, aims at financing the construction of healthcare, sanitation, and educational infrastructure to meet the needs of the growing population in the border region of the Inner Mongolia Province (Freeman and Thompson, 2011). The introduction of the Silk Road Economic Belt and the Maritime Silk Road Initiative by the Chinese government in 2013 aims to strengthen its multilateral cooperation and economic development with neighbouring countries and to promote border trade, tourism, and cultural cooperation (National Development and Reform Commission People's Republic of China, 2015). Such cooperation will not only increase trade opportunities, but will also promote the exchanges of people in the border areas of the two countries through improved transport and communication infrastructures (National Development and Reform Commission of the People's Republic of China, 2015). In addition to Tibet, the economic cooperation policy will attempt to cover all cross-border areas, and China's border towns are likely to experience large inflows of capital alongside rapid urban development and population expansion in the coming decades. These economic activities will heighten public health challenges and create increased opportunities for disease transmissions. Therefore, it is imperative that sufficient resources are allocated to build healthcare infrastructures and strengthen the medical services in these border towns.

Case Study 9.2 Border health on the India–Myanmar border

India's State of Manipur shares a long and porous border with Myanmar. Besides legal cross-border commerce, the area is notorious for the smuggling of narcotics (e.g. heroin) and has a prominent commercial sex industry. The context has contributed significantly to the spread of sexually transmitted diseases (STDs) and HIV/AIDS. Cross-border collaborations between Oxfam and its local partners in the Indian border town of Moreh in Manipur provided health promotion and medical assistance to the vulnerable people, including intravenous drug users, people living with HIV/AIDS and their families, sex workers, and their clients. The organization also worked with church groups situated in Tamu, the Myanmar side of the border, to improve service access and reduce risky behaviours and practices (Oxfam, 2006).

For example, the United States Agency for International Development (USAID) supported the development of several twin-cities programmes in the Greater Mekong Subregion and facilitated cross-border patient referral and to strengthen cross-border collaborations at the working levels of government. Bilingual patient cards were introduced by Cambodia and Thailand in some border regions to help ensure adequate follow-up treatments for the mobile and migrant populations who cross international borders during the course of a treatment (WHO, 2016). In general, health authorities on both sides of a border should maintain close partnerships in order to ensure a functional cross-border health protection system (Freeman and Thompson, 2011).

Safety in water, food, and access to drugs is also influenced by crises (e.g. natural disasters and pollution incidents), as well as standards and regulations of the country across and around the border. For instance, the two bordering towns may face the same problems with their water quality if they share the same water sources. Food quality depends on the agricultural standards (such as the use of fertilizers or pesticides) and environmental factors (floods, droughts, and other disasters). Access to essential drugs and medical treatment might vary significantly for price, quality, and access (e.g. prescribed vs. off-the counter drugs might be different between two countries).

9.1.4 Health promotion

Residents of two neighbouring border cities might originate from the same ethnic group, cultures, traditions, and language which can be different from that of the majority population in their respective country. Education and health promotion strategies in border areas might be different from the rest of the country. To be effective, health education materials should be designed and adapted to the unique geographical locations, cultural structures, languages, and local literacy rates, as well as the socioeconomic context and the migration status (length of stay) of the target population.

Delay in malaria treatment-seeking may result in severe complications and further transmission of the disease. A study at the Thailand–Myanmar border of health-seeking behaviour for malaria found patients' ethnicity was a significant factor for the high prevalence (79.4%) of malaria treatment delay in this area. Although the population is of Thai nationality, it is ethnically identified as part of the 'hill tribes' that include the Karen and Hmong. In terms of their culture, they are very different from other Thais. Language barriers and the difference in belief (e.g. a supernatural cause for illnesses vs. Western scientific basis of disease) are reasons reported for delay treatment. However, to encourage early treatment, health promotion measures should be adapted to local needs that might be different from the majority group of the country (Sonkong *et al.*, 2015).

The following Case Study 9.3 describes how conflicts in border areas can lead to chronic threats to human and health security.

Case Study 9.3 Kashmir dispute between India and Pakistan

Although the Himalayan region of Kashmir may be one of the most scenic landscapes in the world, it is also one of the most militarized zones in the world. India and Pakistan each control about 45% and 35% of the region, respectively, while the China-controlled area, called Aksai Chin and located in the north-east, equals about 20% of the region.

The conflict in Kashmir started in 1947, when Pakistan and India gained independence from British rule. This territory has been partitioned by India and Pakistan, and both countries claim full ownership of the region but only partially control it. The India-controlled part consists of the state of Jammu and Kashmir, which makes up the southern and eastern part of Kashmir. Pakistan controls the northern and western portions, in the areas of Azad Kashmir, Gilgit, and Baltistan. The unresolved dispute has brought Pakistan and India to war on a number of occasions. The situation became more complex when the separatist violence led by Islamic militants began in 1989. A ceasefire agreement was reached by two countries in 2003, although the two sides continued to regularly exchange gunfire across the border. In September 2016, 18 Indian soldiers were killed in an attack by armed militants in the Indian-administered area of Kashmir. Two weeks later, two Pakistani soldiers were killed in a clash with Indian troops across the de-facto border between the two countries.

The case of Kashmir illustrates the fact that the political and military disputes over a border area can bring long-term suffering to the population. In the Indian state of Jammu and Kashmir, although it is a popular place for tourism and contributed significantly to the region's economy, the industry has been hardly hit and disrupted because of the years of unrest. Many non-government agencies are active in the area to support the needs of the people who are directly or indirectly affected by violence there. For example, the European Commission–Humanitarian Aid and Civil Protection (ECHO, 2014) provides psychological care and support, as well as occupational therapy and livelihood support to the population. The humanitarian health needs of the population remain chronic in border towns of the region.

9.1.5 Implications for bottom-up health resilience and disaster risk reduction

Although health protection and disease prevention requires infrastructure, top-down policy, investment, and efforts, effective protection of the well-being of people living in border communities will also depend on the local context and general health literacy towards risks for poor health and disaster preparedness. Border towns attract rural migrant workers and the control of communicable diseases can be challenging for developing countries (see also Chapter 10). Close partnerships between neighbouring countries in disease surveillance and control efforts in border towns are necessary for community health protection and disease prevention.

9.1.6 Conclusion

Border towns face numerous public health challenges. Language and cultural differences, service barriers, risk of disease transmissions, security threats of instability, and complex emergencies are all important issues to be examined if bottom-up health and disaster risk reduction programmes are to be developed.

9.2 Plantations

Key points

- Majority of the world's agricultural and plantation workers are in Asia and the Pacific region. Most of them are living in socioeconomically disadvantaged conditions and are vulnerable to health risk and poor health outcomes.

Agriculture accounts for 31% of global employment and an estimated 1.3 billion people are engaged in agricultural production, among which 500 million are employed on plantations (International Labour Organization [ILO], n.d.-b). Majority of global agricultural workers—over 70%—are in Asia and the Pacific region (International Labour Office, 2000). Agriculture is considered as one of the top three most hazardous sectors (along with construction and mining). Agricultural workers may be exposed to extreme weather and working conditions, which exposes them to increased risks of injury, infectious diseases, and poisonous materials (chemicals and biological products).

Working conditions for agricultural workers vary from place to place and depend on policies and socioeconomic conditions. In general, the most vulnerable agricultural workers include those engaged in family subsistence agriculture, in plantations as daily paid labourers, seasonal and migrant workers, and child labourers (ILO, n.d.-a). Frequently in family subsistence farming, the entire household, including children, pregnant women, and older people, are involved. In many transitional communities, the migration of young men to the city also leaves the agricultural work to the women and children at home (International Labour Office, 2000). Among the estimated 168 million child labourers in the world, Asia and the Pacific region have the largest number, with almost 78 million of them (ILO, n.d.-c). Around 60% of child labourers in the world are found in the plantation and agriculture sector (ILO, n.d.-c).

9.2.1 Physical health

Plantation workers are regularly exposed to occupational hazards such as injury, poisoning, and musculoskeletal disorders. The poor working environment, long working hours, and the lack of policy and regulation protection lead to frequent injuries in plantations (Din *et al.*, 2014; Human Rights Watch, 2016, May 24). Younger farmers have a higher risk of non-fatal injuries, while their older counterparts tend to account for the greatest proportion of fatal injuries (Din *et al.*, 2014). The use of machinery and other sharp tools can cause lacerations, falls, and traumatic limb injuries in the farming environment (Human Rights Watch, 2016, May 24). Heavy machineries, such as tractors and harvesters, cause the highest frequency and fatality rates of injuries (International Labour Office, 2000). Due to poor posture and excessive workload, a lot of farmers also suffer from different musculoskeletal problems, such as back and knee pain (Human Rights Watch, 2016, May 24) (see Case Study 9.4). The occupational use of pesticide is a risk factor for adverse neurological effects and respiratory symptoms (Cha *et al.*, 2012). Many pesticides are toxic to the reproductive health system and can cause fertility and reproductive health issues (Mendola *et al.*, 2008). Tobacco cultivation also threatens the physical health of the workers with acute nicotine poisoning. They can absorb nicotine through the skin while coming into contact with tobacco plants and leaves, which can lead to so-called green tobacco sickness (GTS) (Mendola *et al.*, 2008: Riquinho and Hennington, 2012). Chronic dermal nicotine absorption has been shown to be both toxic to the cardiovascular system and carcinogenic (Mendola *et al.*, 2008). GTS symptoms include vomiting, nausea, dizziness, and headache, and even dehydration in some severe cases (Mendola *et al.*, 2008). Poor management of pesticide-related waste (e.g. bottles) also presents additional occupational health risks and contributes to environmental pollution, especially water and soil contamination. In addition, a study (on two imidazolinone herbicides, imazethapyr and imazaquin) found that the use of pesticide was associated with a statistically significantly higher risk of bladder cancer among farmers (Koutros *et al.* 2016).

9.2.2 Mental health

Poor working environment, long working hours, physically demanding tasks, and the unstable, seasonal nature of the employment could negatively affect the workers' mental well-being. In family-oriented plantations, mono-cropping is the usual practice and the heavy dependence on a single crop as the source of income can threaten the financial stability of a household and, ultimately, affect the mental well-being of the workers. In addition, pesticide toxicity may affect the peripheral and central nervous system (Cha *et al.*, 2012; Din *et al.*, 2014) and in turn affect mental well-being. The use of organophosphate pesticides may undermine the mental health of the workers, causing disorders such as chronic depression, and even contribute to suicidal behaviour (Cha *et al.*, 2012).

9.2.3 Social health

To make a viable profit, many plantations are highly mechanized and a large number of temporary migrant workers are hired only during the harvesting season. Seasonal migrant workers may have to work in various plantations to generate adequate income (Riquinho and Hennington, 2012; Xiang *et al.*, 2000). Continual migration makes it very difficult for them to build a normal residential life and social network. The social well-being of seasonal migration-based plantation workers and those who work in large-scale commercialized plantation farms can suffer from a very poor social health status (Riquinho and Hennington, 2012). Many of these migrant workers may not have access to education and healthcare services and thus their health outcomes suffer significantly as they age.

9.2.4 Child labour

Child labour is another important challenge. Children working in unprotected environments might be exposed to increased risks of diseases and physical and sexual violence (Food and Agriculture Organization of the United Nations [FAO], 2010). The mental health status, social well-being, as well as access to age-appropriate education of children working in agriculture and on plantations should also not be overlooked. According to the Human Rights Watch report on child labour in Indonesia, although most children interviewed said they only worked outside school hours, some reported that they had dropped out of school to work in the tobacco farms to support their families (Human Rights Watch, 2016, May 24). Not being able to attend school may subject young people to social isolation and thus might render them completely invisible in society (FAO, 2010) (see Case Studies 9.4 and 9.5).

9.2.5 Implications for bottom-up health resilience and disaster risk reduction

As highlighted above, plantations are usually located in rural communities and their workers often face high occupational and environmental risks. Increasing health risk awareness and safety practice enhancement programmes in water, soil, and environmental

Case Study 9.4 Health of plantation workers in Indonesia

In Asia, Indonesia is a major producer of agricultural products, including palm oil, natural rubber, rice, and spices. It is also the world's fifth largest tobacco producer and home to more than 500,000 tobacco farms nationwide. Agriculture is the main source of employment in rural areas where poverty is widespread (Quincieu, 2015). It is estimated that over 1.5 million children aged between 10–17 years are working in the agricultural sector in Indonesia, mainly on tobacco, rubber, and palm oil plantations (International Labour Organization, n.d.-d).

Human Rights Watch study on children engagement in farming activities found about half of the child labourers interviewed in Indonesia reported experiencing at least one symptom consistent with acute nicotine poisoning while working in tobacco farming. Many reported multiple symptoms (Human Rights Watch, 2016, May 24). How the health and well-being of plantation workers may be affected by their occupational risks remains under-reported.

Case Study 9.5 Protection of health for plantation workers in China

Cost-effective, low technology-based initiatives may be used to increase the health protection of plantation workers. For example, along the China–Myanmar borders, mobile and migrant people, including workers on plantations and in the forests, are vulnerable to malaria transmission. The distribution of insecticide-treated nets (ITNs) or long-lasting insecticidal nets (LLINs) by organizations would protect against occupational and environmental hazards for working in high malaria risk areas (Liu *et al.*, 2015; Moore *et al.*, 2008).

conservation might reduce health and disaster risk associated with the occupational contexts and socioeconomic limitations (see also the section on climate change in Chapter 8).

9.2.6 Conclusion

The impact of climate change and the problem of food security will continue to change the landscape of the plantation industry in the region. Rural plantation workers often face socioeconomic disadvantages and occupational hazards. Public health efforts and policies should be invested to protect the health and well-being of plantation workers, particularly that of child labourers.

9.3 Nomadic pastoralists

Key points

- Globally, the traditional lifestyle and their harsh living conditions of nomadic people render different health problems and risks when compared with their urban counterparts
- While nomads are decreasing in total number worldwide, they are seriously marginalized and they face huge barriers to accessing basic public facilities, including healthcare services.

In the twenty-first century, global statistics indicate that there are approximately 50–100 million nomads and semi-nomads [2] in the world (UN Economic and Social Commission for Asia and the Pacific, 2014) and over 60% of them live in Africa (Omar, 1992). Nomadic people are generally classified as hunters, collectors, and pastoralists. While hunters and collectors are very few in numbers, nomadic pastoralists are present in the Sahel region of Africa, Central Asia, the Middle East, and India (Zinsstag *et al.*, 2006) (Case Study 9.6).

For centuries, nomadic pastoralists have been living in harsh terrain and extreme climates. With modernization, their seasonal migration lifestyle has made them lag behind settled population in social development in many regions. In general, they have poorer health status, and are at a higher risk of contracting different kinds of infectious diseases and developing health problems.

Case Study 9.6 Nomadic people in the Central Asian plain: Accessibility to healthcare services

Nomads typically live in areas where the climate is not suitable for agriculture but livelihood can be temporarily sustained by grazing animals. In the Central Asian plain, the main nomadic communities include Tibetans, Kazakhs, Mongols, Kyrgyz people, and Tajiks. Their lives are hard and often affected by trauma, conflicts, natural disasters, food shortages, and extreme weather. The nomads migrate seasonally with their families and animals, while semi-nomads frequently move with their livestock between their fixed place of residence and a temporary grazing area. Recently, rapid economic development, climate change and changes in the ecosystem have meant that these nomadic pastoralists can no longer rely on their traditional grazing practice as their prime economic activity. Although only limited literature is available to understand Chinese nomadic peoples, most reports have shared the common health challenges associated with problematic access to healthcare services due to geographical isolation.

9.3.1 Common health problems of nomads

Communicable diseases

Communicable or infectious diseases, such as zoonotic or parasitic diseases, sexually transmitted diseases, and tuberculosis (TB) are commonly found among the nomadic populations (Zinsstag *et al.*, 2006). Due to their close contact with their animals and livestock, there are high prevalence of zoonotic diseases among the nomads. For example, in Tibetan nomadic populations, hydatid cysts were detected in 19% of nomads screened, meaning they were at higher risk of infection than others (Li *et al.*, 2005). Cystic echinococcosis in humans is caused by an infection of the hydatid cyst or the larva of a dog tapeworm. Brucellosis is another zoonosis that threatens the health and livelihood of nomads. In animals, brucellosis mainly affects reproduction and fertility, reduces the survival of newborns, and decreases milk yield. Human brucellosis is commonly caused by exposure to infected livestock and livestock products like raw milk and thus the nomadic pastoralists are highly vulnerable (Zinsstag *et al.*, 2006). The special environment in which nomads live and their lifestyle also causes the high prevalence of diseases such as trachoma and guinea worm (Global Rights, 2008; Nawabi, 2010).

Tuberculosis (TB) is one of the major chronic preventable communicable health problems among nomads. The high prevalence rate of TB among nomads is attributed to their crowded living conditions and poor heath infrastructure (Sheik-Mohamed and Velema, 1999). A study in nomadic districts in Kenya found TB contributed to 28% of all cases registered in Kenya in 1992 while making up only 11% of the total population (van Cleeff *et al.*, 1995). The mobility of nomads makes it extremely difficult to trace TB patients and ensure compliance with the treatment. Studies in a semi-nomadic district in Uganda show that only around half of the TB patients placed on treatment were completely treated (Sheik-Mohamed and Velema, 1999).

Non-communicable diseases (NCDs)

Changes in traditional nomadic lifestyle, and epidemiological and demographic transitions are affecting nomadic communities. Life expectancy increase and livelihood improvement through technological and economic opportunities have changed disease patterns. Gaps exist in the research literature to impede an understanding of the epidemiological patterns of NCDs, ranging from cardiovascular conditions and injury patterns to mental health issues in this population subgroup, and their way of living poses difficulties for long-term disease management.

Access to service of nomadic population with special needs

Nomadic communities often have no or limited access to basic healthcare, education, and services. Nomads commonly manage their health needs by self-care and seek help from traditional healers, but it should not be assumed that they are not interested in modern healthcare (Sheik-Mohamed and Velema, 1999). Mobile clinics together with fixed health centres are situated in strategic locations along the migratory routes (Sheik-Mohamed and Velema, 1999: Zinsstag *et al.*, 2006). Adapted and specific approaches in healthcare provision should be considered, such as an adapted directly observed treatment short course (DOTS) strategy for TB (Sheik-Mohamed and Velema, 1999: Zinsstag *et al.*, 2006). When considering specific strategies for providing healthcare to nomadic populations, a comprehensive and sustainable approach is advocated, which includes the surrounding settled communities in the planning as they are as poor as the nomads (Zinsstag *et al.*, 2006) (Case Studies 9.7 and 9.8).

9.3.2 Implications for bottom-up health resilience and disaster risk reduction

Technology advancement may play a vital role in improving access and information to healthcare for nomadic populations (also see Chapter 10 on technology and health) Integrated biometric fingerprint identification in a geographical information system for mobile pastoralists (Weibel *et al.*, 2008) and the use of mobile phones might facilitate the tracking of nomads and collect data for demographic surveillance (Jean-Richard *et al.*, 2014). Both have proven viable for conducting demographic and health surveillance of

Case Study 9.7 Maternal and child health in the alpine grasslands of the Tibetan Plateau

High rate of miscarriage and infant were reported among Kham Tibetan pastoralists as they had no access to midwives to assist them in pregnancy and delivery (Zinsstag *et al.*, 2006). Women in the alpine grasslands of the Tibetan Plateau had to work during their pregnancy, which was one of the main causes of miscarriage and health problems during pregnancy. It was a problem to which the local community could see no solution. Most of the women delivered at home assisted by a relative (usually their mother), and only 2% were helped by a health worker/doctor (Zinsstag *et al.*, 2006). As there are no traditional midwives, the women have no regular check-ups. Only if there are serious problems during the delivery might they call for a village doctor—who would be male, and probably live far away. All this can spell death from obstructed labour and late post-partum haemorrhage, and the death of newborn infants. These are the most three serious health problems in their community.

Fever, coughing, and diarrhoea were commonly reported childhood illnesses in the alpine grasslands (Zinsstag *et al.*, 2006) and the infant death rate was high, with maternal and child health being significantly affected by the time it takes to obtain water. Although most people live within 15 minutes of a water supply, for a significant proportion of the families it takes over an hour to collect water. Moreover, the lifestyle of moving seasonally and remoteness from the village doctor has significant links with the high morbidity and mortality levels, especially among women and children in pastoral populations (Omar, 1992).

Case Study 9.8 Challenges in health and access to services of nomadic peoples in Afghanistan

The Kuchis are nomadic Afghanistan people, with an estimated number of about 1.5 million (about 6% of the total Afghan population). They are spread across all 34 provinces in the country (Islamic Republic of Afghanistan Ministry of Public Health, 2010). Over the years, many members of the Kuchi ethnic group have permanently settled down in villages or towns (especially in capital Kabul), while close to 18% of them are semi-nomadic and only 2% are still fully nomadic (Afghanistan Independent Human Rights Commission, 2011). Mobile lifestyle and unfavourable living conditions of Kuchis leave them at a higher risk of TB; there is a lack of ventilation in the Kuchi tents and infection can easily be transmitted within the whole family (Islamic Republic of Afghanistan Ministry of Public Health, 2010). In a survey on domestic abuse conducted among 4,700 households across Afghanistan, an overwhelming majority (87%) of the interviewed women reported at least one form of physical, sexual, or psychological violence. Among them were all of the Kuchi women (from 101 households) settled in or at the outskirts of Kabul (Global Rights, 2008). Of those who settled, reports of the lack access to services, including drinking water, and discrimination by the local population were common (Foschini, 2013; Minority Rights Group International, 2015).

The nomadic Kuchi children have lower vaccination rates compared with other children in urban or rural areas. Around 31% of Kuchi children had not received any dose of vaccine, compared to 15% and 7% for rural and urban children (ICON Institute, 2009). [3] According to the National Risk and Vulnerability Assessment (2007–2008), only 13% of Kuchi children had received full immunization (DTP3) compared to 33% among rural children and 63% among urban children. Kuchi women are also more vulnerable than general Afghan women as the maternal care for Kuchi women is very limited. In Afghanistan, 76% of the deliveries assisted by urban skilled health personnel while that in rural areas is only 33%; for Kuchi women, it is only 13%. Most women are also deprived of tetanus toxoid (TT) coverage to protect themselves and their babies. Some 84% did not receive any injection at all during their last pregnancy, while the national average was below 60% (Islamic Republic of Afghanistan Central Statistics Organization, 2014).

Barriers to healthcare

Literacy rates among nomads in Afghanistan remain among the lowest in the world (Afghanistan Independent Human Rights Commission, 2011; UNHCR, 2016). The overall literacy rate in the population aged 15 years and over was 31% in 2011–2012, with 54% and 25% among the urban and rural populations, whereas among Kuchis adult literacy is as low as 7% (Islamic Republic of Afghanistan Central Statistics Organization, 2014). The low literacy rates and education level may pose barriers for nomadic people to understand health information. In addition, the time it takes to reach health facilities is widely different among urban, rural, and Kuchi populations. While the urban population has virtually universal access to healthcare of any type within two hours, the access time is less favourable for rural and Kuchi populations (Islamic Republic of Afghanistan Central Statistics Organization, 2014).

Conflicts and tension between the nomadic and settled communities are common and they can be caused by disputes over land or competition for resources and assistance distribution in, for example, those areas where Kuchis are settled at the same location with another internally displaced person (IDP) group (Samuel Hall Consulting, 2014). The situation of Kuchis has grown worse since the 2001 United States-led invasion of Afghanistan (Nawabi, 2010) and the nomadic population's access to healthcare is further hampered in the ongoing wars and conflicts.

Mines continue to kill and injure Afghan citizens throughout the country. Scattered or buried beside roads, on mountainsides, in pasture land, on the banks of rivers and irrigation systems, inside houses, and elsewhere, mines still claim victims daily (MSF, 1997). Many medical non-governmental organizations, such as Médecins Sans Frontières (MSF), are witnessing the daily impact of mines in Afghanistan. MSF clinics regularly provide the first line of emergency treatment to mine victims before referral to surgical hospitals. As a consequence of decades of war, there are many minefields in and around villages, towns, and cities. These are the priority areas to be cleared but, as there are simply too many minefields in Afghanistan overall, the assumption that it will never be totally cleared is taken as a concrete and accepted fact by the international community. For this reason, it is imperative that Afghans know how to live with the mines which surround them and that they have the knowledge and skills to protect themselves. Because of their lifestyle, it is extremely difficult to confer mine awareness information to nomadic Kuchis and location messages might also fail to reach them. Roaming for hundreds of kilometres over the hills and plains of Afghanistan with their camels, donkeys, dogs, and herds of sheep and goats, Kuchis have often fallen outside the scope of mine awareness training. Handicap International attempted to build mine awareness training around Kandahar by tracing the traditional migration patterns of the Kuchis in order to disseminate information related to landmine risk to communities that travel along those routes (Handicap International, n.d.).

---

these hard-to-reach communities. This could lead to improved planning and healthcare provision for both nomadic humans and their animals.

Given the intimate relationship between nomads and their domesticated animals, nomadic communities are important target groups to ensure health risk reduction and adverse health outcome protection in the notion of 'One Health' (Kamani *et al.*, 2015). Animal health may serve as an ideal entry point for the provision of human health services (Majok and Schwabe, 1996) and the merging of public health and veterinary services may provide co-benefits to both human and animals. Joint human and animal vaccination campaigns carried out previously in conflict settings have proved successful (Schelling *et al.*, 2005) and such campaigns can be replicated and expanded to other health services.

9.4 Conclusion

With modernization and urbanization, nomads will continue to decrease in number and remain a very small proportion of the world's population. Nevertheless, the health needs and well-being of nomads should not be forgotten in the twenty-first century (Sheik-Mohamed and Velema, 1999; Zinsstag *et al.*, 2006).

Notes

1. The countries in the Greater Mekong Subregion include Thailand, Vietnam, Myanmar, Cambodia, Laos, and China's Yunnan Province.
2. Semi-nomads practice some non-pastoral activities such as small-scale businesses and farming while retaining migration and livestock herding as their basic economic activities (Sheik-Mohamed and Velema, 1999).
3. The figures were not updated in the latest NRVA 2011–2012 report.

References

Afghanistan Independent Human Rights Commission (AIHRC) (2011). *Fifth Report: Situation of Economic and Social Rights in Afghanistan*. Kabul, Afghanistan: AIHRC.

Baidu Baike (n.d.-a). [The initiative of developing the border and enriching the border people]. Available at: http://baike.baidu.com/view/4774511.htm (accessed 29 October 2015) (Chinese) [Online].

Baidu Baike (n.d.-b). [The strategy of revitalisation of the old industrial base in Northeast China]. Available at: http://baike.baidu.com/view/3221085.htm (accessed 29 October 2015) (Chinese) [Online].

Buursink, J. (2014). The binational reality of border-crossing cities. *Geo Journal*, **54**, 7–19.

Centers for Disease Control and Prevention (2014). U.S.–Mexico cross-border health. Available at: http://www.cdc.gov/healthcommunication/toolstemplates/entertainmented/tips/us-mexico-health.html (accessed 26 January 2017) [Online].

Cha, E. S., Lee, Y. K., Moon, E. K., *et al.* (2012). Paraquat application and respiratory health effects among South Korean farmers. *Occup Environ Med*, **69**, 398–403.

Constitution of Afghanistan (2004). Available at: http://www.refworld.org/docid/404d8a594.html (accessed 14 January 2017) [Online].

Cotter, C., Sturrock, H. J., Hsiang, M. S., *et al.* (2013). The changing epidemiology of malaria elimination: new strategies for new challenges. *Lancet*, **382**, 900–11.

Des Jarlais, D. C., Johnston, P., Friedmann, P., *et al.* (2005). Patterns of HIV prevalence among injecting drug users in the cross-border area of Lang Son Province, Vietnam, and Ning Ming County, Guangxi Province, China. *BMC Public Health*, **5**, 89.

Din, N. C., Ghazali, S. E., Ibrahim, N., *et al.* (2014). Health needs assessment of older people in an agricultural plantation. *Int J Gerontol*, **8**, 120–6.

Edwards, H. M., Canavati, S. E., Rang, C., *et al.* (2015). Novel cross-border approaches to optimise identification of asymptomatic and Artemisinin-resistant Plasmodium infection in mobile populations crossing Cambodian borders. *PLoS One*, **10**, e0124300.

European Commission–Humanitarian Aid and Civil Protection (ECHO) (2014). *ECHO Factsheet: India*. Available at: http://reliefweb.int/sites/reliefweb.int/files/resources/ECHO%20Factsheet%20-%20January%202014%20-%20India.pdf [Online].

Food and Agriculture Organization (FAO) of the United Nations (2010). *Breaking the rural poverty cycle: getting girls and boys out of work and into school* (Gender and Rural Employment Policy Brief No. 7). Available from: http://www.fao.org/docrep/013/i2008e/i2008e07.pdf (accessed 10 February 2017) [Online].

Foschini, F. (2013). *The Social Wandering of the Afghan Kuchis: Changing patterns, perceptions and politics of an Afghan community*. Afghanistan Analysts Network (AAN). Available at: http://www.afghanistan-analysts.org/wp-content/uploads/2013/11/20131125_FFoschini-Kuchis.pdf (accessed 8 February 2017) [Online].

Freeman, C. (2011). Fragile edges between security and insecurity: China's border regions. In: Guo, R. & Freeman, C. (eds), *Managing Fragile Regions: Method and Application*, pp. 23–46. New York, NY: Springer-Verlag.

Freeman, C. & Thompson, D. (2011). *China on the Edge: China's Border Provinces and Chinese Security Policy*. Washington, DC: The Center for the National Interest and Johns Hopkins SAIS.

Global Rights (2008). *Living with violence: a national report on domestic abuse in Afghanistan*. Available at: https://www.humanitarianresponse.info/en/operations/afghanistan/document/living-violence-national-report-domestic-abuse-afghanistan-global [Online].

Griffiths, S., Jewell, T., & Donnelly, P. (2005). Public health in practice: the three domains of public health. *Public Health*, **119**, 907–13.

Handicap International (n.d.). Afghanistan. Available at: https://www.handicap-international.org.uk/country/afghanistan (accessed 7 February, 2017) [Online].

Hu, Y. & Guo, A. (2014). Yunnan takes action to stem spread of HIV/AIDS. *China Daily*. Available at: http://usa.chinadaily.com.cn/epaper/2014-02/21/content_17297789.htm (accessed 26 January 2017) [Online].

Human Rights Watch (2016, May 24). 'The Harvest is in My Blood': Hazardous child labor in tobacco farming in Indonesia. Available at: https://www.hrw.org/report/2016/05/24/harvest-my-blood/hazardous-child-labor-tobacco-farming-indonesia (accessed 10 February 2017) [Online].

ICON Institute (2009). *National Risk and Vulnerability Assessment (NRVA) 2007/8: A profile of Afghanistan*. Kabul, Afghanistan. Available at: http://www.unodc.org/documents/afghanistan/EUGovtofAFG_NRVA_2007-8_report.pdf (accessed 8 February 2017) [Online].

International Labour Office (2000). *Safety and Health in Agriculture*. Available at: http://www.ilo.org/wcmsp5/groups/public/---ed_protect/---protrav/---safework/documents/publication/wcms_110193.pdf (accessed 10 February 2017) [Online].

International Labour Organization (ILO) (n.d.-a). Agriculture: a hazardous work. Available at: https://www.ilo.org/safework/areasofwork/hazardous-work/WCMS_110188/lang--en/index.htm (accessed 30 December 2016) [Online].

International Labour Organization (ILO) (n.d.-b). Agriculture; plantations; other rural sectors. Available at: https://www.ilo.org/global/industries-and-sectors/agriculture-plantations-other-rural-sectors/lang--en/index.htm (accessed 30 December 2016) [Online].

International Labour Organization (ILO) (n.d.-c). Child labour. Available at: https://www.ilo.org/global/topics/child-labour/lang--en/index.htm (accessed 30 December 2016)

International Labour Organization (ILO) (n.d.-d). Child labour in plantation. Available at: www.ilo.org/jakarta/areasofwork/WCMS_126206/lang--en/index.htm?ssSourceSiteId=global/lang--en/index.htm (accessed 30 December 2016) [Online].

Islamic Republic of Afghanistan Ministry of Public Health (2010). *National Guidelines for Tuberculosis Control Program in Afghanistan*. Kabul, Afghanistan: Islamic Republic of Afghanistan Ministry of Public Health.

Islamic Republic of Afghanistan Central Statistics Organization (2014). *National Risk and Vulnerability Assessment 2011–12: Afghanistan Living Condition Survey*. Kabul, Afghanistan: CSO.

Jean-Richard, V., Crump, L., Daugla, D. M., *et al.* (2014). The use of mobile phones for demographic surveillance of mobile pastoralists and their animals in Chad: proof of principle. *Glob Health Action*, 7, 23209.

Kamani, T. M., Kazwala, R., Mfinanga, S., *et al.* (2015). One Health: a concept led by Africa, with global benefits. *Vet Rec*, **176**, 496–7.

Kamel, W. W. (2009). Health in border areas. In: Mansourian, P. B. (ed.), *Global Perspective in Health* (Vol. II, Encyclopedia of Life Support Systems series), pp. 326–43. Paris, France: UNESCO-EOLSS.

Koutros, S., Silverman, D. T., Alavanja, M. C., *et al.* (2016). Occupational exposure to pesticides and bladder cancer risk. *Int J Epidemiol*, **45**, 792–805.

Li, T., Qiu, J., Yang, W., *et al.* (2005). Echinococcosis in Tibetan populations, Western Sichuan Province, China. *Emerg Infect Dis*, **11**, 1866–73.

Majok, A. A. & Schwabe, C. W. (1996). *Development Among Africa's Migratory Pastoralists*. Westport, CA: Greenwood Publishing Group

Médecins Sans Frontières (MSF) (1997). *Living in a Minefield: The Landmine Problem in Afghanistan*. Available at: http://www.doctorswithoutborders.org/news-stories/special-report/living-minefield-landmine-problem-afghanistan (accessed 7 February 2017) [Online].

Mendola, P., Messer, L. C., & Rappazzo, K. (2008). Science linking environmental contaminant exposures with fertility and reproductive health impacts in the adult female. *Fertil Steril*, **89**(2, Supplement), e81–94.

Minority Rights Group International (2015). State of the world's minorities and indigenous peoples 2015—Afghanistan. Available at: http://www.refworld.org/docid/55a4fa6915.html (accessed 8 February 2017) [Online].

Moore, S. J., Min, X., *et al.* (2008). Border malaria in China: knowledge and use of personal protection by minority populations and implications for malaria control: a questionnaire-based survey. *BMC Public Health*, **8**, 344.

National Development and Reform Commission of the People's Republic of China (2015). Vision and actions on jointly building silk road economic belt and 21st-century maritime silk road. Available at: http://en.ndrc.gov.cn/newsrelease/201503/t20150330_669367.html (accessed 26 Jan 2017) [Online].

Nawabi, K. (2010). *Fractured Relationships: Understanding Conflict Between Nomadic and Settled Communities in Wardak's Pastureland*. Kabul, Afghanistan: Cooperation for Peace and Unity.

Omar, M. A. (1992). Health care for nomads too, please. *World Health Forum* **13**, 307–10.

Oxfam (2006). *HIV/AIDS work across borders*. Available at: http://policy-practice.oxfam.org.uk/publications/hivaids-work-across-borders-129046 (accessed 10 February 2017) [Online].

Quincieu, E. (2015). *Summary of Indonesia's Agriculture, Natural Resources, and Environment Sector Assessment* (ADB Papers on Indonesia No. 08). Available at: https://www.adb.org/sites/default/files/publication/177036/ino-paper-08-2015.pdf (accessed 10 February 2017) [Online].

Riquinho, D. L. & Hennington, E. A.. (2012). Health, environment and working conditions in tobacco cultivation: a review of the literature. *Ciência & Saúde Coletiva*, **17**, 1587–600.

Samuel Hall Consulting (2014). *Displacement Dynamics: IDP Movement Tracking, Needs and Vulnerability Analysis: Herat and Helmand Afghanistan*. Commissioned by the International Organization for Migration (IOM). Kabul, Afghanistan: IOM

Schelling, E., Wyss, K., Béchir, M., *et al.* (2005). Synergy between public health and veterinary services to deliver human and animal health interventions in rural low income settings. *BMJ*, **331**, 1264–7.

Sheik-Mohamed, A. & Velema, J. P. (1999). Where health care has no access: the nomadic populations of sub-Saharan Africa. *Trop Med Int Health*, **4**, 695–707.

Sonkong, K., Chaiklieng, S., Neave, P., & Suggaravetsiri, P. (2015). Factors affecting delay in seeking treatment among malaria patients along Thailand-Myanmar border in Tak Province, Thailand. *Malaria Journal*, **14**, 3.

Thailand Bureau of Epidemiology (2011). *Annual Epidemiological Surveillance Report*. Bankok, Thailand: Ministry of Public Health.

Thompson, D. (2009). Border burdens: China's response to the Myanmar refugee crisis. *WSI China Secur*, **5**, 13–23.

United Nations (UN) Economic and Social Commission for Asia and the Pacific (2014). *Statistical yearbook for Asia and the Pacific 2014*. Available at: http://www.unescap.org/sites/default/files/ESCAP-SYB2014_0.pdf (accessed 14 January 2017) [Online].

United Nations High Commissioner for Refugees (UNHCR) (2016). *Eligibility guidelines for assessing the international protection needs of asylum-seekers from Afghanistan*. Available at: http://www.refworld.org/docid/570f96564.html [Online].

van Cleeff, M. R. A., Becx-Bleumink, M., Bosman, M. J., *et al.* (1995). Tuberculosis control in North and South: four strategies for different socio-economic situations, In: van der Velden, J. *et al.* (eds), *Health Matters: Public Health in North–South Perspective*, pp. 217–41. Amsterdam, Netherlands: Royal Tropical Institute.

Weibel, D., Schelling, E., Bonfoh, B., & Zinsstag, J. (2008). Demographic and health surveillance of mobile pastoralists in Chad: integration of biometric fingerprint identification into a geographical information system. *Geospatial Health*, **3**, 113–24.

World Health Organization (WHO) (2016). *Approaches for Mobile and Migrant Populations in the Context of Malaria Multi-Drug Resistance and Malaria Elimination in the Greater Mekong Subregion*. Geneva, Switzerland: WHO.

World Heart Federation (n.d.). Rheumatic heart disease (RHD). Available at: www.world-heart-federation.org/what-we-do/rheumatic-heart-disease-rhd/ (accessed 6 January 2017) [Online].

Xiang, H., Wang, Z., Stallones, L., Keefe, T. J., Huang, X. U., & Fu, X. (2000). Agricultural work-related injuries among farmers in Hubei, People's Republic of China. *Am J Public Health*, **90**, 1269.

Xiao, Y., Kristensen, S., Sun, J., *et al.* (2007). Expansion of HIV/AIDS in China: lessons from Yunnan province. *Soc Sci Med*, **64**, 665–75.

Yang, W. (2015). Yunnan battles new strain of HIV. *China Daily Asia*. Available at: http://usa.chinadaily.com.cn/epaper/2015-09/16/content_21894087.htm (accessed 26 January 2017) [Online].

Zinsstag, J., Taleb, M. O., & Craig, P. S. (2006). Health of nomadic pastoralists: new approaches towards equity effectiveness. *Trop Med Int Health*, **2**, 563–8.

Chapter 10

Special topics in rural health III

Older persons, migration, and technology

This chapter provides a brief discussion of how ageing, migration, and technology may influence health needs and outcomes in rural Asia.

10.1 Older persons

Key points

- Population ageing is a global phenomenon. The growth in the number of older people is faster in developing regions than developed countries.
- Older people living in rural areas in developing nations are experiencing changes that are associated with sociodemographic development, such as empty nesters and grandparents raising grandchildren.
- With the rapid population ageing, societies are facing the pressure of healthcare provision and maintaining quality of life for older people.

Increased longevity and reduction in fertility rates have led to an overall global growth in the number of older people. According to the United Nations (UN), older people are defined as people aged 60 or over. In 2015, there were 901 million people aged 60 or above in the world and the number is projected to grow to 1.4 billion by 2030. The growth is more significant in developing regions than in developed regions. Over the next 15 years, the number of older people is expected to grow fastest in Latin America and the Caribbean—with a projected 71% increase—followed by Asia where the number is set to grow by 66% from 508 million. In 2030, Asia's share of the world's older people is projected to increase to 60% (from 56% in 2015) when a projected 845 million people aged 60 years or over will live in the region (UN, 2015). Well-being management of older persons has become a major emerging challenge for communities and policy makers in the coming century.

10.1.1 Physical health

Ageing is usually associated with a decrease in physical well-being. The increased difficulties of carrying out activities of daily living (ADLs) and instrumental activities of daily living (IADLs) are measures of that difficulty. ADLs are the basic self-care daily skills such as bathing, eating, getting out of bed or a chair, dressing or undressing, moving about the house, and using the toilet (Zhang *et al.*, 2005), while IADLs are activities necessary for independent living such as using a telephone, shopping, preparing a hot meal, doing housework, taking medication, managing financial matters, getting to places beyond walking distance, and doing laundry (Li *et al.*, 2006). ADL disability can vary greatly among the elders in the same age group, but it generally increases with age. As functional limitations and difficulties with ADLs and IADLs worsen, the need for assistance from caregivers becomes increasingly necessary (HelpAge International, 2015).

As ageing is usually accompanied by deteriorating physiological functioning and various diseases. The WHO Global Burden of Disease estimate for 2012 also found stroke, malignant neoplasms, ischaemic heart disease, respiratory diseases, diabetes mellitus, mental health conditions, and hypertensive heart diseases to be the leading contributors to disease burden among older people in China (WHO, 2015). In rural China, 'stroke, cancer or malignant tumor, cataracts or glaucoma are the three most common serious diseases that have major effects on activities of daily living (ADL) of the elderly' (Zhang *et al.*, 2005). Other common chronic diseases include: heart disease, cerebrovascular disease, osteoporosis, arthritis/rheumatism, high blood pressure, polio, bronchitis or other respiratory ailments, and gastric ulcers or other stomach ailments (Zhang *et al.*, 2005; Zheng *et al.*, 2011). Usually, older people suffer from multiple chronic diseases, also known as multimorbidity or co-morbidity.

Less effective immune responses can also lead to an increased risk of contracting infectious diseases such as shigellosis, a bacterial infectious disease leading to diarrhoea, fever, and stomach cramps for approximately a week (Centers for Disease Control and Prevention, 2015). A 2002 survey showed the incidence rate of shigellosis among the elders in Hubei province was 7/1,000/year, the population subgroup with the highest rate after children under five years (Wang *et al.*, 2015).

One of the key determinants for the quality of life of older people is to delay functional deterioration and thereby prolong and maintain autonomy. Autonomy is, defined as 'the perceived ability to control, cope with and make personal decisions about how one lives on a day-to-day basis, according to one's own rules and preferences' and independence, or 'the ability to perform functions related to daily living . . . with no and/or little help from others' (HelpAge International, 2014). On a practical level, if the community can provide age-friendly, accessible infrastructure for older people to improve the mobility of the ageing elderly population, they may be able to better integrate into their society and prolong their ability to carry out their daily activities independently.

10.1.2 Mental health

Good mental health has a positive effect on physical health. As people age, they may face changes in 'personality, mental functioning (such as memory, learning and intelligence), and sensory and perceptual processes' (Phillips *et al.*, 2010); and 'Cognitive disability gradually replaces chronic diseases as the main cause of the decline in ADLs' (Zhang *et al.*, 2005). The mental well-being of older people affects their quality of life. Numerous studies have found a positive relationship between social support and the psychological well-being of older people. Most elderly parents find maintaining contact with children who move out of the household contributes to their social and emotional well-being (HelpAge International, 2015). Case 10.1 shows that the situation of loneliness will affect both social and mental health.

10.1.3 Social health

An individual's social health and well-being may be determined by the quality of the individual's social interaction and participation and his/her interpersonal relationship with the social cycle. Measurements of social health of older people may include: relationships quality with family/friends/neighbours; availability of help when needed; co-residence with family members; frequency of relatives visiting; and community participation in religious or senior activities (Chen *et al.*, 2005). Loneliness, isolation, and lack of support become more significant with increasing age, because the 'decreased health status of the elderly makes social contacts difficult' (Liu and Guo, 2007).

The following case studies describe the health issues experienced by older people living in rural areas of China (see Case Study 10.1) and Thailand (see Case Study 10.2).

10.1.4 Implications for bottom-up health resilience and disaster risk reduction

Rural health programmes have traditionally emphasized the improvement of well-being. These programmes have frequently placed emphasis on the reduction of health risks for maternal and child health, and improvement of water, sanitation, and livelihoods. With population ageing and the demographic changes with migration in rural communities (see also Chapter 9 on migration), new approaches to address older people's needs and their health and disaster risk reduction will be important (see also Chapter 8 on natural disasters).

10.1.5 Conclusion

Population ageing around the world is occurring more dramatically than last century. For example, France had almost 150 years to adapt to a rise in the proportion of its older population from 10% to 20%. However, a number of Asian countries, e.g. China and Thailand, will have only slightly more than 20 years to adjust to a similar demographic change (WHO, 2015, September). The health systems of these countries have to be prepared for these changes. Policies, research, evidence-based interventions, strong legal protection, and the development of an age-friendly infrastructure are needed to support older people, especially those living in rural context, to optimize their quality of life, and follow the World Health Organization's (WHO) concept of 'active ageing' (WHO, 2002).

Case Study 10.1 Older people's issues in rural China

The United Nations and China's Elderly Protection Law define 'elderly' or 'older' people as aged 60 years or older (Baidu Baike, n.d.; WHO, 2002). In China, the elderly population is projected to grow from 10% of the total population in 2000 to 30% in 2050 (UN, 2007). According to HelpAge International (2005), China has one of the 'highest rates of population ageing at present' in the Asia–Pacific region, with a 15% rate. 'In 1998, there were more than six working-age adults (15–59 years) for every one elderly person (aged 60 and older) in the Chinese population; by 2040, there will be only two working-age adults for every one elderly person' (Zimmer and Kwong, 2003). Large-scale surveys such as the China Health and Retirement Longitudinal Study (CHARLS), the Chinese Longitudinal Healthy Longevity Survey (CLHLS), WHO's Study on Global Ageing and Adult Health (SAGE), and the Longitudinal Study of the Elderly in Anhui Province have been ongoing to track the socioeconomic, health, and living conditions of China's older population.

Rural versus urban older people in China

China was a predominately rural population until the first decade after the millennium. In 2015, 43.90% of China's population was still living in rural areas, downed from 46.27% in 2013 (National Bureau of Statistics of the People's Republic of China [PRC], 2014; 2016). However, according to a 2001 article on population and policy, the 'proportion of elderly in rural areas and poor regions will be higher than in the urban areas and rich regions' (Yi, 2001). This is largely a result of the urban migration trend where adult children relocate from rural to urban areas for employment and leave behind their parents. There is an increasing number of so-called empty-nest older persons who have to tend to their households or family farms on their own due to the urban migration of their adult children. The three major differences between the urban and rural older people are: living arrangements, sources of support, and work/retirement.

Older people used to live in traditional three-generational family households, but because of modernization and urban migration, this practice has become less common. The older people in urban areas tend to favour living independently of children (Silverstein *et al.*, 2006) and have seen a larger decline in living in intergenerational households (Lei *et al.*, 2011). By 2000, only 15.9% of urban households were three-generational, compared with the 22.2% of rural households (Zeng and Wang, 2003). In rural China, there is also an increasing prevalence of skipped-generation households, where the elders take care of their grandchildren since the parent generation is absent due to migration or other circumstances (Silverstein *et al.*, 2006); 18% of older people lived in skipped-generation households in a survey of Anhui Province, a province with higher than average rates of out-migration (Silverstein *et al.*, 2006).

In terms of the primary source of support, 45.4% of the urban older people depends mostly on pensions, however, 'lack of a pension system for the rural elderly' (Giles and Mu, 2007) causes the majority (54.1%) to rely on family support (Cai *et al.*, 2012). Because adult children are often the main source of support for older people in rural areas (Zimmer and Kwong, 2003), the well-being of the rural older people is affected by family structure changes. Zimmer and Kong's (2003) study of 12 provinces showed that 'having more than one child increases the probability of receiving support from children' for both the rural and urban older people. The effects of the one-child policy enacted in 1980 and beginning to be phased out in 2015 would be significant for the coming few decades. Although the one-child policy was relaxed in 1988 to enable rural families to have a second child (if their first was a daughter) (Ruan and Lau, 2001), the reduced numbers of the next generation will still put a strain on the adult children to provide their parents with the needed economic support.

The urban and rural older people also differ when it comes to work and retirement, with 37.9% of rural older people depending on labour income as their primary source of support, as opposed to 13% of the urban ones (Cai *et al.*, 2012). While the urban Chinese retire early, at age 50 for women and 60 for men (Hvistendahl, 2013), the rural population does not. In a survey of 60 rural villages in China, 67.6% of the elders aged 60–69 and 19% of those aged 70-plus remained in the formal workforce (Pang *et al.*, 2004). Rural-to-urban migration further provokes these circumstances. It was found that time allocated to farm work and domestic work both increased when one household member moved, and the time increased 'to a greater extent for elderly women, than for elderly men' (Chang *et al.*, 2011). Elderly women devoted an average of 34% (197 hours) more time to farm work annually and 23% more to domestic work daily (Chang *et al.*, 2011). The rural old people continue to work, not only to ensure support for themselves, but also 'to allow adult children to increase family income through employment outside the village' (Giles and Mu, 2007).

Mental health

A 2005 study found the prevalence of depression among older people in rural China (6.0%) to be lower than that of older people in Western countries, even Chinese emigrants in the United Kingdom (13.0%) (Chen *et al.*, 2005). Although the region surveyed was generally poor, a lower risk of depression was associated with social support, as well as a subjective view of a very satisfactory or satisfactory family income (33.3% of participants) (Chen *et al.*, 2005). The study concluded that when compared with the United Kingdom, 'fewer older people in China lived alone, and more of them visited children or other relatives and participated in community activities' (Chen *et al.*, 2005).

Some of the indicators for positive mental well-being are life satisfaction and happiness. These internal subjective evaluations of well-being are often dependent on external circumstances. For example, a study of older people in Anhui Province results showed that older parents with stronger emotional connections to their children had better psychological well-being (Silverstein *et al.*, 2006). Numerous studies have found a positive relationship between social support and psychological well-being of older people (Poulin *et al.*, 2014). Good mental health also has a positive effect on physical health. A study in Chaohu in central Anhui showed that 'intergenerational emotional closeness is beneficial to the ADLs of the elderly, with a greater effect on the functional status of men than on that of women' (Zhang *et al.*, 2005).

Social health

This change in family structure can lead to less interaction with family members and caring for the older people, i.e. filial piety, a culturally important source of support. Loneliness is a growing issue with an increasing number of older people living alone instead of in a traditional three-generation household. However, the at-risk population groups include not only the empty nesters (those whose children have left home), but also those who never married and the widowed, divorced, and childless. A sample in Hubei province showed a significantly higher than average level of loneliness among the elder empty nesters (10.9% moderately high) when compared with the non-empty nesters (6.3% moderately high) (Liu and Guo, 2007). In Anhui Province, 81% of elderly empty nesters were shown to have 'moderate to high levels of loneliness' (Wu *et al.*, 2010), with a significant negative association with social support and satisfaction with family relationships. A study found that not only did the elderly empty nesters experience a higher than average degree of loneliness, but also lower physical and mental scores compared with those who were living with their children (Liu and Guo, 2007). Although the childless older people are a small proportion of China's total elderly population (data from the CLHLS 2002 reports 4.6% out of 13,447 older people), this subgroup has a higher level of loneliness than those with children, even when sociodemographic variables are controlled (such as age, gender, and education) (Zhang and Liu, 2007).

Associated with loneliness and lower levels of social support is the risk of the mistreatment or abuse (Dong and Simon, 2013) of older people. Particularly in rural areas, negligence about care can happen easily since family members are primarily responsible for the economic and social support of elders. Older people may face mistreatment or abuse by family members or caregivers, leading to adverse health outcomes (Wu *et al.*, 2012). A study of rural older people in Hubei province reported a 36.2% prevalence rate of elder mistreatment, which was higher than rates found in Western countries (2–10%) (Wu *et al.*, 2012). The most common forms were psychological mistreatment and caregiver neglect (Wu *et al.*, 2012). In seeking to address these issues, the government enacted laws on the Protection of the Rights and Interests of the Elderly, specifically stating in Article 3 that 'Discriminating against, insulting, maltreating or forsaking the elderly is forbidden' (National People's Congress of the PRC [NPC], 2012) and requiring family members to provide economic support. In addition, a new amendment in 2012 seeks to prevent social negligence, stating in Article 17: 'Children who do not live with their elderly parents must visit or greet them often' (NPC, 2012). However, the awareness level and enforcement of these laws have not been studied sufficiently, particularly among older people living in rural China, after the amendment.

Regardless of old age, many older people in China still contribute to their families. Not only do a significant number of the rural older people work past retirement age and help sustain themselves and/or their families (Benjamin *et al.*, 2003), but also, according to HelpAge International, 'enable their adult children to migrate in search of better work opportunities, often minding the grandchildren, farming the family land, and maintaining the family house and assets' (HelpAge International & Shaanxi Provincial Committee on Ageing, 2010). A survey of Zhejiang province showed that taking care of children and doing housework were the major leisure activities for the rural older people (Su *et al.*, 2006). Involvement in the lives of grandchildren is quite high among older people in rural China. When asked whether they had taken 'care of their grandchildren last year', 58% of grandparents in China agreed, compared with about 50% in the United States and Europe, and 6–13% in Korea (no difference was found between the urban and rural grandparents in China) (Ko and Hank, 2014).

At the community level, more of the rural older people participate in social visiting than their urban counterparts during their leisure time, visiting friends or neighbours in the community (Su *et al.*, 2006). However, more of them also spend time idling/doing nothing compared with their urban counterparts (Su *et al.*, 2006). This reflects 'the relatively low availability of recreational resources and less choice for alternative activities for rural elderly residents' (Su *et al.*, 2006). One of the available resources provided by the PRC government is older people's associations. At the end of 2010, China had over 400,000 older people's associations, with over 43,890,000 people participating (Wei, 2011, November 25). These associations provide a space for older people to meet up, spend time chatting, or engage in recreational activities (Xia and Yang, 2015, February 26). Through them they can form a network to support one another, celebrate cultural festivities, engage in community service, and preserve cultural traditions (Wang and Liu, 2014). Some older people's associations also provide welfare assistance and starting from 2009, poverty alleviation and health promotion, through a project by HelpAge International and China National Committee on Ageing (2007). Through these arrangements, older people can also have a large influence on the direction of community health.

Case Study 10.2 Ageing situation in rural Thailand

In Asia, Thailand has one of the highest proportion of older people in its population. In 2015, there were 10.7 million people aged 60 or above and this age subgroup accounts for 16% of its total population. The proportion of the older population in Thailand is projected to increase to 37% by 2050 (UN, 2015). Of note, more than 70% of Thailand's older persons live in rural areas (HelpAge International, 2014; WHO, n.d.-b).

Physical health

Ageing can be defined as a gradual deterioration of the physiological functioning of the organs and systems of the human body. The development of the non-communicable diseases (NCDs) is a common characteristic of older people. In Thailand, strokes, diabetes, ischaemic heart disease, and chronic obstructive pulmonary disease (COPD) were the leading diseases in 2013. The percentage of NCD deaths among the elderly population compared to the younger generation is expected to increase from 74% in 2015 to 80% in 2025 (International Health Policy Program, 2015). The main causes of mortality among the elderly Thai population over the next few decades are predicted to be related to cancer, cardiovascular disease, diabetes mellitus, and COPD (International Health Policy Program & Ministry of Public Health, Thailand, 2016; WHO Regional Office for South-East Asia, 2016).

A national survey (2014) on the older persons in Thailand shows that functional limitations and difficulties with self-care and other daily living activities increase sharply with age. Overall, about 40% of the respondents experience at least one of these difficulties and women were more likely to report their difficulties than men (HelpAge International, 2015). As physical capabilities decline, maintaining autonomy and independence remains one of the key determinants for the quality of life of older people (WHO, 2002) and giving practical help by providing suitable facilities to assist in mobility and integration.

Mental health

Study of older people in a rural area of western Thailand showed almost 30% of the respondents indicated they suffered from depression. The results also showed that infirmity (such as breathlessness, arthritis, weakness, hearing difficulties), disability (including understanding and communicating with the world, getting around, self-care, getting along with people), and serious life events (such as illness, lack of contact with children, financial problems) had a significant effect on the incidence of depression (Haseen and Prasartkul, 2011). Contrary to common belief and fears, studies have found that the increasing number of younger people moving out of rural areas in Thailand does not appear to cause a greater risk of depression for the 'empty-nest' parents (Abas *et al.*, 2013). Instead, older parents usually benefit from material/financial support from their children working in urban areas, while technological development, like the widespread use of mobile phones, greatly helps maintain social/family contacts (Knodel *et al.*, 2010).

Social health

Over the last 25 years, co-residence with children has steadily declined while more older people are living alone or only with their spouse. The increased migration of younger adults, especially from the rural areas, has led to greater geographic dispersion and social health consequences. The proportion of children living outside their parents' province increased from 28% to 39% between 1995 and 2011. However, results from surveys show that among the older parents whose children are all outside their province, the majority (over 90%) had social contact, received monetary support or both from at least one child, and thus appeared not to be abandoned. It is believed that the contacts between the older parents and their children have been largely facilitated by the expansion of the transport system and ownership of mobile phones. A 2014 survey shows approximately 22% of older parents have no son or daughter in the same village and 14% have no offspring in the same province. These changes have raised concerns about the extent of the sense of desertion of the empty-nest older people and their well-being (HelpAge International, 2015).

It is very common for older Thai people to provide intergeneration support and care for their grandchildren on behalf of their co-resident or non-co-resident children. In most of these cases, the grandparents are the main carers of the grandchildren. Overall, 15% of older people have at least one young co-resident grandchild with absent parents. The percentage is higher in rural areas than in urban areas, probably because the grandchild's parents have moved to other provinces for better work opportunities.

Study results also showed that more older people in rural communities engage in work, compared to those who live in urban areas. This could reflect the fact that there is a higher tendency for rural people to be engaged in self-employed agricultural activities and there is no age limit for retirement. Participation in community activities is also a way for older people to remain engaged and experience social support. According to the 2014 Survey of Older Persons in Thailand, many older people participate in some form of community activity such as National Elderly Day events, Thai New Year celebrations, and religious ceremonies. Participation is higher among the elders in their 60s and 70s and drops among those aged 80 years or over probably because of declining health (HelpAge International, 2015). The majority of the population in Thailand is Buddhist and Thais appear to engage more in religious activities when they are older (Cowgill, 1968).

The Thai government has supported the establishment of senior citizen clubs as self-help organizations for older people. These elderly clubs are registered with, and supervised by, the National Senior Citizen Council. As of 2013, there were over 25,000 registered senior citizen clubs with more than 1.6 million members outside Bangkok and about 280 older people's associations in Bangkok (HelpAge International, 2015).

Access to health services

All Thai nationals, including the older people, have access to free government health services. Moreover, the Old Age Allowance programme was expanded in 2009 to become a universal social pension scheme for all persons aged 60 and above. There have been different community-based initiatives launched by the government in recent years. One example is the nationwide establishment of centres for the quality of life development and occupational promotion for older persons in 2013. The main purpose of the centres is to provide comprehensive services to older persons to improve their quality of life, including healthcare promotion, lifelong learning activities, and the promotion of volunteer caregivers among older people. As of 2014, these centres were established in 878 subdistricts throughout the country (HelpAge International, 2015).

Although all Thai citizens are covered by health protection schemes, significant gaps exist in non-medical costs and social support to facilitate access to and utilization of healthcare services. The dependence of elderly patients on the availability of carers and relatives to bring them to a health facility appears to be a key reason for their low utilization of health services. In addition, according to a World Bank Group report (Osornprasop and Sondergaard, 2016), the lack of public and affordable transport is the most important barrier to accessing health services among elders in rural areas. Older people without private cars who reside outside of Greater Bangkok and major cities are unlikely to have access to taxis and need to rely on public buses or renting private cars. The report said that many elderly interviewees who do not have access to public buses identified the cost of renting private vehicles as a major impediment to their regular access to health and emergency services.

10.2 Migration

Key points

- Majority of global migrants are moving from rural to urban areas.
- The demographic pressure of migration brings major challenges to both urban and rural areas (e.g. putting pressure on healthcare and health systems).

Human mobility has reached unprecedented levels across the globe by the twenty-first century. People on the move include migrants moving within their countries of origin and those moving abroad. The number of international migrants worldwide has continued to grow rapidly over the past 15 years and reached 244 million in 2015, the highest on record (International Organization for Migration [IOM], 2016). Human migration can also be further divided into voluntary migration (in which people choose to migrate), and involuntary migration (in which they are forced to move to other places). Refugees and internally displaced persons (IDPs) are examples of forced migrants who have to flee conflicts, violence, and environmental pressure.

Globally, both internal and international migrants have a tendency to move to urban areas. In the Asia–Pacific region, an estimated 120,000 people are migrating to cities every day. The proportion of the population living in urban areas in the region is expected to rise to 63% by 2050 (UN Economic and Social Commission for Asia and the Pacific, 2014). Apart from the rural–urban migratory flow, there is also relocation of population from urban to rural areas. They may be economic migrants moving back to their rural hometowns by choice or when they get old, sick, or disabled.

10.2.1 Migration and rural communities

Migration brings both risks and opportunities and to the rural areas, cities, and governments (IOM, 2015). Among the migrants, the most vulnerable are those who are not entitled to any legal protection. The cases of Nepal (see Case Study 10.3) and China (see Case Study 10.4) discuss the healthcare challenges experienced by migrants in the contexts.

10.2.2 Implications for bottom-up health resilience and disaster risk reduction

Migration is one of the major reasons for rural depopulation and it exacerbates the pace of ageing. Programmes that improve health resilience and reduce disaster risk should examine periodically how migration patterns might have changed the demographic composition, economic capacity, behavioural practices, and health beliefs of their community of interest to ensure their activities might be relevant and appropriate to address real health needs and disaster risks. Bottom-up measures which improve health management of

---

Case Study 10.3 Internal and international migration in Nepal

According to the 2011 census, one in every four households (25.42%; 1.38 million households) in the country reported that at least one member was living out of the country and the total number of emigrant population was found to be 1.9 million, among whom almost 71% cited private and institutional jobs abroad as the reasons for migration (Government of Nepal, 2012). While remittance from migrant workers accounts for about 28% of Nepal's total GDP during the fiscal year 2013/14, the total number of migrant workers who died during foreign employment between the fiscal years 2008/09 and 2014/15 as reported to the government was 4,322 and almost one-third a result of cardiovascular diseases (Government of Nepal, 2016). Nepal faces many obstacles and challenges in addressing migrant health issues. Demographic data showed that internal migrants made up nearly 30% (1.28 million) of the total native born population in urban areas, 84% of whom from rural areas (Government of Nepal, 2012). The country is particularly hampered in any bid to demand the protection of Nepali migrants as major conventions related to migration were not ratified and there is a lack of leverage and authority in the international community[1]. Uninsured migrant workers also do not have easy access to healthcare services in host countries due to the high medical and hospital fees. Greater efforts are needed to protect the health and well-being, labour rights, and human rights of migrant workers from Nepal and other South Asian nations.

Case Study 10.4 Migrants returning from cities to villages and the health challenges in China

China has been experiencing a huge flow of rural– urban migration since the 1980s. There are major implications for the healthcare system, disease prevention, and service provisions to address this demographic pattern. With the continuous rural–urban flow of younger migrants, older migrants are forced to leave the workforce in the cities and return to their hometowns. Majority of these migrants have lower education levels and have been working in unskilled and physically demanding jobs such as construction work. They have been suffering higher risk of workplace injuries that may result in disability and as a result they are it more likely to return to their rural homes without working ability (Zheng *et al.*, 2011). These returnees face challenges in terms of retirement and healthcare.

Official statistics from the Chinese authorities in 2014 showed the participation rate of the rural-to-urban migrants in the basic pension insurance was only 16.4% and in medical insurance the rate was 18.2%. In the construction industry, which employs many middle-aged to elderly migrants, the participation rates in the basic pension insurance and the medical insurance were only 3.9% and 5.4% (National Bureau of Statistics of the PRC, 2015). Studies found as workers experience welfare programme access issues (Xu *et al.*, 2011), a lot of them may choose to return to their hometowns to start their own business with the experience and capital they have acquired and accumulated in the cities (Ma, 2001). There are also migrants who return to the villages for family reasons. Some female migrants choose to get married in their hometowns (Ma, 2005; Wang and Fan, 2006).

Although the returnees from the cities bring back incomes, skills, and new ideas, they may also bring more diseases and health risks (Hansen, 2001; Mou *et al.*, 2013). The rural-to-urban migrants usually live in a very densely populated environment in the cities which increases their likelihood to contact infectious diseases such as TB. Their return to the rural areas, if not carefully managed, may lead to disease transmission (Huang and Manderson, 2005; Jia *et al.*, 2008).

migrants include electronic health record systems and the improvement of health literacy that will facilitate self efficacy in maintenance of well-being of this migrant population.

10.2.3 **Conclusions**

Migration has changed considerably the demographic and epidemiological disease patterns and health needs of rural community. With the rapid urbanization and the pace of population movements across the world, health needs in rural communities should be reviewed periodically to ensure the migration patterns and dynamics are truly reflected and considered in the setting.

10.3 **Technology**

Key points

- Science and technology have far-reaching impact on human life in the twenty-first century.
- Although the use of information and communication technology has a great potential to improve the healthcare coverage in rural areas, considerations must be taken for ethics, and applicability of the context.

In the twenty-first century, science and technology advancements have facilitated socioeconomic development and access to healthcare in developing countries. 'Digital' or 'smart' technologies are often used to improve the weather forecasting, disease surveillance, disaster risk reductions, crisis monitoring, and clinical disease management. The application of technology in rural communities can overcome geographical barriers and improving access to information, education, and medical services for populations living in poor and remote settings. The implications of technology are felt across the pathway of care (see also Chapter 2) and have benefitted communities from disease prevention, health protection, and health promotion, to diagnoses, treatments, rehabilitation, and palliative care.

10.3.1 The use of information and communication technology in healthcare

The development and popularization of communication technology has transcended geographical limitations and has greatly narrowed the distance between urban and rural areas. Telemedicine is the medicine provision via advanced communication technology, allows both medical and public health services to be provided without face-to-face contact. Instead of the traditional, face-to-face consultation approach, telemedicine uses information and communication technology (ICT) to provide healthcare from a distance (Smith *et al.*, 2005) and allows patients and medical staff, or other medical professionals, to communicate at their convenience through phones, radio, emails, videotelephony, or any other form supported by ICT. It also shows how technology may improve healthcare to underserved and difficult-to-reach communities.

10.3.2 Application of technology across the pathway of care

Disease prevention, health protection, and health promotion

Traditionally, health promotion relies mostly on poster display, leaflet distribution or face-to-face communication, but these methods have limited reach and are not cost-effective. However, the growing popularity of mobile devices has made wireless technology an increasingly important channel for the dissemination of health information and enable access to information and services. Study findings indicate that short reminder messages transmitted by mobile phones can effectively improve the health service participation and utilization rate (World Vision India, 2013, 2015) and may effectively guide recipients to adopt more healthy lifestyles, e.g. weight loss and smoking cessation (Free *et al.*, 2013; Gurol-Urganci *et al.*, 2013; World Vision International, 2014, June). Technology was also shown to be able to support disaster warning and preparedness in rural communities (Gow *et al.*, 2007; Samarajiva and Waidyanatha, 2009)

Diagnoses and treatments

Telemedicine is adopted and used for remote clinical diagnosis, disease management, medical research, and continuing medical education simultaneously in diverse locations (WHO, 2009). eHealth (electronic health) is a term which describes the health practices supported by electronic processes and ICT (WHO, n.d.-a). An important concept and application of eHealth is mHealth (mobile health). mHealth is composed of medical and public health practices that are supported by mobile communication devices, such as mobile phones, tablet computers, patient monitoring devices, personal digital assistants (PDAs), and other wireless devices (WHO, 2011).

The rapid development of mobile technologies has enabled the advancement of innovative applications designed for healthcare in developing countries. In many low- and middle-income countries, the penetration of mobile network services are so high that they sometimes even surpass the availability of other infrastructures, such as paved roads and electricity. The rapid development of mobile phone networks has also enabled remote and continuous transmission of data regarding patients' health in rural areas. Portable sensors and remote technology have been widely used in researchand rehabilitation to monitor a number of bodily functions such as sleeping, physical activities, and other rehabilitative activities (Appelboom *et al.*, 2014). However, with the current cost associated with technology, mobile devices with built-in sensors may not become widely used in Asian developing countries. The Swinfen Charitable Trust, an organization based in the United Kingdom, has been operating a telemedicine network since 1999 and its network links healthcare workers in developing countries to an international pool of specialist medical consultants. Through emails and other enhanced communication messaging systems, volunteer specialists may provide clinical advice and support through referring physician networks to support different clinical needs (Smith *et al.*, 2005). This technical support is particularly beneficial to the physicians working in remote regions where there is limited access to diagnostic testing, as they can receive a second opinion on specific medical cases from an available tele-specialist (WHO, 2009).

Technology also allows access to specialized healthcare in rural and remote settings. The application of mHealth programmes aims to address needs in these areas with poor resources (WHO, 2011). India, for instance, has more than one billion mobile phone subscribers in the country (Bloomberg, 2015). Apart from the use of ICT, there are other innovative and technological developments that are being employed to improve diagnoses and treatment methods, especially in situations where there are serious geographical and logistic constraints. The following are three examples in India, Papua New Guinea, and Nepal (see Case Studies 10.5, 10.6, and 10.7; see also Case Study 10.8).

10.3.3 Rehabilitation and palliative care

According to WHO, palliative care refers to the the quality of life improvement for terminally ill patients and their families by preventing and alleviating their suffering (WHO, n.d.-e). Although the main purpose of palliative care is not to cure the disease, it enables the patient to live comfortably during the last stage of life, and to die with dignity.

Telemedicine provides an opportunity for patients in palliative care to receive treatment at home while maintaining communication with medical staff. Through video conferencing or other means of communication, patients may spend their last stage of life at home and be spared the stress of travelling to hospital and healthcare facilitates. Medical staff can continue to monitor patients via different devices and applications. Study results

Case Study 10.5 mHealth in India

World Vision India, an international non-governmental organization (NGO), started integrating mHealth into its programmes in 2011, in the Melghat area with a maternal, newborn, and child health monitoring system (World Vision India, 2013); and later in Narsinghpur District in the state of Madhya Pradesh (World Vision India, 2015). Both regions are located in rural India, where the population suffers from poverty.

Maternal and child health

In collaboration with the local health authorities, World Vision provided training to the village community health workers on the use of a mobile application called CommCare to manage and monitor the health records of children and pregnant women, as well as to support diagnoses and treatment methods, collect real-time data, and refer complicated cases. For example, the medical records collected by CommCare facilitate the health workers in disseminating health messages to specific groups of villagers, such as pregnant women. Meanwhile, the district and national health authorities also have access to real-time data that is collected to help monitor the health situation in these areas. The usefulness of mobile applications has also been proven by the ability to collect more complete sets of data from the patients. For instance, in these World Vision project locations, the data completeness has been increased from 67% with paper-based systems to 84% with CommCare. The mobile system has also supported an up to a 48% improvement in the knowledge retention among community healthcare workers (World Vision International, 2014, 2014, June).

Diabetic care

mhealth also enables disease prevention efforts. The burden of diabetes is especially high in India, where it is estimated that more than 60 million people live with diabetes and one million may die from the disease each year. Indians often get diabetes in their 30s and 40s—a much younger age than the population in Western countries. If left untreated, diabetes can lead to heart disease, blindness, amputations, and kidney failure. According to the World Health Organization (WHO), a healthy lifestyle can greatly help in the prevention of diabetes (Arogya World, n.d.; Pfammatter *et al.*, 2016).

mDiabetes is a large diabetes prevention mHealth programme run by Arogya World, a global nonprofit health organization based in India. Through mDiabetes, text messages which encourage the health behaviours that will help to prevent diabetes are sent to the participants in the programme. In 2012, a total of 56 culturally adapted messages were sent to more than one million participants across India, in 12 different dialects. The effectiveness of this programme has been evaluated by phone interviews with the participants. From this, it was discovered that there has been an increase in the awareness of diabetes, as well as a trend for some behavioural changes: an 11% increase in daily exercise; a 15% increase in the intake of 2–3 servings of fruit each day, and an 8% increase in the intake of 2–3 servings of vegetables each day (Arogya World, n.d.; Pfammatter *et al.*, 2016).

suggest virtual visits facilitated by video conferencing technology also enhance the communication level, as well as the engagement and satisfaction of the patients (Holland *et al.*, 2014; WHO, 2011; World Vision, 2015).

10.3.4 Controversial issues and challenges in using technology for healthcare

With advancement in medical diagnoses and treatment methods, how health and medical services may be provided along the care pathway will continue to evolve and the

Case Study 10.6 Tackling tuberculosis with a new technology in Papua New Guinea

The prevalence of tuberculosis (TB) in Papua New Guinea (PNG) is among the highest in the world, and it ranks second among the leading causes of death in the country (WHO, n.d.-c). The global emerging problem of multidrug-resistant TB (MDR-TB) is of particular concern. In the fight against this epidemic, an early diagnosis and the timely delivery of treatment to the patient is essential. However, many rural parts of PNG remain highly inaccessible, and more than 80% of the country's population lives in rural areas (WHO, n.d.-c). This poses a huge logistic challenge for the health workers who wish to effectively manage the transportation of test samples.

Médecins Sans Frontières (MSF), an international medical humanitarian organization, has run a TB project in Kerema, a gulf province of PNG, since mid-2014. The MSF laboratory in the Kerema General Hospital is the only one in the area with functioning microscopy and the diagnostic tools needed to analyse the sputum samples of suspected TB patients. There are six health centres in the peripheral area of the hospital and three of these are only accessible by boat. To reach out to the village health facilities, the health workers running the project are confronted with a massive swamp, as well as a dangerous and treacherous sea, rivers infested with crocodiles, and muddy roads during the rainy seasons (MSF, n.d., 2014, November 14; Soesilo, 2016, September 29)

To explore the solutions to overcome these barriers, MSF engaged in a pilot project in 2014 that used unmanned aerial vehicles (UAVs), commonly known as drones, to transport the diagnostic samples from the remote health centres to the Kerema hospital for testing. Working closely with Matternet, a technology company based in the United States, MSF selected a health clinic near Malalaua for the pilot study. The distance between the Kerema hospital and the clinic is 63 km by road and takes four hours to travel by car. However, with the UAVs, operated through a smartphone, the travel time was reduced to 55 minutes. During the tests, the UAVs carried a light load and travelled at speeds of up to 60 km per hour, with a maximum range of 28 km in good weather conditions. After the trial, MSF concluded that UAVs had been proven to shorten the transportation time of the test samples. The organization regarded UAVs, even though it was in its development stage, could be useful in supporting the remote and inaccessible health facilities (MSF, n.d., 2014, November 14; Soesilo, 2016, September 29).

Case Study 10.7 Screening of rheumatic heart disease in Eastern Nepal

Rheumatic heart disease (RHD) is a preventable, treatable form of cardiovascular disease that affects over 33 million people worldwide in 2017 and claims 320,000 lives annually. Although RHD has been almost eradicated in developed countries, it remains a public health concern for the world's poorest, most vulnerable populations. If left untreated, RHD can lead to heart valve damage, strokes, heart failure, and death (World Heart Federation, n.d.). South Asia and some African countries have a very high prevalence of this disease (Rothenbuler *et al.*, 2014), and RHD is the most commonly acquired heart disease in young people below 25 years of age. Although a sole clinical auscultation cannot detect the silent form of RHD, an ultrasound can (Rothenbuler *et al.*, 2014). Research conducted in Eastern Nepal found that RHD affects 1 in 100 schoolchildren in the region, and is primarily clinically silent. Among the nearly 5,500 schoolchildren who were screened, 80% of them live in rural areas. The screening was done through a cardiac auscultation and transthoracic echocardiography (Shrestha *et al.*, 2016).

Early detection of these silent RHD cases might prevent their progression to severe valvular damage (Shrestha *et al.*, 2016). The development of a handheld echocardiography (HAND) device, or point-of-care ultrasound (POCUS), has greatly increased the practicality of organizing RHD screening for the children in rural areas. Studies have shown that such screening programmes can be even led by non-experts, which offers a potential solution to the financial and workforce barriers face in RHD-endemic countries (Ploutz *et al.*, 2016). This could also be advanced as a method of screening refugees and migrant children fleeing war-torn countries in either the location where they are in transit, or at their final destinations (Rossi and Lee, 2016a, 2016b).

Case Study 10.8 Use of the Internet and health in rural China

China has made significant advancement in both development and application of science and technology for the past decade. As was reported by the Ministry of Industry and Information Technology of the PRC (MIIT; 2015, August a, b), China's mobile phone users comprised close to 1.3 billion people in 2015, with a mobile phone penetration rate of 94.5%; mobile Internet users number close to 950 million, with a penetration rate of about 68.9%; and there are more than 200 million people with access to Internet broadband services, with a penetration rate of 15.3%.

The impact of science and technology on public health has far-reaching consequences. Some important examples of medical and health technologies include: medicines; anaesthesia; surgery and equipment; instruments to be implanted in the body; equipment for diagnostic tests; and the use of medical tools (Gurol-Urganci *et al.*, 2013; Tinnelly *et al.*, 2000). A study conducted in the rural areas of Zhejiang showed technology could improve the availability and accessibility of public health services in rural areas (Free *et al.*, 2013; Ren *et al.*, 2015). It is also important to emphasize that the application of technology is not only limited to the diagnosis of a disease. They can be used throughout the whole process of healthcare, including: (1) disease prevention, health protection, and health promotion; (2) diagnoses; (3) treatment; (4) rehabilitation; and (5) palliative treatment.

Screening: Heart disease screening

Another example of the technology used in rural China involves remote heart disease screening. According to data from WHO, China's urban and rural mortality rates in 2010 from heart disease were 154.8/100,000 and 163.1/100,000, respectively, accounting for 20.9% of the total urban and rural deaths. In September 2011, a project entitled the Mobile Heart Health Program (Ni *et al.*, 2014; WHO, 2012) was conducted in some of the resource-poor communities located in Shandong Province, Anhui Province, Sichuan Province, and Chongqing Municipality. The project involved the use of a cardiovascular disease monitoring system deployed in the community health service centre, and a mobile phone with the built-in electrocardiogram sensing function that can be applied to the user's hand. The user only needs to hold the mobile phone for 30 seconds, and the ECG data can then be sent through a real-time transmission to a heart specialist in Beijing. As of 2014, the programme had provided more than 10,000 users with screening services, of which 1,700 were referred to higher-level hospitals.

Diagnoses: Tuberculosis

Tuberculosis is the second largest killer among the infectious diseases in China. The average mortality rate from tuberculosis in China from 1990 to 2010 was about 8.6% (Li *et al.*, 2011). Additionally, the number of tuberculosis cases in China accounts for 11% of the global number, ranking second only to India in the world (Appelboom *et al.*, 2014). The recently recorded morbidity and prevalence rates were 100/10,000 and 208/100,000, respectively, of which 5% were the multidrug-resistant type of tuberculosis, which is resistant to a variety of antimicrobial agents (China Internet Network Information Center, 2015).

The prevalence of tuberculosis in rural China is about twice that found in urban areas, and it is one of the major diseases that restricts the development of rural areas (China Internet Network Information Center, 2015; Jackson *et al.*, 2006; WHO, n.d.-d). An early diagnosis and regular treatment are the keys to fighting tuberculosis. The commonly used methods of diagnosing tuberculosis include tuberculosis sputum smears and tuberculosis cultures, as well as chest X-rays and biopsies. However, due to the low sensitivity of the sputum tuberculosis smear test, the fact that a bacterial culture takes a long time, and the challenges presented by some of the advanced technology because the required equipment is expensive, professionals are needed to operate the equipment, and diagnosis is difficult to perform widely in China's rural and poor areas with a high incidence of tuberculosis. Technology has enabled a technique known as the isothermal nucleic acid amplification system could be a simple, economical, and accurate way of rapidly diagnosing pulmonary tuberculosis, as the technology presents a simple manner for the detection of pulmonary tuberculosis DNA using a portable instrument. As mentioned in the Emerging Health Technologies Program launched by WHO in 2011, the test results could be available in two hours, and the sensitivity and specificity are 99% and 94% (Holland *et al.*, 2014; WHO, 2012). The operator of the technology only requires simple training and can operate the test in the clinics of rural areas or in primary hospitals. The potential implementation in China of such technology will be valuable to the mobile rural migrant workers in the country (see Case Study 10.4).

Treatment and rehabilitation

The introduction of appropriate medical equipment and technologies will enhance capacity in disease management in the rural community (Li *et al.*, 2011; Maxwell, 1984). The assessment of a bodily function's status is an important indicator of the progress taking place in the rehabilitation of patients, and is also the basis for healthcare workers in formulating the next stage of the rehabilitation programme. Therefore, the ability to collect time-sensitive data, such as the body temperature, blood pressure, heart rate, and blood sugar, and so on, helps healthcare workers to accurately track these functions, and respond to and monitor the rehabilitation progress of the patients. The technology is also able to remind patients to complete the functional training in the rehabilitation process.

In fact, the monitoring of bodily functions by portable sensors and remote technology has been widely used abroad in both research and rehabilitation, including during sleep, physical activity, and other rehabilitation activities (Appelboom *et al.*, 2014).

The rapid development of mobile phone networks in rural areas provides the possibility for remote and continuous transmissions of a patient's bodily functions even in rural areas, the introduction of medical technology may not be able to benefit rural residents. Wireless mobile devices with built-in sensors, despite their superior performance, may not be suitable for use in rural China due to their high price. An alternative would be for the hospitals to remind patients to perform their rehabilitation activities, or measure a physical indicator on time, through a mobile application or a short message. The patient may also be helped by using a relatively inexpensive electronic measurement and transmission device.

Palliative treatment

In China, the concept of palliative care is still in its initial development stage for both citizens and its service providers. With new medical diagnoses and treatment discoveries which may prolong life expectancy and survival, it is uncertain how the healthcare system may be willing to provide and cater for palliative treatment to patients who require such support (Appelboom *et al.*, 2014; Maxwell, 1984, 1992; Rossi and Lee, 2016b).

Conclusion

Opportunities, as well as uncertainties, have been identified in the application of science and technology in the rural areas of China. In addition to technical considerations, the availability of support facilities, service maintenance, and relevant training are all pertinent questions that will remain to be answered to maximize the benefit which rural residents may obtain from the modern technological revolution.

---

accompanied technological requirements will become more sophisticated. However, the multifaceted pursuit of advances in science and technology may potentially be counter-productive to the benefit of mankind. While there is a lot of potential for the application of science and technology to protect human health and improve the well-being of

Case Study 10.9 Overdiagnosis and misdiagnosis with technology

While working in the remote Hui minority-based villages on the Loess Plateau, CCOUC came across local women who expressed major concerns about the high incidence of breast cancer in the community. Upon investigation, the CCOUC team learned that the local women had minimal health education and knowledge about the disease, together with the limited medical training of local health providers, misdiagnoses of medical conditions (e.g. breast cancer) with a newly acquired ultrasound machine were reported. This example showed that the introduction of a technology without relevant community health literacy knowledge and training to health service providers will inevitably be accompanied by many problems (CCOUC, 2011).

populations, a number of controversial issues are also involved. Long-term safety, true efficacy, and implication of how technology (e.g. the large-scale development of transgenic foods, in vitro fertilization (IVF), and gene therapy) may impact human well-being are still inconclusive. In addition, some of the science and technologies have yet to bring practical benefits to the identification of debilitating diseases (such as Huntington's disease). Yet, even with the availability of disease screening tools, without relevant referral and treatment options, these tools (e.g. diagnosis equipment) may increase patients' psychological burden. Investment and maintenance of equipment, and manpower capacity upgrading will be needed to ensure the effectiveness of application of technology to improve health. Case Study 10.9 describes the unfortunate situations when technology might be misused in diagnosis and care.

Application of technology in healthcare also involved challenges to maintain security and privacy. For example, although there are benefits of the use of electronic patient records or sensor networks for in-home patient monitoring, the risks concerning the security of the patients' records and the potential compromises to patients' privacy remain.

10.3.5 Implications for bottom-up health resilience and disaster risk reduction

Although technology has improved well-being and disaster risk reduction in rural communities, as illustrated by some of the case examples, certain levels of technological literacy of both the providers and users are expected to maximize such potential of technology. Health education initiatives may bridge this gap by improving technology literacy (e.g. train older age groups how to access smart technology and the Internet) and building the technology platforms to help and empower rural communities to outreach to health services and information. In addition, technology may provide a training platform to upgrade technical skills, thus promoting health staff retention in rural and remote areas as it allows professional workers to continue their training virtually anywhere in the world.

10.4 Conclusion

The application of science and technology in rural areas shows promise but there are also challenges. In addition to technical considerations, the availability of support facilities, service maintenance, and training are all pertinent questions that will need to be examined and addressed in the rural communities that might have an interest in benefiting from the modern technological revolution.

Note

1. Nepal has not ratified the major conventions related to migration: the Convention on the Protection of the Rights of All Migrant Workers and Members of Their Families, and the UN Protocol to Prevent, Suppress, and Punish Trafficking in Persons. Also, Nepal has not ratified either of the two International Labour Organization conventions.

References

Abas M. A., Tangchonlatip, K., Punpuing, S., *et al.* (2013). Migration of children and impact on depression in older parents in rural Thailand, Southeast Asia. *JAMA Psychiatry*, **70**, 226–34.

Appelboom, G., Yang, A. H., Christophe, B. R., *et al.* (2014). The promise of wearable activity sensors to define patient recovery. *J Clin Neurosci*, **21**, 1089–93.

Arogya World (n.d.). mDiabetes: the largest diabetes prevention mHealth program in the world. Available at: https://www.arogyaworld.org/mdiabetes [Online].

Baidu Baike (n.d.). [The elderly population]. Available at: http://baike.baidu.com/link?url=6H724T1gL_eL2mW-mJBceYKxm-hTHcsYbwWeOVl4hIbfYgOCQWWlbAUoyCg3fiWsbkqFzGexo3CvF79Xvls3Oa (accessed 9 October 2015) (Chinese) [Online].

Benjamin, D., Brandt, L., & Fan, J.-Z. (2003). Ceaseless toil? Health and labor supply of the elderly in rural China (William Davidson Institute Working Paper Number 579). Available at: https://papers.ssrn.com/sol3/papers.cfm?abstract_id=417820&rec=1&srcabs=1368540&alg=7&pos=6 (assessed 8 February 2017) [Online].

Bloomberg (2015, December 30). India becomes mobile-phone market with a billion subscribers. Available at: https://www.bloomberg.com/news/articles/2015-12-30/india-becomes-seond-phone-market-to-cross-1-billion-subscribers (accessed 6 January 2017) [Online].

Cai, F., Giles, J., O'Keefe, P., Wang D (2012). *The Elderly and Old Age Support in Rural China.* Washington, DC: World Bank Publications.

Centers for Disease Control and Prevention (2015). Shigella—shigellosis. Available at: http://www.cdc.gov/shigella/ (assessed 26 October 2015) [Online].

Chang, H., Dong, X., & MacPhail, F. (2011). Labor migration and time use patterns of the left-behind children and elderly in rural China. *World Dev*, **39**, 2199–210.

Chen, R., Wei, L., Hu, Z., Qin, X., Copeland, J. R., & Hemingway, H. (2005). Depression in older people in rural China. *Arch Intern Med*, **165**, 2019–25.

China Internet Network Information Center (2015). *The 36th Statistical Report on Internet Development in China.* Available at: http://cnnic.com.cn/IDR/ReportDownloads/201601/P020160106496544403584.pdf (accessed 10 February 2017) [Online].

Collaborating Centre for Oxford University and CUHK for Disaster and Medical Humanitarian Response (CCOUC) (2011). *Field trip—Datan village, Maluxiang, Zhangjia County (Huizu), Tianshui City, Gansu* (Activity Report). Hong Kong, China: CCOUC.

Constitution of the World Health Organization, 22 July 1946, T.I.A.S. No. 1,808.

Cowgill, D. (1968). The social life of the ageing in Thailand. *Gerontologist*, **8**(3 Part 1), 159–63.

Dong, X. & Simon, M. A. (2013). Urban and rural variations in the characteristics associated with elder mistreatment in a community-dwelling Chinese population. *J Elder Abuse Negl*, **25**, 97–125.

Free, C., Phillips, G., Galli, L., *et al.* (2013). The effectiveness of mobile-health technology-based health behaviour change or disease management interventions for health care consumers: a systematic review. *PLoS Med*, **10**, e1001362.

Giles, J. & Mu, R. (2007). Elderly parent health and the migration decisions of adult children: evidence from rural China. *Demography*, **44**, 265–88.

Government of Nepal, National Planning Commission Secretariat Central Bureau of Statistics (2012). *National Population and Housing Census 2011 (National Report)*. Available at: http://cbs.gov.np/image/data/Population/National%20Report/National%20Report.pdf (accessed 14 July 2017) [Online].

Government of Nepal, Ministry of Labour and Employment (2016). *Labour Migration for Employment: A Status Report for Nepal: 2014/2015*. Available at: http://www.ilo.org/wcmsp5/groups/public/---asia/---ro-bangkok/---ilo-kathmandu/documents/publication/wcms_500311.pdf (accessed 14 July 2017) [Online].

Gow, G., Anderson, P., & Waidyanatha, N. (2007). *Community-Based Hazard Warnings in Rural Sri Lanka: Performance of Alerting and Notification in a Last-Mile Message Relay*. Available at: https://ssrn.com/abstract=1572329 (accessed 14 July 2017) [Online].

Gurol-Urganci, I., de Jongh, T., Vodopivec-Jamsek, V., Atun, R., & Car, J. (2013). Mobile phone messaging reminders for attendance at healthcare appointments. *Cochrane database Syst Rev*, **12**, CD007458.

Hansen, P. (2001). Long march, bitter fruit: the public health impact of rural-tourban migration in the People's Republic of China. *Stanford J East Asian Aff*, **1**, 75–85.

Haseen, F. & Prasartkul, P. (2011). Predictors of depression among older people living in rural areas of Thailand. *Bangladesh Medical Research Council Bulletin*, **37**, 51–6.

HelpAge International (2014). Ageing population in Thailand. Available at: www.ageingasia.org/ageing-population-thailand1/#keyfacts (accessed 29 December 2016) [Online].

HelpAge International (2015). *The Situation of Thailand's Older Population: An Update Based on the 2014 Survey on Older Persons in Thailand*. Available at: http://www.psc.isr.umich.edu/pubs/pdf/rr15-847.pdf [Online].

HelpAge International, China National Committee on Ageing (2007). Older people's associations and poverty alleviation in rural areas: the experience in China. Available at: https://www.ageinternational.org.uk/Documents/OPA%20in%20China.pdf (accessed 8 February 2017) [Online].

HelpAge International, Shaanxi Provincial Committee on Ageing (2010). *A snapshot of older people's lives in rural Shaanxi*. Available at: https://www.ageinternational.org.uk/Documents/A%20snapshot%20of%20older%20people's%20lives%20in%20rural%20Shaanxi.pdf (assessed 8 February 2017) [Online].

Holland, D. E., Vanderboom, C. E., Ingram, C. J., *et al.* (2014). The feasibility of using technology to enhance the transition of palliative care for rural patients. *Comput Inform Nurs*, **32**, 257–66.

Huang, Y.-X. & Manderson, L. (2005). The social and economic context and determinants of schistosomiasis japonica. *Acta Trop*, **96**(2-3), 223–31.

Hvistendahl, M. (2013). Can China age gracefully? A massive survey aims to find out. *Science*, **341**(6148), 831–2.

International Health Policy Program, Thailand (2015). *The report on burden of disease and injuries in Thailand 2011*. Available at: http://bodthai.net/%E0%B8%A3%E0%B8%B2%E0%B8%A2%E0%B8%87%E0%B8%B2%E0%B8%99%E0%B8%A7%E0%B8%B4%E0%B8%88%E0%B8%B1%E0%B8%A2/ (assessed 8 February 2017) [Online].

International Health Policy Program; Ministry of Public Health, Thailand (2016). *Burden of Disease Project 2013*. Available at: http://bodthai.net/%E0%B8%A3%E0%B8%B2%E0%B8%A2%E0%B8%8

7%E0%B8%B2%E0%B8%99%E0%B8%A7%E0%B8%B4%E0%B8%88%E0%B8%B1%E0%B8%A2/ (assessed 8 February 2017) [Online].

International Organization for Migration (IOM) (2015). *World Migration Report 2015: Overview.* Available at: http://www.iom.int/sites/default/files/country/docs/syria/IOM-World-Migration-Report-2015-Overview.pdf (accessed 14 January 2017) [Online].

International Organization for Migration (IOM) (2016). *Global Migration Trends Factsheet 2015.* Available at: http://publications.iom.int/books/global-migration-trends-factsheet-2015 (accessed 10 February 2017) [Online].

Jackson, S., Sleigh, A. C., Wang, G. J., & Liu, X. L. (2006). Poverty and the economic effects of TB in rural China. *Int J Tuberc Lung Dis*, **10**, 1104–10.

Jia, Z. W., Jia, X. W., Liu, Y. X., *et al.* (2008). Spatial analysis of tuberculosis cases in migrants and permanent residents, Beijing, 2000–2006. *Emerg Infect Dis*, **14**, 1413–20.

Knodel, J., Kespichayawattana, J., Saengtienchai, C., & Wiwatwanich, S. (2010). How left behind are rural parents of migrant children? Evidence from Thailand. *Ageing & Society*, **30**, 811–41.

Ko, P. C. & Hank, K. (2014). Grandparents caring for grandchildren in China and Korea: findings from CHARLS and KLoSA. *J Gerontol B Psychol Sci Soc Sci*, **69**, 646–51.

Lei, X., Strauss, J., Tian, M., & Zhao, Y. (2011). *Living Arrangements of the Elderly in China: Evidence from CHARLS* (RAND Labor and Population Working Paper Series Number WR-866). Available at: http://www.rand.org/content/dam/rand/pubs/working_papers/2011/RAND_WR866.pdf (accessed 8 February 2017) [Online].

Li, C., Wu, W., Jin, H., *et al.* (2006). Successful aging in Shanghai, China: definition, distribution and related factors. *Int Psychogeriatr*, **18**, 551–63.

Li, P., San, J., Yang, Y. H., Liu, Y. H., & Yang, W. X. (2011). [Evaluation on Promotion and Application of Appropriate Technology for Rural Health in Tianjin]. *Chinese General Practice*, **25**(Septemer), 2940–2 (Chinese).

Liu, L.-J. & Guo, Q. (2007). Loneliness and health-related quality of life for the empty nest elderly in the rural area of a mountainous county in China. *Qual Life Res*, **16**, 1275–80.

Ma, E. (2005). 'Naked' bodies: experimenting with intimate relations among migrant workers in South China. *Int J Cult Stud*, **8**, 307–28.

Ma, Z. (2001). Urban labour-force experience as a determinant of rural occupation change: evidence from recent urban-rural return migration in China. *Environment and Planning A*, 237–55.

Maxwell, R. J. (1984). Quality assessment in health. *Br Med J (Clin Res Ed)*, **288**(6428), 1470–2.

Maxwell, R. J. (1992). Dimensions of quality revisited: from thought to action. *Qual Health Care*, **1**, 171–7.

Médecins Sans Frontières (n.d.). New technology for an old disease: UAVs for tuberculosis sample transport in Papua New Guinea [Youtube]. Available at: https://www.youtube.com/watch?v=XpsGay6n8cM [Online].

Médecins Sans Frontières (2014, November 14). Papua New Guinea: Innovating to reach remote TB patients and improve access to treatment. Available at: https://www.msf.org/en/article/papua-new-guinea-innovating-reach-remote-tb-patients-and-improve-access-treatment (accessed 6 January 2017) [Online].

Ministry of Industry and Information Technology of the People's Republic of China (2015, August a). [Fulfilment of the key indicators in the communication industry I]. Available at: http://www.miit.gov.cn/n1146312/n1146904/n1648372/c4324192/content.html (accessed 12 November 2015) (Chinese) [Online].

Ministry of Industry and Information Technology of the People's Republic of China (2015, August b). [Fulfilment of the key indicators in the communication industry II]. Available at: http://www.

miit.gov.cn/n1146312/n1146904/n1648372/c4324197/content.html (accessed 11 November 2015) (Chinese) [Online].

Mou, J., Griffiths, S. M., Fong, H., & Dawes, M. G. (2013). Health of China's rural-urban migrants and their families: a review of literature from 2000 to 2012. *Br Med Bull*, **106**, 19–43.

National Bureau of Statistics of the People's Republic China (2014). *China Statistical Yearbook 2014: Population and its Composition*. Beijing, China: China Statistics Press. Available at: http://www.stats.gov.cn/tjsj/ndsj/2014/indexeh.htm [Online].

National Bureau of Statistics of the People's Republic of China (2015). [Investigational and monitoring report of Chinese migrant workers 2014]. Available at: http://www.stats.gov.cn/tjsj/zxfb/201504/t20150429_797821.html (accessed 10 February 2017) (Chinese) [Online].

National Bureau of Statistics of the People's Republic China (2016). *China Statistical Yearbook 2016: Population and its Composition*. Beijing, China: China Statistics Press. Available at: http://www.stats.gov.cn/tjsj/ndsj/2016/indexeh.htm [Online].

National People's Congress of the People's Republic of China (2012). Elderly protection law. Available at: http://www.npc.gov.cn/npc/xinwen/lfgz/flca/2012-07/06/content_1729109.htm [Online].

Ni, Z., Wu, B., Samples, C., & Shaw, R. J. (2014). Mobile technology for health care in rural China. *Int J Nurs Sci*, **1**, 323–4.

Osornprasop, S. & Sondergaard, L. M. (2016). *Closing the health gaps for the elderly: promoting health equity and social inclusion in Thailand*. Washington, DC: World Bank Group. Available at: http://documents.worldbank.org/curated/en/148431468299339382/Closing-the-health-gaps-for-the-elderly-promoting-health-equity-and-social-inclusion-in-Thailand (accessed 8 February 2017) [Online].

Pang, L., de Brauw, A., & Rozelle, S. (2004). Working until you drop: the elderly of rural China. *China J*, **52**, 73–94.

Pfammatter, A., Spring, B., Saligram, N., *et al.* (2016). mHeath intervention to improve diabetes risk behaviors in India: a prospective, parallel group cohort study. *JMIR*, **18**(8), e207.

Phillips, J. E., Ajrouch, K. J., & Hillcoat-Nalletamby, S. (2010). *Key Concepts in Social Gerontology*. Thousand Oaks, CA: Sage Publications.

Ploutz, M., Lu, J. C., Scheel, J., *et al.* (2016). Handheld echocardiographic screening for rheumatic heart disease by non-experts. *Heart*, **102**, 35–9.

Poulin, J., Houser, L., & Deng, R. (2014). The life satisfaction of elderly Chinese widows living alone and those living with adult children. *China J Soc Work*, **7**, 119–30.

Ren, J., Liu, C., Gao, Q.-S., Yang, L., Huang, X., & Guo, Q. (2015). Use of appropriate healthcare technologies: a cross-sectional study in rural Zhejiang of China. *BMC Health Serv Res*, **15**, 295.

Rossi, G. & Lee, V. S. (2016a). Assessing the burden of rhematic heart disease among refugee children: a call to action. *J Glob Health*, **6**, 020305.

Rossi, G. & Lee, V. S. (2016b). Call for preventive care for rheumatic heart disease in refugee children. *BMJ*, **353**, i2312.

Rothenbuler, M., O'Sullivan, C. J., Stortecky, S., *et al.* (2014). Active surveillance for rheumatic heart disease in endemic regions: a systematic review and meta-analysis of prevalence among children and adolescents. *Lancet Glob Health*, **2**, e717–26.

Ruan, F. & Lau, M. P. (2001). China: demographics and a historical perspective. In: Francoeur, R. T. (ed.), *The International Encyclopedia of Sexuality*. New York, NY: The Continuum Publishing Company.

Samarajiva, R. & Waidyanatha, N. (2009). Two complementary mobile technologies for disaster warning, *info*, **11**, 58–65. Available at: https://doi.org/10.1108/14636690910941885 (accessed 14 July 2017) [Online].

Shrestha, N. R., Karki, P., Mahto, R., *et al.* (2016). Prevalence of subclinical rheumatic heart disease in Eastern Nepal: a school-based cross-sectional study. *JAMA Cardiology*, **1**, 89–96.

Silverstein, M., Cong, Z., & Li, S. (2006). Intergenerational transfers and living arrangements of older people in rural China: consequences for psychological well-being. *J Gerontol B Psychol Sci Soc Sci*, **61**, S256–66.

Smith, A. C., Bensink, M., Armfield, N., Stillman, J., & Caffery, L. (2005). Telemedicine and rural health care applications. *J Postgrad Med*, **51**, 286–93.

Soesilo, D. (2016, September 29). How drones helped fight tuberculosis in Papua New Guinea [blog]. Available at: www.droneblog.com/2016/09/29/how-drones-helped-fight-tuberculosis-in-papua-new-guinea/ (accessed 9 February 2017) [Online].

Su, B., Shen, X., & Wei, Z. (2006). Leisure life in later years: differences between rural and urban elderly residents in China. *J Leis Res*, **38**, 381–97.

Tinnelly, K., Kristjanson, L. J., McCallion, A., & Cousins, K. (2000). Technology in palliative care: steering a new direction or accidental drift? *Int J Palliat Nurs*, **6**, 495–500.

United Nations (UN) (2007). World population ageing: 1950–2050. Available at: http://www.un.org/esa/population/publications/worldageing19502050/ [Online].

United Nations (UN) Economic and Social Commission for Asia and the Pacific (2014). *Statistical Yearbook for Asia and the Pacific 2014*. United Nations. Available at: www.unescap.org/sites/default/files/ESCAP-SYB2014_0.pdf (accessed 14 January 2017) [Online].

United Nations (UN), Department of Economic and Social Affairs, Population Division (2015). *World Population Ageing 2015* (ST/ESA/SER.A/390).

Wang, W. W. & Fan, C. C. (2006). Success or failure: selectivity and reasons of return migration in Sichuan and Anhui, China. *Environ Plan A*, **38**, 939–58.

Wang, X.-Y., Du, L., Von Seidlein, L., *et al.* (2015). Occurrence of shigellosis in the young and elderly in rural China: results of a 12-month population-based surveillance study. *Am J Trop Med Hyg*, **73**, 416–22.

Wang, Z. & Liu, L. (2014). [A study of the function of rural older people's associations in a 'rite-custom society' perspective]. *China Agric Univ J Soc Sci Ed*, **31**, 98–106. Available at: http://zgnydxsk.cnjournals.net/ch/reader/create_pdf.aspx?file_no=20140316002&flag=1 (accessed 3 November 2015) (Chinese) [Online].

Wei, M. (2011, November 25). [More than 40 million older people participate in social development through older people's associations at various levels]. *Xinhua News Agency*. Available at: http://www.gov.cn/jrzg/2011-11/25/content_2003626.htm (accessed 4 November 2015) (Chinese) [Online].

World Health Organization (WHO) (n.d.-a). eHealth. Available at: www.who.int/topics/ehealth/en/ (accessed 6 January 2017) [Online].

World Health Organization (WHO) (n.d.-b). *Older Population and Health System: A profile of Thailand*. Available at: http://www.who.int/ageing/projects/intra/phase_one/alc_intra1_cp_thailand.pdf (accessed 7 February 2017) [Online].

World Health Organization (WHO) (n.d.-c). Papua New Guinea: WHO statistical profile. Available at: www.who.int/countries/png/en/ (accessed 6 January 2017) [Online].

World Health Organization (WHO) (n.d.-d). Tuberculosis in China. Available at: http://www.wpro.who.int/china/mediacentre/factsheets/tuberculosis/en/ (accessed 11 November 2015) [Online].

World Health Organization (WHO) (n.d.-e). WHO definition of palliative care. Available at: http://www.who.int/cancer/palliative/definition/en/ (accessed 11 November 2015) [Online].

World Health Organization (WHO) (2002). *Active Ageing: A Policy Framework*. Available at: http://apps.who.int/iris/bitstream/10665/67215/1/WHO_NMH_NPH_02.8.pdf (accessed 8 February 2017) [Online].

World Health Organization (WHO) (2009). *Telemedicine: Opportunities and developments in Member States: report on the second global survey on eHealth*. Geneva, Switzerland: WHO.

World Health Organization (WHO) (2011). *mHealth: New horizons for health through mobile technologies: second global survey on eHealth*. Geneva, Switzerland: WHO.

World Health Organization (WHO) (2012). *Compendium of New and Emerging Health Technologies*. Geneva, Switzerland: WHO.

World Health Organization (WHO) (2015). *China country assessment report on ageing and health*. Geneva, Switzerland: WHO.**World Health Organization (WHO) Regional Office for South-East Asia** (2016). Health system responses to population ageing and noncommunicable diseases in Asia. *Comparative Country Studies*, **2**(2). Available at: http://apps.who.int/iris/bitstream/10665/252738/1/apo-ccs-ageing5b.pdf [Online].

World Heart Federation (n.d.). Rheumatic Heart Disease (RHD). Available at: https://www.world-heart-federation.org/programmes/rheumatic-heart-disease/ (accessed 14 July 2017) [Online].

World Vision India (2013). mHealth India. Available at: http://www.wvi.org/health/publication/mhealth-india [Online].

World Vision India (2015). mHealth India. Available at: http://www.wvi.org/health/global-mhealth-report [Online].

World Vision International (2014). *More than numbers: why better data adds up to saving the lives of women and children? A Child Health Now policy briefing*. Available at: http://www.wvi.org/sites/default/files/More%20Than%20Numbers.English.Summary_0.pdf [Online].

World Vision International (2014, June). *Harnessing mHealth to reach every woman, every child. mHealth Policy Brief*. Available at: http://www.wvi.org/sites/default/files/mHealth%20Policy%20Brief.FINAL_.pdf [Online].

Wu, L., Chen, H., Hu, Y., *et al.* (2012). Prevalence and associated factors of elder mistreatment in a rural community in People's Republic of China: a cross-sectional study. *PLoS One*, **7**(3), e33857.

Wu, Z.-Q., Sun, L., Sun, Y.-H., Zhang, X.-J., Tao, F., & Cui, G.-H. (2010). Correlation between loneliness and social relationship among empty nest elderly in Anhui rural area, China. *Aging Ment Health*, **14**, 108–12.

Xia, Z. & Yang, C. (2015, February 26). [A tale of home returning: older people's associations and older people's recreation centres well run]. *Guanchazhewang*. Available at: http://www.guancha.cn/XiaZhuZhi/2015_02_26_310317_s.shtml (accessed 3 November 2015) (Chinese) [Online].

Xu, Q., Guan, X., & Yao, F. (2011). Welfare program participation among rural-to-urban migrant workers in China. *Int J Soc Welf*, **20**, 10–21

Yi, Z. (2001). The main features of population aging and policy considerations in China. *Popul Econ*, 05. Available at: http://en.cnki.com.cn/Article_en/CJFDTOTAL-RKJJ200105000.htm (accessed 6 October 2015) [Online].

Zeng, Y. & Wang, Z. (2003). Dynamics of family and elderly living arrangements in China: new lessons learned from the 2000 census. *China Rev*, **3**, 95–119.

Zhang, W., Li, S., & Feldman, M. W. (2005). Gender differences in activity of daily living of the elderly in rural China: evidence from Chaohu. *Journal of Women & Aging*, **17**, 91–106

Zhang, W. & Liu, G. (2007). Childlessness, psychological well-being, and life satisfaction among the elderly in China. *J Cross Cult Gerontol*, **22**, 185–203.

Zheng, X., Chen, G., Song, X., *et al.* (2011). Twenty-year trends in the prevalence of disability in China. *Bull World Health Organ*, **89**, 788–97.

Zimmer, Z. & Kwong, J. (2003). Family size and support of older adults in urban and rural China: Current effects and future implications. *Demography*, **40**, 23–44.

Epilogue

Global population has finally transited from rural- to urban-based settlement patterns in 2010 (UN-Habitat, 2008). Nevertheless, although urbanized living is the predominant lifestyle for the twenty-first century, 'rural living' remains a significant mode of living in our world in the coming decades. With the global commitments in sustainable development, disaster risk reduction, and climate change mitigation efforts (see Chapter 6), more examples and scientific evidence should be available to support top-down rural-based interventions to protect the well-being of people in the world.

Yet, as this book has highlighted, there are community needs that may require bottom-up solutions to address and reduce health and disaster risks to support resilience enhancement efforts. The case examples and experience shared in this book may at best show some of the humble efforts to address health and disaster efforts in the ever-growing challenges in the rural-based context. More lessons learnt and examples should be documented and made available to allow global learning of bottom-up efforts and to maximize the possibilities of rural community empowerment and engagement process. (Walley and Wright, 2011; Chan, 2013, 2017).

References

Chan, E. Y. Y. (2013). Bottom-up disaster resilience. *Nature Geoscience*, **6**, 327–8.

Chan, E. Y. Y. (2017). *Public Health Humanitarian Responses to Natural Disasters* (Routledge Humanitarian Series). London, UK: Routledge.

UN-Habitat. (2008). *State of the World's Cities 2010/2011- Cities for All: Bridging the Urban Divide.* London, UK: Earthscan.

Walley, J. & **Wright, J.** (2010). *Public Health: An Action Guide to Improving Health*, 2nd Edition. Oxford, UK: Oxford University Press.

Appendix 1

Basic knowledge and skills of Chinese citizens on health literacy

Health literacy refers to the ability of a person in accessing and understanding basic health information and services, along with their ability to utilize and apply them in making correct judgements and decisions. Health literacy is used to empower individuals, promoting and maintaining their health. On 4 January 2008, the Ministry of Health of the People's Republic of China issued a trial policy paper on the basic knowledge and skills of health literacy for Chinese citizens. It is one of the global pioneer attempts for the government to outline the scope and content of its expected level of citizens' health literacy. There are 66 concepts which Chinese government regards as essential for health literacy for the twenty-first century. Although some of these concepts might be country/context specific, there are nevertheless meaningful health communication/education messages for promotion in rural and remote contexts. The following section lists the translated 66 concepts.

A1.1 Basic knowledge and concepts

1. Health is not just the absence of disease or infirmity, it is a state of complete physical, mental, and social well-being.
2. Every person has the responsibility to maintain both their personal and social well-being, which can be promoted through the adoption and practice of a healthy lifestyle.
3. A healthy lifestyle includes four main areas, namely a balanced diet, adequate exercise, smoking cessation with limited alcohol intake, and psychological balance.
4. A balance of work and rest needs to be considered together. A person should get seven to eight hours of sleep per day.
5. Both active and passive smoking can increase the risk of cancer, cardiovascular diseases, respiratory diseases, and other illnesses.
6. Quit smoking; the sooner the better, although it is never too late to quit.
7. Dietary supplements are not a substitute for medications.
8. Health and the environment are closely related; protecting the environment promotes health.
9. Promote free blood donation, as blood donation can really help others.
10. Normal systolic and diastolic blood pressure for an adult is less than 140 mmHg and 90 mmHg, respectively; armpit body temperature is normally 36–37°C; resting

respiratory rate should be between 16–20 breaths per minute; pulse rate should be between 60–100 beats per minute.

11. Avoid unnecessary injections and infusions, and ensure that during injections, one person has one needle and one tube (i.e. do not share needles).
12. Workers engaging in toxic and hazardous work should be guaranteed the right to occupational protection.
13. Immunization or vaccination is the most effective and economical way to prevent some infectious diseases.
14. Tuberculosis is an infectious disease that spreads mainly through the air, via droplets produced when a patient coughs, sneezes, or talks loudly.
15. Tuberculosis needs be checked if a patient presents with a cough with or without sputum for more than two weeks, or if the patient has haemoptysis (bloody sputum).
16. Most cases of tuberculosis can be cured as long as patients adhere to regular and proper treatment.
17. AIDS, hepatitis B, and hepatitis C can be transmitted in three ways, through sexual contact, blood/fluid and/or from mother to child (perinatal transmission). They are not spread via human contact at work or in people's daily lives.
18. Mosquitoes, flies, rats, cockroaches, and other vector animals can spread diseases.
19. Abnormal mass, intraluminal haemorrhage, and unintentional weight loss are important early warning signs of cancer.
20. CPR (cardiopulmonary resuscitation) may be performed as an emergency first-line assistance for the sick or wounded suffering from breathing difficulties and/or cardiac arrest.
21. People with psychological problems should take the initiative to seek help, as it is important to pay attention to and maintain one's mental health status.
22. Everyone should be caring and helpful towards others, without discriminating against the sick and disabled.
23. Having an influenza vaccination before the flu season can reduce both the risk and symptoms of influenza.
24. Toxic substances (such as pesticides, medicines, and so on) should be properly stored and kept away from children.
25. Traumatic or severe haemorrhage should be immediately bandaged to stop bleeding; wounded patients with fractures should not be moved unless when necessary.

A1.2 Healthy lifestyle and behaviour

26. Wash hands frequently, take showers or baths often, but do not share towels and toiletries.

27. Brush your teeth every day, and use mouthwash after eating a meal to protect your teeth.
28. Cover your nose and mouth when sneezing or coughing, and do not spit.
29. Do not smoke in public places, and respect the right of non-smokers in avoiding passive second-hand smoke.
30. Reduce alcohol intake, prevent alcoholism.
31. Do not abuse sedatives, hypnotics, analgesics, and other addictive drugs.
32. Refuse drugs.
33. Use sanitary latrines and have good management of manure and other human wastes.
34. Pay attention to the safety and cleanliness of drinking water, be aware of drinking water health.
35. Open windows often to improve and maintain indoor ventilation.
36. A proper diet should be mainly comprised of grains, fruits, vegetables and potatoes, although it is important to pay attention to the balance between meat and vegetables.
37. Milk, beans, and related products should be regularly consumed.
38. A healthy dietary requirement includes low sodium and fat.
39. Maintain a normal body weight, avoid being overweight or obese.
40. After falling ill, it is important to receive treatment as soon as possible, cooperate with doctors' treatments, and follow any doctor-prescribed medication schedule and dosage.
41. Do not abuse the use of antibiotics.
42. Meals should be cooked properly, while fruits and vegetables should be washed properly before consumption.
43. Raw food and cooked food should be stored and processed separately.
44. Do not eat spoiled food or food that has exceeded the specified shelf life.
45. After getting pregnant, women should attend hospital physical examinations in a timely manner, with at least five check-up visits during the pregnancy, while also ensuring delivery in hospital.
46. Infants should be breastfed as soon as possible, and it is suitable to add food supplements after the child is six months old.
47. To prevent the occurrence and development of myopia, children and adolescents should develop good eye care habits.
48. Workers need to understand the hazards associated with their work, abide by working rules, pay attention to personal safety and protection, while also developing good working habits.
49. Children should receive vaccination according to the planned immunization programme.

50. Correct use of condoms can reduce the risk of AIDS and sexually transmitted diseases (STDs).
51. Discovery of dead poultry needs to be reported, while sick or contaminated poultry and livestock should not be processed and eaten.
52. Domestic dogs should receive a rabies vaccination. If someone is scratched or bitten by cats or dogs, the wound should be washed immediately and disinfected thoroughly, while the patient should obtain an antiserum and rabies vaccine injection as soon as possible.
53. Avoid contact with infected water in schistosomiasis epidemic areas. If someone contacts the infected water, they should take preventative medication immediately.
54. To prevent iodine deficiency disorders, consume qualified or medically recognized iodized salt.
55. Undergo a health check or physical examination once a year.
56. Reduce road traffic injuries by wearing seatbelts (or helmets), not speeding, and not driving under the influence of alcohol or drugs.
57. Prevent drowning by keeping children away from dangerous waters.
58. Store pesticides safely, according to pesticide-use instructions.
59. Beware of gas poisoning when using winter heating, pay attention to ventilation.

A1.3 Basic skills

60. Call 120 (emergency services hotline in China) when emergency medical assistance is required.
61. Understand the labels and instructions for food, medicine, cosmetics, and health products.
62. Measure armpit body temperature.
63. Correctly measure pulse.
64. Keep away from danger. Be able to identify and distinguish between common risk identification labels, such as high pressure, flammable, explosive, toxic, radioactive, biological and chemical safety, and so on.
65. When rescuing a patient suffering from electric shock, first cut off the power; do not touch the body of the patient directly.
66. In the case of fire, be able to protect oneself by using a wet towel to cover the nose and mouth, and while escaping use the safe posture (being on all fours; low posture), while also be able to call 119 (fire alarm).

Appendix 2

Semi-structured questions for in-depth interviews with village heads (using rural China as an example)

- Record information about villagers' routines using Tables A2.1 and A2.2.

A2.1 Guided questions with village head

1. How long have you been the village head?
2. How long has this village been established?
3. How many households are there in the village currently? How many households have moved away in the past year? (If there are subvillages, ask the number of households in each subvillages)
4. How are the households distributed? How many minutes does it take to reach the farthest household on foot?
5. How many people are there in a household on average? What is the generally family structure?
6. How many villagers are in the village? How many of them usually reside here?
7. What is the average age of the villagers? What is the male-to-female ratio? How about the ratio of the majority national ethnic group to the ethnic minorities?
8. What is the daily routine of the villagers? When do they usually wake up, go to work, and come home?
9. Which seasons or months are the busiest for farming? What are the main crops in the village?
10. What are the important festivals in the village?
11. Is there any disaster in the village? What are the main hazards?
12. What has been done in disaster preparation and disaster reduction in the village?
13. What do you think about the hygiene conditions of the village? (e.g. the conditions of toilets and pollution)
14. How do the villagers manage the domestic waste? Is there any fixed site for disposal or burning?
15. Overall, what is the main problem in the village?

Table A2.1 Seasonal calendar

Month **Activity**	**Jan**	**Feb**	**Mar**	**Apr**	**May**	**Jun**	**Jul**	**Aug**	**Sep**	**Oct**	**Nov**	**Dec**
Farming												
Festivals												
Working in towns or cities as migrant labour												
Other activities												

Table A2.2 Daily timetable

Hours Activity	1	2	3	4	5	6	7	8	9	10	11	12	13	14	15	16	17	18	19	20	21	22	23	0
Farming																								
Meals																								
Rest																								
Other activities																								

A2.2 Guided questions with village doctor

1. How long have you been the village doctor?
2. When was this village clinic established?
3. What training have you received?
4. How many patients do you see per day?
5. Do the patients have specific characteristics, for example of a particular age group or gender?
6. What are the main problems of the patients in general?
7. When you encounter some diseases or problems that cannot be handled in the clinic, what would you do?
8. How many newborns were there in the village last year?
9. Apart from seeing the patients, what are your daily tasks?
10. How is the work of chronic disease management going in the village?
11. Was there any health or disaster preparedness education conducted last year? If so, what were the contents?
12. Is there any health knowledge that many villagers are concerned about but lacks promotion?
13. Overall, what is the main health problem in the village?

Appendix 3

Example of focus group discussion questions (using rural China as an example)

Hello everyone, I am [**name**] from [**organization**]. Today, I would like to have a brief discussion with you to learn more about your living conditions. Your participation in this study is completely voluntary and you are free to join in or not as you wish. We hope that you will speak up, as your opinions and ideas are really important in our planning of future services. Anything you say will be kept strictly confidential and, please, also respect each other's shared thoughts and opinions. In the next hour or so, we will be discussing your lifestyle and physical and mental health, as well as the way you receive healthcare services. If you have any queries, do feel free to call [**telephone number**] and contact [**name**] at [**name of organization**].

Before we start, does anyone have any question? If not, let us begin with a round of introductions. Could you please briefly introduce yourself?

A3.1 Community health

- How long have you been living in this village?
- Have there been any new villagers moving into the village recently?
  - If so, how many? What fraction of the village population do they make up?
  - What do you think about the new villagers?
- How would you describe the relationship among people within the village?
- Who would you ask if you are in need of help?
- How is your current health?
  - Good (% of all respondents): In what aspect(s)?
  - Poor (% of all respondents): In what aspect(s)? What have you done to improve your health?
- How is your family's current health condition? [Children under five years, older people (how many have chronic illnesses?), females, males]
- What are the major diseases suffered by the village? Why do you have this impression?

A3.2 Healthcare services

- Where do you seek healthcare services when you have MINOR illnesses? How do you get there? How long does it take?

  Hint: Village doctor (%) | *City/provincial hospital (%)*
  Township hospital/clinic (%) | *Herbalist/bonesetter (%)*
  County hospital (%) | *Others (%)*

- Where do you seek healthcare services when you have MAJOR illnesses? How do you get there? How long does it take?

  Hint Village doctor (%) | *City/provincial hospital (%)*
  Township hospital/clinic (%) | *Herbalist/bonesetter (%)*
  County hospital (%) | *Others (%)*

- What factors will you consider before seeking healthcare services?

  Hint: Fees/charges (%) | *Trustworthiness (%)*
  Distance/proximity(%) | *No other choice (%)*
  Quality (%) | *Others (%)*

- What would you do if you had a sudden illness or serious accident?
- Where do you obtain information about health?

  Hint: Government (%) | *Village chief (%)* | *Family member (%)*
  Friend (%) | *Neighbour (%)* | *TV/radio (%)*
  Newspaper (%) | *Internet (%)* | *Clinic (%) School (%)*

A3.3 Disaster preparedness

- Do you think you are living in an area of high disaster risk? If so, what disaster are you at risk of?

  Hint: Natural disasters: earthquake, forest fire, mudslide, flooding, rainstorm, cyclone
  Man-made disasters: household fires, traffic accident, accident in handling machinery

- Have you experienced a disaster before?

  If so, when: ______________________

  What was the type of disaster?

  Hint: Natural disasters: earthquake, forest fire, mudslide, flood, rainstorm, cyclone
  Man-made disasters: household fires, traffic accident, accident in handling machinery

- Have you been injured in a disaster?
- Have your family members been injured in a disaster?
- Did you suffer from any property loss? *Hint: housing, crops, livestock, tools for work*

- Do you think you or your family have the ability to protect your health and safety? Why?
- Do you think you are well prepared for disaster in general?
- Have you ever thought of packing a disaster preparedness kit? Why?
- Have you or your family already got a disaster preparedness kit?

  If so, when did you get the kit?

  What should a disaster preparedness kit include? (Do NOT prompt)

  ____

  ____

  If not, why not?
- Will you consider packing a disaster preparedness kit?
  - Yes (%)
  - No (%) Why?
- Do you think it important to bring your regular medications along when a disaster strikes?
- Have you prepared any medications to bring along with you? If so, what kinds of medication?

  ____

  ____

  If not, why not?

A3.4 Conclusion

In addition to the topics mentioned above, are there any important issues related to your life or your health that you would like to share with us? If not, I would like to thank everyone for sharing their ideas. If you would like to talk to us alone about important issues, you are welcome to contact us. Thank you very much once again for your help!

Note: Texts in italics are answer prompts designed to provide respondents with possible ideas for their answers. It is not necessary to read out these hints when asking the questions. Note down the percentage of respondents giving a particular answer.

Appendix 4

Basic information of focus group interviewees (using China as an example)

Use the form provided in Table A4.1 to collect basic information about focus group interviewees.

Table A4.1 Interviewee information collection form

Personal information	
Name:	
Gender (please circle one):	Male/Female
Age:	
Subvillage:	
Ethnicity:	
Language use:	
Occupation:	
Number of household members:	
Annual family income (please select one of the options)	
Local currency (e.g. RMB):	
1.	Less than 500
2.	501–1,000
3.	1,001–1,500
4.	1,501–2,000
5.	2,001–2,500
6.	2,501–3,000
7.	Over 3,000
8.	Unspecified
Main source of income (please select one of the options)	
1.	Plant/sale of crops
2.	Livestock and poultry breeding/sale
3.	Employed labour
4.	Doing business
5.	Village public services (e.g. village doctor)
6.	No clear source of income
7.	Other:
Level of education (please select the highest level the interviewee has attained)	
1.	Illiterate
2.	No formal education but can read
3.	Primary school
4.	Junior high school
5.	High school/secondary school
6.	Tertiary college
7.	University and above

Appendix 5

A sample of a health and disaster response survey research questionnaire in rural China

The following questionnaire serves as an example of a tool to collect information related to health status and needs. The sample survey should be adjusted according to specific local environment and culture. For example, if the village of interest is of Hui/Muslim ethnic group, the section of the question referring to pigs (question HC 9) should be skipped and if drinking alcohol is strictly prohibited in the area, alcohol-related questions should also be omitted.

Sample

The Chinese University of Hong Kong JC School of Public Health and Primary Care
Health and Disaster Response Survey Research Questionnaire

Name of organization:[]　　**Research Period:** 20YY/MM/DD - 20YY/MM/DD
Name of village:[]

Hello! We are conducting a survey to learn more about your life, health, and hygiene conditions. We would like to conduct an interview with either the head of your household, or an adult household member who knows the household well. This interview will take around 30 minutes, and our conversation will be kept strictly confidential. The information, data, and details collected in the interview will only be used for our research and will not be disclosed to others. Participation is completely voluntary and can be stopped any time if you would like to withdraw from the interview. Are you willing to participate?

☐ Yes, I am willing to participate in the interview. (Complete the basic survey about the household, then start the interview.)
☐ No, I am not willing to do the interview. (Note down the response in a household questionnaire summary table.)

Note: Each household should complete a questionnaire, preferably by the head of the household. If the head of the household is not available, the questionnaire should be completed by an *adult* household member who is well-informed about the composition, basic information, and economic status of the household.

Household survey information	
HS1 Interview date (YYYY/MM/DD): 201__ / ___ / ____	**HS2 Name of interviewer:**
HS3 Subvillage number / name:	**HS4 House number:**
HS5 House number on map / Characteristic feature of house location (for ease of return visit):	**HS6 Respondent information:** ☐ 1. Interviewee is the head of the household or an adult household member who knows the household situation the best. ☐ 2. Interviewee is the only adult at home. ☐ 3. Interviewee is the only household member in the household willing to participate/able to communicate in the interview.
HS7 Start **time of interview** (hh:mm): ____: ____	**HS8** End **time of interview** (hh:mm): ____: ____

Respondent background

RB1 Name of respondent:_________ ☐ 997. Don't know ☐ 998. Refuse to answer

RB2 Gender: ☐ 1. Male ☐ 2. Female

RB3 Age:_________ ☐ 997. Don't know ☐ 998. Refuse to answer

RB4 Ethnicity: ☐ 1. Main ethnic group of the village ☐ 2. Others, please specify_____
☐ 997. Don't know ☐ 998. Refuse to answer

RB5 Is the respondent the head of the household?
☐ 1. Yes ☐ 2. No ☐ 997. Don't know ☐ 998. Refuse to answer

RB6 Respondent's highest level of education attained (Have you ever attended school? If so, what education level have you attained?):
☐ 1. Illiterate ☐ 2. No formal education, but can read
☐ 3. Some primary school education ☐ 4. Completed primary school
☐ 5. Some junior high school education ☐ 6. Completed junior high school
☐ 7. Some high school/vocational school education ☐ 8. Completed high school/ vocational school
☐ 9. Some tertiary/university education ☐ 10. Completed tertiary school/ university or above
☐ 997. Don't know ☐ 998. Refuse to answer

RB7 Respondent's current occupation (which main household income derived from)
☐ 1. Farming ☐ 2. Doing business ☐ 3. Employed work
☐ 4. Student ☐ 5. Temporary work ☐ 6.Others, please specify ____________
☐ 997. Don't know ☐ 998. Refuse to answer

Household characteristics

HC1 How many people are there in your household? ___________ ☐ 997. Don't know ☐ 998. Refuse to answer

List of household members: I would like to know about each member of your household, including their age, education level, and health status.

HM1 Serial no.	HM2 Relationship with respondent*	HM3 Gender 1. M 2. F	HM4 Age	HM5 Highest level of education**	HM6 Health and medical condition							HM7 Personal health habits		HM8 Over the past year, did you leave the village to work in the town/city?***	HM9 Do you own a mobile phone? ***
					A. Has the doctor diagnosed you with any of the following diseases?				B. Are you taking any long-term medication?***	C. Do you have a stable supply of required medication? ***	D. Over the past year, how many times have you visited the doctor? If none, write 0	A. Do you have a smoking habit? ***	B. Do you have a drinking habit ? ***		
					A1. Hypertension***	A2. Diabetes ***	A3. Rheumatism***	A4. Please specify if you have any other diseases or disability conditions, including self-diagnosed illnesses.							
1															
2															
3															
4															
5															
6															
7															
8															
9															
10															
11															
12															

1	*__Relationship with respondent:__	**1** Respondent **2** Spouse **3** Parent **4** (Parent) In-law **5** Children **6** Son/Daughter-in-law 7 Grandson/granddaughter **8** Grandson/granddaughter-in-law **9** Sibling **10** Spouse of sibling **11** Nephew/niece **12** Other relatives **13** Other non-relatives
2	**__Highest education level:__	**1** Illiterate **2** No formal education, but can read **3** Some primary school education **4** Completed primary school **5** Some junior high school education **6** Completed junior high school **7** Some high school/vocational school education **8** Completed high school/vocational school **9** Some tertiary/university education **10** Completed tertiary school/university or above **997** Don't know **998** Refuse to answer
3	***__General code:__	**1** Have/need/yes **2** Don't have/need not/no **888** N/A **997** Don't know **998** Refuse to answer

Fill in **HC2–HC6** based on the above List of household members. If the information in the list is incomplete, please ask follow-up questions.		
HC2 Number of people within each age group in the household (enter 0 if no member of the particular age group)		
A. Under 5: _____	☐ 997. Don't know	☐ 998. Refuse to answer
B. Aged 60 or above: _____	☐ 997. Don't know	☐ 998. Refuse to answer
C. Under 15: _____	☐ 997. Don't know	☐ 998. Refuse to answer
D. 15 to 64 years old: _____	☐ 997. Don't know	☐ 998. Refuse to answer
E. Aged 65 or above: _____	☐ 997. Don't know	☐ 998. Refuse to answer
HC3 Are the children at home between the ages of 7 and 14 all studying in school? ☐ 1. Yes ☐ 2. No ☐ 888. N/A (No children between 7-14) ☐ 997. Don't know ☐ 998. Refuse to answer		
HC4 Is there at least one person in the household who has completed 6 years of education? ☐ 1. Yes ☐ 2. No ☐ 997. Don't know ☐ 998. Refuse to answer		
HC5 In the past year, **how many household members went out to work in town or city?** (If none, write 0):______ ☐ 997. Don't know ☐ 998. Refuse to answer		
HC6 How many people at home have a cell phone? (If none, write 0):______ ☐ 997. Don't know ☐ 998. Refuse to answer		

HM10 Completion of household member list:

☐ 1. Completed (All household members have been listed)
☐ 2. Partially completed (interviewee information listed at least)

Please continue the questionnaire . . .

HC7 How many acres of agricultural land does the household own?
(If none, write 0):______acres
☐ 997. Don't know ☐ 998. Refuse to answer

HC8 Are there any livestock or poultry at home?
☐ 1. Yes ☐ 2.No
☐ 997. Don't know ☐ 998. Refuse to answer

HC9 If the household has livestock or poultry at home, please list both the variety and quantity (If none, write 0):

A. Cattle		□ 997. Don't know	□ 998. Refuse to answer
B. Horse, donkey, mule		□ 997. Don't know	□ 998. Refuse to answer
C. Goat		□ 997. Don't know	□ 998. Refuse to answer
D. Pig		□ 997. Don't know	□ 998. Refuse to answer
E. Chicken, duck, goose		□ 997. Don't know	□ 998. Refuse to answer

HC10 What is the main source of income of your household? (Choose the most important one)

□ 1. Farming/Selling crops □ 2. Breeding/Selling livestock and poultry
□ 3. Employed work □ 4. Doing business
□ 5. Village service work (e.g. village doctor) □ 6. No clear source of income
□ 7. Others, please specify: ___________
□ 997. Don't know □ 998. Refuse to answer

HC11 What is the total annual household income? __________
□ 888. Not applicable (No fixed income)
□ 997. Don't know □ 998. Refuse to answer

HC12 Does anyone at home have regular access to the Internet?
□ 1. Yes □ 2. No
□ 997. Don't know □ 998. Refuse to answer

HC13 What are your main purposes of regularly using the Internet? (Choose the 3 most important purposes and place them in order of importance)
□ 1. Browsing the news/social information (e.g. weather information)
□ 2. Practical information (e.g. government policies, daily information)
□ 3. Learning
□ 4. Using social media
□ 5. Recreation
□ 6. Work-related purposes
□ 7. Others, please specify: ___________
□ 997. Don't know □ 998. Refuse to answer

Health and healthcare

Fill in **HH1** to **HH5** using information directly from **HM6** of the List of household members above. If the information in the list is incomplete, please ask follow-up questions.
HH1 How many people in the household suffer from chronic illness? (If none, write 0): ______ ☐ 997. Don't know ☐ 998. Refuse to answer
HH2 How many people in the household are suffering from two or more chronic illnesses concurrently? (If none, write 0):______ ☐ 997. Don't know ☐ 998. Refuse to answer
HH3 How many people in the household require long-term medication? (If none, write 0): ______ ☐ 888. N/A ☐ 997. Don't know ☐ 998. Refuse to answer
HH4 Do the people requiring long-term medication in the household have a stable supply of drugs? ☐ 1. Yes (All people with long-term medication have a stable drug supply.) ☐ 2. No (There are people without a stable drug supply.) ☐ 888. N/A (No one needs long-term medication.) ☐ 997. Don't know ☐ 998. Refuse to answer
HH5 In the past year, **how many people in the household went to consult a doctor?** (If none, write 0): ______ ☐ 997. Don't know ☐ 998. Refuse to answer

Please continue . . .

HH6 In general, how would you describe your current health status?

☐ 1. Very poor ☐ 2. Poor ☐ 3. Ordinary ☐ 4. Good ☐ 5. Very good
☐ 997. Don't know ☐ 998. Refuse to answer

HH7 Compared with 1 year ago, you think your current health status is:

☐ 1. A lot better ☐ 2. Better ☐ 3.Similar ☐ 4.Worse ☐ 5. A lot worse
☐ 997. Don't know ☐ 998. Refuse to answer

HH8 How many elderly aged over 60 in the household have had a tetanus vaccination?
(If none, write 0): ______
☐ 888. N/A (No elderly over 60 in the household)
☐ 997. Don't know ☐ 998. Refuse to answer

HH9 In the past month, **did any child under 5 in the household experience diarrhoea?**
(Note: Diarrhoea refers to having 3 times or more of loose or watery stool in one day.)
☐ 1. Yes ☐ 2. No ☐ 888. N/A (No child under 5 in the household)
☐ 997. Don't know ☐ 998. Refuse to answer

HH10 In the past month, **has any other household members (excluding children under 5) experienced diarrhoea?** (Note: Diarrhoea refers to having 3 times or more of loose or watery stool in one day.)
□ 1. Yes □ 2. No □ 997. Don't know □ 998. Refuse to answer

HH11 If someone in the household has diarrhoea, how would it be dealt with generally? (Note: Diarrhoea refers to having 3 times or more of loose or watery stool in one day.)
□ 1. Do nothing and allow natural recovery □ 2. Self-medication (Herbal medicine/over the counter)
□ 3. Consult the doctor □ 4. Others, please specify ______
□ 888. N/A (The household never had diarrhoea.)
□ 997. Don't know □ 998. Refuse to answer

HH12 In the past year, **how was the overall situation of diarrhoea in the household?** (Note: Diarrhoea refers to having 3 times or more of loose or watery stool in one day.)
□ 1. Remained the same □ 2. Increased □ 3. Decreased
□ 997. Don't know □ 998. Refuse to answer

HH13 Have you ever heard that you can take a solution formed by mixing salt and sugar in clean water to prevent dehydration after diarrhoea?
□ 1. Yes, heard before □ 2. Never heard before
□ 997. Don't know □ 998. Refuse to answer

HH14 In the past year, **did anyone in the household experience food poisoning?**
□ 1. Yes □ 2. No □ 997. Don't know □ 998. Refuse to answer

HH15 In the past year, **did anyone in the household experience pesticide poisoning?**
□ 1. Yes □ 2. No □ 997. Don't know □ 998. Refuse to answer

HH16 In the past year, **did you or your household members encounter a situation where you did not go to see the doctor because you could not afford it?**
□ 1. Yes □ 2. No □ 888. N/A (No need to consult doctor in the past year)
□ 997. Don't know □ 998. Refuse to answer

HH17 If anyone in the household needs to see a doctor, where would you usually go to?
□ 1. City hospital □ 2. County hospital
□ 3. Town/township hospital □ 4. Village clinic/village doctor
□ 5. Others, please specify ________ □ 888. N/A (No need to consult doctor)
□ 997. Don't know □ 998. Refuse to answer

HH18 How many people in the household have participated in the national medical insurance scheme (e.g. 'New Rural Cooperative Medical Scheme' in China)?
(If none, write 0): ____ □ 997. Don't know □ 998. Refuse to answer

Health-related behaviours

Fill in **HB1–HB4** directly using the information from **HM7** of the List of household members above. If the information in the list is incomplete, please ask follow-up questions.
HB1 How many people in the household have a smoking habit? (If none, write 0):______ ☐ 997. Don't know ☐ 998. Refuse to answer
HB2 How many people in the household under 18 years old have a smoking habit? (If none, write 0):______ ☐ 888. N/A (No one under 18 in the household) ☐ 997. Don't know ☐ 998. Refuse to answer
HB3 How many people in the household have a drinking habit? (If none, write 0): ______ ☐ 997. Don't know ☐ 998. Refuse to answer
HB4 How many people in the household under 18 years old have a smoking habit? (If none, write 0): ______ ☐ 888. N/A (No one under 18 in the household) ☐ 997. Don't know ☐ 998. Refuse to answer

Please continue . . .

HB5 If someone at home has a drinking habit, what type of alcohol do they usually drink?

☐ 1. Beer ☐ 2. Distilled liquor ☐ 3. Both beer and distilled liquor
☐ 4.Others: ______ ☐ 997. Don't know ☐ 998. Refuse to answer

HB6 Do you think excessive drinking has a negative impact on your health?

☐ 1.Yes ☐ 2. No ☐ 997. Don't know ☐ 998. Refuse to answer

HB7 How often does anyone smoke inside your home (indoor smoking)?

☐ 1. Everyday ☐ 2. Occasionally (at least once a month) ☐ 3. Never
☐ 997. Don't know ☐ 998. Refuse to answer

HB8 Do you think smoking has a negative effect on the health of smokers?

☐ 1. Yes ☐ 2. No ☐ 997. Don't know ☐ 998. Refuse to answer

HB9 Do you think smoking has a negative effect on the health of non-smokers who are around the smokers?

☐ 1. Yes ☐ 2. No ☐ 997. Don't know ☐ 998. Refuse to answer

HB10 Do you usually wash your hands before having your meal?
☐ 1. Most of the time ☐ 2. Sometimes ☐ 3. Usually don't wash
☐ 997. Don't know ☐ 998. Refuse to answer

HB11 Do you usually wash your hands after going to the toilet?
☐ 1. Most of the time ☐ 2. Sometimes ☐ 3. Usually not
☐ 997. Don't know ☐ 998. Refuse to answer

HB12 Do your household members have the habit of brushing their teeth?
☐ 1. Yes, every household member has the habit.
☐ 2. Yes, some household members have the habit.
☐ 3. No one in the household has the habit.
☐ 997. Don't know ☐ 998. Refuse to answer

Food and safety

FS1 Where does most of the food your household eat come from? Is it mainly self-grown, purchased, or from other sources? (Choose only the most important option.)
☐ 1. Self-grown ☐ 2. Purchased ☐ 3. Others, please specify: ________
☐ 997. Don't know ☐ 998. Refuse to answer

FS2 Does your household usually have enough food for all members?
☐ 1. Enough ☐ 2. Barely enough/so-so
☐ 3. Not enough ☐ 997. Don't know ☐ 998. Refuse to answer

FS3 If there are leftovers after a meal, how do you usually deal with them?
☐ 1. Refrigerate the leftovers ☐ 2. Leave them at room temperature to eat next time
☐ 3. Feed to livestock/poultry ☐ 4. Throw away
☐ 5. Others, please specify: _____ ☐ 888. N/A (Usually no leftovers)
☐ 997. Don't know ☐ 998. Refuse to answer

FS4 Do you usually check the shelf-life before buying packaged food?
☐ 1. Usually ☐ 2. Sometimes
☐ 3. Usually not ☐ 888. N/A (Never eats or buys packaged food)
☐ 997. Don't know ☐ 998. Refuse to answer

FS5 Have you ever heard of or noticed the nutrition labelling on food packages?
☐ 1. Yes ☐ 2. No
☐ 997. Don't know ☐ 998. Refuse to answer

FS6 What is the main source of fuel for cooking in the household? (If more than one source of fuel is used, note down only the most commonly used one.)
☐ 1. Electricity ☐ 2. Firewood ☐ 3. Coal ☐ 4. Charcoal
☐ 5. Straws of crops ☐ 6. Animal waste ☐ 7. Others, please specify: _____
☐ 888. N/A (Don't cook at home)
☐ 997. Don't know ☐ 998. Refuse to answer

Water and sanitation

WS1 What is the main source of drinking water in your home?
☐ 1. Tap water ☐ 2. Tubular/Piped well ☐ 3. Dug water well
☐ 4. Spring water ☐ 5. Rainwater (collected by tanks/reservoirs)
☐ 6. River/Stream/Lake/Pond/Canal
☐ 7. Bottled water ☐ 8. Others, please specify: __________
☐ 997. Don't know ☐ 998. Refuse to answer

WS2 How long does it take to obtain drinking water?
☐ 1. Instantly (tap water) ☐ 2. Within 5 minutes ☐ 3. Within 30 minutes
☐ 4. Over 30 minutes
☐ 997. Don't know ☐ 998. Refuse to answer

WS3 How stable is the drinking water supply?
☐ 1. Very stable, always have water ☐ 2. Stable, with occasional water shortage
☐ 3. Unstable, water shortage occurs often
☐ 997. Don't know ☐ 998. Refuse to answer

WS4 In general, is there enough drinking water for the household?
☐ 1. Enough ☐ 2. So-so/Just enough ☐ 3. Not enough
☐ 997. Don't know ☐ 998. Refuse to answer

WS5 Do you worry about the quality of the drinking water?
☐ 1. Yes ☐ 2. No
☐ 997. Don't know ☐ 998. Refuse to answer

WS6 If worried, what are you worried about? (Please write down directly):

____

☐ 888 N/A (Not worried) ☐ 997. Don't know ☐ 998. Refuse to answer

WS7 Do you usually drink the water from the water source directly, or treat the water before drinking?
☐ 1. Drink directly ☐ 2. Treat the water before drinking
☐ 3. Sometimes treat before drinking and sometimes drink directly
☐ 997. Don't know ☐ 998. Refuse to answer

WS8 If you treat the water, which of the following method(s) do you use? (Can choose more than one option.)

A. Boil	☐ 1. Yes	☐ 2. No	☐ 888. N/A (Don't treat the water)	☐ 997. Don't know	☐ 998. Refuse to answer
B. Add disinfectant	☐ 1. Yes	☐ 2. No	☐ 888. N/A (Don't treat the water)	☐ 997. Don't know	☐ 998. Refuse to answer
C. Filter	☐ 1. Yes	☐ 2. No	☐ 888. N/A (Don't treat the water)	☐ 997. Don't know	☐ 998. Refuse to answer
D. Others, please specify: _______			☐ 888. N/A (Don't treat the water)	☐ 997. Don't know	☐ 998. Refuse to answer

WS9 What are the main source(s) of water for domestic use other than drinking (e.g. non-drinking water sources for washing hands, vegetables, clothes, etc.)?
☐ 1. Tap water ☐ 2. Tubular/Piped well ☐ 3. Dug water well
☐ 4. Spring water ☐ 5. Rainwater (collected by tanks/reservoirs)
☐ 6. River/Stream/Lake/Pond/Canal
☐ 7. Others, please specify: ___________
☐ 997. Don't know ☐ 998. Refuse to answer

WS10 Are there any places or containers for the storage of water at home (e.g. water vaults, pools, tanks, buckets, etc.)**?**
☐ 1. Yes ☐ 2. No ☐ 997. Don't know ☐ 998. Refuse to answer

WS11 How much does water cost your household a month? (use RMB as an example)
☐ 1. No need to pay ☐ 2. < RMB 50
☐ 3. RMB 50 to 100 ☐ 4. > RMB 100
☐ 997. Don't know ☐ 998. Refuse to answer

WS12 In general, where do your household members go to urinate and defaecate?
☐ 1. Toilet at home ☐ 2. Public toilet in village ☐ 3. Out on the field
☐ 4. Others, please specify: _____
☐ 997. Don't know ☐ 998. Refuse to answer

Waste management

WM1, WM2: The main garbage type and treatment method

Begin by asking about the main types of garbage (WM1). No need to read out the options. Simply circle the appropriate option(s) answered by the respondent. More than one option can be circled. At the same time, observe the household environment and make further enquiries where necessary. Based on the respondent's answer to WM1, ask about how the respondent deals with each type of garbage.

WM1 What are the main types of garbage in the household?				**WM2 In general, how do you manage / treat the waste?** (Only one treatment method for each type of garbage)										
	Yes	No	Refuse to answer	Don't know how to manage the waste	Discard at will	Incinerate / burn	Store together/ centrally	Bury	Feed live-stock	Sell	Others, please specify	N/A	Don't know	Refuse to answer
A. Agricultural waste (straw, etc.)	1	2	998	0	1	2	3	4	5	6	7.____	888	997	998
B. Kitchen waste (leftovers, etc.)	1	2	998	0	1	2	3	4	5	6	7.____	888	997	998
C. Waste paper (books, newspapers, cartons, etc.)	1	2	998	0	1	2	3	4	5	6	7.____	888	997	998
D. Plastic (bottles, bags, packaging, etc.)	1	2	998	0	1	2	3	4	5	6	7.____	888	997	998

E. Glass (bottles, jars, etc.)	1	2	998	0	1	2	3	4	5	6	7._____	888	997	998
F. Metal (cans, etc.)	1	2	998	0	1	2	3	4	5	6	7._____	888	997	998
G. Fabric (clothing, towels, etc.)	1	2	998	0	1	2	3	4	5	6	7._____	888	997	998
H. Pesticide containers	1	2	998	0	1	2	3	4	5	6	7._____	888	997	998
I. Used/waste batteries	1	2	998	0	1	2	3	4	5	6	7._____	888	997	998
J. Medical waste (expired drugs/ syringes/needles, etc.)	1	2	998	0	1	2	3	4	5	6	7._____	888	997	998
K. Others, please specify: ______	1	2	998	0	1	2	3	4	5	6	7._____	888	997	998

WM3 If burning / incineration is a method used to deal with the garbage, where does it usually take place?

☐ 1. Indoors ☐ 2. Outdoors ☐ 3. Sometimes indoors, sometimes outdoors
☐ 4. Others, please specify: _____ ☐ 888. N/A (Don't burn garbage)
☐ 997. Don't know ☐ 998. Refuse to answer

WM4 Does your household use pesticides? (If pesticide container is answered in WM1, option 1 can be chosen without asking the question, then continue with the next question.)

☐ 1. Yes ☐ 2. No
☐ 997. Don't know ☐ 998. Refuse to answer

WM5 (If pesticides are used) **How do the household members usually handle pesticide packages or containers?**

☐ 1. Discard casually ☐ 2.Burn/incinerate ☐ 3. Store centrally ☐ 4. Bury
☐ 5. Reuse as containers for other things
☐ 6. Others, please specify: ______ ☐ 888. N/A (Don't use pesticides)
☐ 997. Don't know ☐ 998. Refuse to answer

WM6 (If pesticides are used) **Do you usually read and understand the label on the packaging before using the pesticide?**

☐ 1. Usually ☐ 2. Sometimes ☐ 3.Usually not
☐ 888. N/A (Don't use pesticides)
☐ 997. Don't know ☐ 998. Refuse to answer

WM7 Are you satisfied with the garbage disposal situation in the village?

☐ 1. Yes ☐ 2. No ☐ 997. Don't know ☐ 998. Refuse to answer

WM8 If not satisfied, what aspects are you not satisfied with? (Open-ended question, please write down relevant points): ______________

☐ 888. N/A (Satisfied with garbage disposal situation)
☐ 997. Don't know ☐ 998. Refuse to answer

WM9 Are you worried that the current garbage disposal method(s) will affect you and your household members' health?

☐ 1. Yes ☐ 2. No ☐ 997. Don't know ☐ 998. Refuse to answer

<u>Disaster preparedness</u>

DP1 Do you think the area you live in is susceptible to the impact of disasters (including natural disasters and manmade incidents)**?**

☐ 1.Yes ☐ 2. No ☐ 997. Don't know ☐ 998. Refuse to answer

DP2 (If susceptible) **What is the most common type of natural or manmade disaster here?** (Select one only)

☐ 1. Earthquakes ☐ 2. Forest fires ☐ 3. Mudslides ☐ 4. Floods
☐ 5. Rain storms ☐ 6. Wind storms ☐ 7. Droughts
☐ 8. Sand/dust storms ☐ 9. Home fires
☐ 10. Traffic accidents ☐ 11. Machine accidents
☐ 12. Others, please specify: _____ ☐ 888. N/A (Not susceptible to disaster)
☐ 997. Don't know ☐ 998. Refuse to answer

DP3 Have you or your household members experienced any disasters?

☐ 1.Yes ☐ 2. No ☐ 997. Don't know ☐ 998. Refuse to answer

DP4 (If a disaster has been experienced) **When did the disaster which had the** <u>greatest impact</u> **on your household occur?** ________

☐ 888. N/A (Never experienced a disaster)
☐ 997. Don't know ☐ 998. Refuse to answer

DP5 (If a disaster has been experienced) **What was the type of disaster which had the** <u>greatest impact</u> **on your household?**

☐ 1. Earthquakes ☐ 2. Forest fires ☐ 3. Mudslides ☐ 4. Floods
☐ 5. Rain storms ☐ 6. Wind storms ☐ 7. Droughts
☐ 8. Sand/dust storms ☐ 9. Home fires
☐ 10. Traffic accidents ☐ 11. Machine accidents
☐ 12. Others, please specify: _____ ☐ 888. N/A (Not susceptible to disaster)
☐ 997. Don't know ☐ 998. Refuse to answer

DP6 Did anyone in your household get injured or killed in the disaster which had the <u>greatest impact</u> **on your home?**

☐ 1. Yes ☐ 2. No ☐ 888. N/A (Never experienced a disaster)
☐ 997. Don't know ☐ 998. Refuse to answer

DP7 Did your household suffer from any economic/financial losses (e.g. housing/crops/livestock/business) in the disaster which had the <u>greatest impact</u> **on your household?**

☐ 1. Yes ☐ 2. No ☐ 888. N/A (Never experienced a disaster)
☐ 997. Don't know ☐ 998. Refuse to answer

DP8 If there is a disaster in the future, do you think your household members have the ability to protect their own health and safety?

☐ 1. Yes ☐ 2. No ☐ 997. Don't know ☐ 998. Refuse to answer

DP9 If someone in the household is sick and requires long-term medication, do you think it is important to carry the medication in the event of a disaster?

□ 1. Important □ 2. Not important
□ 997. Don't know □ 998. Refuse to answer

DP10 In the event of a disaster, do you think it necessary to carry a disaster preparedness kit? (Please explain the concept of a disaster preparedness kit first if the respondent does not know what it is: include its basic contents related to food and water, warmth, and protection, hygiene, and information, as well as its purpose of facilitating self-help and helping neighbours while waiting for outside assistance during a disaster.)

□ 1. Yes (necessary) □ 2. No (not necessary)
□ 997. Don't know □ 998. Refuse to answer

DP11 Do you have a disaster preparedness kit at home?

□ 1. Yes □ 2. No □ 997. Don't know □ 998. Refuse to answer

DP12 Do you know what items should be put in a disaster preparedness kit?

□ 1. Yes □ 2. No □ 3. Not sure □ 998. Refuse to answer

DP13 What would you put in your disaster preparedness kit? (Don't read out the options. Just note down the respondent's response by selecting from the following options):

□ **A.** Soap □ **B.** A towel □ **C.** A sealable water container (e.g. a water bottle)
□ **D.** An emergency blanket □ **E.** A handheld torch
□ **F.** A multipurpose tool/knife □ **G.** A flint □ **H.** A whistle
□ **I.** First-aid supplies (wound dressings, gauze bandages, etc.)
□ **J.** General medications (medicines for cold and painkillers) □ **K.** A family photo
□ **L.** Identification cards or documents of household members (originals/photocopies/photos)
□ Others: ______________________________
□ 997. Don't know □ 998. Refuse to answer

DP12 Regarding the disaster preparedness kit, do you have any questions?

____

<u>Climate change</u>

CC1 Do you think the weather has been unusual in recent years?

□ 1. Yes □ 2. No □ 997. Don't know □ 998. Refuse to answer

CC2 In what way do you think the weather has been unusual?

□ 1. Temperature □ 2. Rainfall □ 3. Frequency of natural disasters
□ 4. Others
□ 888. N/A (Don't think weather is unusual)
□ 997. Don't know □ 998. Refuse to answer

CC3 Do you know what global climate change is?

☐ 1.Yes ☐ 2. No ☐ 997. Don't know ☐ 998. Refuse to answer

CC4 Generally speaking, do you think you have the ability to cope with the impact of unusual weather conditions?

☐ 1.Yes ☐ 2. No ☐ 997. Don't know ☐ 998. Refuse to answer

CC5 Do you think your acts will affect the weather?

☐ 1.Yes ☐ 2.No ☐ 997. Don't know ☐ 998. Refuse to answer

CC6 Do you think climate change has any impact on health?

☐ 1.Yes ☐ 2. No ☐ 997. Don't know ☐ 998. Refuse to answer

Environment assessment

Take photos of six places (the water source, toilet, kitchen, outlook of the house, indoor wall decorations, and shed for poultry and livestock) while observing the environment. Please obtain consent from the respondents before taking photos.

EA1 The main flooring material used in the house is (Choose only one type which covers most of the house floor):

☐ 1. Natural soil/sand ☐ 2. Raw woods/bamboos

☐ 3. Wood floor boards ☐ 4. Cement/masonry ☐ 5. Tiles ☐ 6. Plastics

☐ 7. Others, please specify: ____________________

EA2 The main material of the house's exterior wall is (Choose only the most important option):

☐ 1. Wood ☐ 2. Bamboo ☐ 3. Stone ☐ 4. Brick

☐ 5. Cement ☐ 6. Ram/soil

☐ 7. Others, please specify: ____________________

EA3 The main fuel for heating the house during winter is:

☐ 1. Electricity ☐ 2. Firewood ☐ 3. Coal ☐ 4. Charcoal

☐ 5. Straws of crops ☐ 6. Animal waste ☐ 7. Others, please specify: _____

EA4 Does the household have the following equipment or devices? (Ask only if the object cannot be observed)

1	Electricity supply	☐ 1. Yes	☐ 2. No	☐ 3. Unable to judge
2	Radio	☐ 1. Yes	☐ 2. No	☐ 3. Unable to judge
3	Television set	☐ 1. Yes	☐ 2. No	☐ 3. Unable to judge
4	Landline telephone	☐ 1. Yes	☐ 2. No	☐ 3. Unable to judge
5	Refrigerator	☐ 1. Yes	☐ 2. No	☐ 3. Unable to judge
6	Electric rice cooker	☐ 1. Yes	☐ 2. No	☐ 3. Unable to judge

7	Washing machine	☐ 1. Yes	☐ 2. No	☐ 3. Unable to judge
8	Air conditioning	☐ 1. Yes	☐ 2. No	☐ 3. Unable to judge
9	Computer	☐ 1. Yes	☐ 2. No	☐ 3. Unable to judge
10	Satellite antenna	☐ 1. Yes	☐ 2. No	☐ 3. Unable to judge
11	Car/motorcycle/agricultural vehicle	☐ 1. Yes	☐ 2. No	☐ 3. Unable to judge
12	Solar energy equipment (stoves, water heaters, etc.)	☐ 1. Yes	☐ 2. No	☐ 3. Unable to judge
13	Stairs	☐ 1. Yes	☐ 2. No	☐ 3. Unable to judge

EA5 Observe the water source for the household and take a photo. **From observation, is the water source protected?**

☐ 1. Yes ☐ 2. No

☐ 3. Unable to observe (the water source is too far away from the household)

☐ 4. Unable to determine if the water source is protected or not

☐ 888. N/A

EA6 If there is a water storage container at home, observe if there is a cover on the container.

☐ 1. Yes ☐ 2. No ☐ 888. N/A (No water storage device at home)

EA7 Is there a place for handwashing at home? (Where do your household members wash their hands? Can you show me the place?)

☐ 1. Yes (can be seen) ☐ 2. No

☐ 3. Yes, but too far away and cannot be seen ☐ 997. Unable to judge

EA8 If there is a place for handwashing at home, observe if water can be found there. (Check water taps, basins, etc.)

☐ 1. Yes ☐ 2. No

☐ 888. N/A (No place for handwashing at home) ☐ 997. Unable to judge

EA9 If there is a place for handwashing at home, observe if cleaning agents (e.g. soap and detergent) can be found there. (If this cannot be observed directly, ask respondent if there is cleaning agent before further observation.)

☐ 1. Yes, can be observed directly ☐ 2. Yes, observed after asking respondent

☐ 3. No

☐ 888. N/A (No place for handwashing at home) ☐ 997. Unable to judge

EA10 If there is cleaning agent for handwashing, note down related observations below:

A. Solid soap	□ 1. Yes	□ 2. No	□ 888. N/A
B. Liquid soap	□ 1. Yes	□ 2. No	□ 888. N/A
C. Other cleaning agents (washing powder, dishwashing liquid, detergent, etc.)	□ 1. Yes	□ 2. No	□ 888. N/A
D. Others, please specify: ________________			□ 888. N/A

EA11 Is there a place for bathing at home?

□ 1. Yes □ 2. No □ 997. Unable to judge

EA12 If there is a toilet at home, <u>take a photo</u>, observe and note down the facilities of the toilet below:

□ 1. Flush – directly to a septic tank/pipe system/pit
□ 2. Flush – to nearby places (river, street, open ditches, etc.)
□ 3. Flush – flushed to an unknown place
□ 4. Dry toilet – with partitions
□ 5. Dry toilet – without partitions
□ 6. Others, please specify ________________
□ 888. N/A (No toilet at home)

EA13 Condition of toilet at home:

A. Are faeces directly visible?	□ 1. Yes	□ 2. No	□ 3. Can't distinguish	□ 888. N/A (No toilet)
B. Is there a noticeable odour?	□ 1. Yes	□ 2. No	□ 3. Can't distinguish	□ 888. N/A (No toilet)
C. Are there lots of flies or mosquitoes?	□ 1. Yes	□ 2. No	□ 3. Can't distinguish	□ 888. N/A (No toilet)

EA14 Where is the place for cooking at home? <u>Please take a photo</u> (including hearth, stove, fireplace, etc.)

□ 1. A separate room □ 2. No separate kitchen (indoors, as a part of the living room)
□ 3. Outdoors
□ 4. Others, please specify ________________
□ 888. N/A (Don't cook at home)

EA15 If cooking takes place indoors, is the room ventilated (e.g. with windows, vents, etc.)?
☐ 1. Yes ☐ 2. No ☐ 3. Difficult to judge, please explain ________ ☐ 888. N/A (Don't cook indoors)

EA16 If cooking takes place indoors, the condition of indoor ventilation is:
☐ 1. Good ☐ 2. Moderate ☐ 3. Poor
☐ 4. Difficult to judge, please explain ______
☐ 888. N/A (Don't cook indoors)

EA17 Observe the exterior of the house and take a photo. **Evaluate the quality of the house in comparison to other houses in the village:**
☐ 1. A lot better than average ☐ 2. Slightly better than average
☐ 3. Similar to other houses ☐ 4. Slightly poorer than average
☐ 5. Significantly poorer than average

EA18 Household environment: Are the following descriptions of the house and its surroundings correct?

1	There are lots of flies and mosquitoes around the house or in the yard (evidently more than 5 flies or mosquitoes).	☐ 1. Yes	☐ 2. No	☐ 3. Can't tell	☐ 888. N/A
2	It is clean, neat, and tidy around the house or in the yard.	☐ 1. Yes	☐ 2. No	☐ 3. Can't tell	☐ 888. N/A
3	Still water can be observed on the ground around the house or in the yard.	☐ 1. Yes	☐ 2. No	☐ 3. Can't tell	☐ 888. N/A
4	Mosquitoes or larvae are visible on the surface of still water.	☐ 1. Yes	☐ 2. No	☐ 3. Can't tell	☐ 888. N/A
5	There are designated places for keeping livestock and poultry (e.g. pig sheds). Please take a photo.	☐ 1. Yes	☐ 2. No	☐ 3. Can't tell	☐ 888. N/A
6	Livestock and poultry are free to enter the house where people live.	☐ 1. Yes	☐ 2. No	☐ 3. Can't tell	☐ 888. N/A
7	The interior of the house is neat and orderly.	☐ 1. Yes	☐ 2. No	☐ 3. Can't tell	☐ 888. N/A

8	The interior of the house is bright (i.e. able to read the questionnaire without the need for lights during daytime).	☐ 1. Yes	☐ 2. No	☐ 3. Can't tell	☐ 888. N/A
9	There are human faeces or animal manure in the house or the yard.	☐ 1. Yes	☐ 2. No	☐ 3. Can't tell	☐ 888. N/A
10	There are visible piles of rubbish in the house or the yard (i.e. rubbish is scattered everywhere without being cleared away).	☐ 1. Yes	☐ 2. No	☐ 3. Can't tell	☐ 888. N/A
11	There are photos, posters, awards, or other decorations hanging or stuck on the wall. Please take a photo.	☐ 1. Yes	☐ 2. No	☐ 3. Can't tell	☐ 888. N/A
12	Recyclable glass bottles (e.g. beer bottles) are **disposed of casually** around the house.	☐ 1. Yes	☐ 2. No	☐ 3. Can't tell	☐ 888. N/A
13	Recyclable glass bottles (e.g. beer bottles) are **collected in one place** outside the house.	☐ 1. Yes	☐ 2. No	☐ 3. Can't tell	☐ 888. N/A
14	There are stray dogs around the house (not raised by the household).	☐ 1. Yes	☐ 2. No	☐ 3. Can't tell	☐ 888. N/A
15	The house is shared by two or more families (e.g. brothers, relatives, etc.)	☐ 1. Yes	☐ 2. No	☐ 3. Can't tell	☐ 888. N/A
16	There is an odour in the house due to poor ventilation.	☐ 1. Yes	☐ 2. No	☐ 3. Can't tell	☐ 888. N/A
17	There are visible cracks or damage in the house.	☐ 1. Yes	☐ 2. No	☐ 3. Can't tell	☐ 888. N/A

Feedback

FB1 Respondent's lingua franca proficiency:
☐ 1. Very good – no difficulty in communication
☐ 2. Moderate – generally able to communicate
☐ 3. Poor – interpretation required

FB2 Degree of openness and cooperation of respondent:
☐ 1. Fully cooperative
☐ 2. Somewhat reserved/evasive
☐ 3. Very resistant/uncooperative

FB3 Were family members, friends, or neighbours present during the interview?
☐ 1. Yes ☐ 2. No

FB4 Did the other people present during the interview sometimes help or get involved in responding to the questions?
☐ 1. Yes ☐ 2. No ☐ 888. N/A (No other people present during the interview)

FB5 Name of interpreter for the interview: ____________________
☐ 888. N/A (No interpreter involved)

FB6 Comments/Special issues:

____

End of questionnaire

Please note down the time for the end of the interview on the first page.

Index

Note: figures, tables, and boxes are indicated by *f*, *t*, and *b* after the page number

The manufacturer's authorised representative in the EU for product safety is Oxford University Press España S.A. of el Parque Empresarial San Fernando de Henares, Avenida de Castilla, 2 – 28830 Madrid (www.oup.es/en or product.safety@oup.com). OUP España S.A. also acts as importer into Spain of products made by the manufacturer.

www.ingramcontent.com/pod-product-compliance
Lightning Source LLC
LaVergne TN
LVHW080019210926
848481LV00011B/3062
* 9 7 8 0 1 9 8 8 0 7 1 7 9 *